Chinese Medicine: A Comprehensive Guide

Chinese Medicine: A Comprehensive Guide

Edited by
Roberto Forbes

Larsen & Keller
www.larsen-keller.com

Chinese Medicine: A Comprehensive Guide
Edited by Roberto Forbes
ISBN: 978-1-63549-065-7 (Hardback)

☰ Larsen & Keller

Published by Larsen and Keller Education,
5 Penn Plaza,
19th Floor,
New York, NY 10001, USA

Cataloging-in-Publication Data

Chinese medicine : a comprehensive guide / edited by Roberto Forbes.
     p. cm.
Includes bibliographical references and index.
ISBN 978-1-63549-065-7
1. Medicine, Chinese. 2. Traditional medicine--China. 3. Alternative medicine--China. I. Forbes, Roberto.
R602 .C45 2017
610.951--dc23

The publisher's policy is to use permanent paper from mills that operate a sustainable forestry policy. Furthermore, the publisher ensures that the text paper and cover boards used have met acceptable environmental accreditation standards.

Printed and bound in the United States of America.

For more information regarding Larsen and Keller Education and its products, please visit the publisher's website www.larsen-keller.com

Table of Contents

Permissions

Index

Preface

Chinese medicine or traditional Chinese medicine is an alternate form of treatment. It uses techniques like massage, herbal medicine, exercise, acupuncture, cup therapy, Chinese food therapy, gua sha, and dietary therapy to treat various diseases like asthma, migraine, neurogenic bladder dysfunction, diarrhea, infertility, etc. The book studies, analyses and upholds the pillars of Chinese medicine and its utmost significance in modern times. Some of the diverse topics covered in it address the varied branches that fall under this category. The topics covered in this text offer students new insights in this field. Coherent flow of topics, student-friendly language and extensive use of examples make this textbook an invaluable source of knowledge.

To facilitate a deeper understanding of the contents of this book a short introduction of every chapter is written below:

Chapter 1- Chinese medicine is almost 2500 years old; and traditional Chinese medicine includes herbal medicine, acupuncture, massages (tui na) and exercises (qigong). This traditional form of medicine is still widely preferred in China for it is herbal and organic and not chemically manufactured.

Chapter 2- Chinese herbology or herbal therapy are an undocumented school of alternate medicine that uses ancient and modern medicinal recipes, derived from plant extracts, animal parts and other elements. Different regions of China have different approaches to Chinese herbology. The chapter strategically encompasses and incorporates the major components and key concepts of Chinese herbology, providing a complete understanding.

Chapter 3- Herbs are an important component of Chinese medicine and certain herbs such as Camellia sinensis and liquorice are used in an everyday sense in cooking, for instance. These herbs contain medicinal properties that can benefit the human body. The major categories of Chinese medicinal plants are dealt with great details in the chapter.

Chapter 4- In order to completely understand Chinese traditional medicine, it is necessary to understand acupuncture. The insertion of needles in the skin or muscles of a person is known as acupuncture, in traditional Chinese medicine it aims at affecting the flow of Qi. According to the tradition it eases pain and treats various diseases.

Chapter 5- Cupping therapy, Chinese food therapy, Tui na and qigong are important therapeutic approaches and techniques discussed in this chapter. Tui na is a form of acupressure where instead of using oils, thumb presses or rubbing is involved whereas qigong is a form of exercise and meditation that combines breathing with focused awareness and helps in the balance of qi. This chapter closely examines all the therapeutic approaches to provide an extensive understanding of the subject.

Chapter 6- This chapter explains to the reader the significance of the body in traditional Chinese medicine. Qi, meridian, zang-fu and other principles are the functional entities used by the Chinese tradition. Such methods of treatment evolved much before the Enlightenment and scientific medical practice and are still practiced in many parts of the world.

Chapter 7- Chinese traditional medicine has a strong philosophical background. Some of the philosophical beliefs are yin and yang, wu xing, deng shui, the eight principles and the three treasures. Disease is perceived as an imbalance in the functions of yin and yang, qui, meridians or an imbalance in the interaction between the human body and the environment. The aspects elucidated in this chapter are of vital importance, and provide a better understanding of traditional Chinese medicine.

I owe the completion of this book to the never-ending support of my family, who supported me throughout the project.

Editor

Introduction to Chinese Medicine

Chinese medicine is almost 2500 years old; and traditional Chinese medicine includes herbal medicine, acupuncture, massages (tui na) and exercises (qigong). This traditional form of medicine is still widely preferred in China for it is herbal and organic and not chemically manufactured.

Traditional Chinese Medicine

Traditional Chinese medicine (TCM; simplified Chinese: 中医; traditional Chinese: 中醫; pinyin: *Zhōngyī*) is a style of traditional Asian medicine informed by modern medicine but built on a foundation of more than 2,500 years of Chinese medical practice that includes various forms of herbal medicine, acupuncture, massage (tui na), exercise (qigong), and dietary therapy. It is primarily used as a complementary alternative medicine approach. TCM is widely used in China and is becoming increasingly prevalent in Europe and North America.

One of the basic tenets of TCM "holds that the body's vital energy (*chi* or *qi*) circulates through channels, called *meridians*, that have branches connected to bodily organs and functions." Concepts of the body and of disease used in TCM reflect its ancient origins and its emphasis on dynamic processes over material structure, similar to European humoral theory. Scientific investigation has found no histological or physiological evidence for traditional Chinese concepts such as *qi*, meridians, and acupuncture points. [a] The TCM theory and practice are not based upon scientific knowledge, and its own practitioners disagree widely on what diagnosis and treatments should be used for any given patient. The effectiveness of Chinese herbal medicine remains poorly researched and documented. There are concerns over a number of potentially toxic plants, animal parts, and mineral Chinese medicinals. There are also concerns over illegal trade and transport of endangered species including rhinos and tigers, and the welfare of specially farmed animals including bears. A review of cost-effectiveness research for TCM found that studies had low levels of evidence, but so far have not shown benefit outcomes. Pharmaceutical research has explored the potential for creating new drugs from traditional remedies, with few successful results. A *Nature* editorial described TCM as "fraught with pseudoscience", and said that the most obvious reason why it hasn't delivered many cures is that the majority of its treatments have no logical mechanism of action. Proponents propose that research has so far missed key features of the art of TCM, such as unknown interactions between various ingredients and complex interactive biological systems.

The doctrines of Chinese medicine are rooted in books such as the *Yellow Emperor's Inner Canon* and the *Treatise on Cold Damage*, as well as in cosmological notions such as yin-yang and the five phases. Starting in the 1950s, these precepts were standardized in the People's Republic of China, including attempts to integrate them with modern notions of anatomy and pathology. In the 1950s, the Chinese government promoted a systematized form of TCM.

TCM's view of the body places little emphasis on anatomical structures, but is mainly concerned with the identification of functional entities (which regulate digestion, breathing, aging etc.). While health is perceived as harmonious interaction of these entities and the outside world, disease is interpreted as a disharmony in interaction. TCM diagnosis aims to trace symptoms to patterns of an underlying disharmony, by measuring the pulse, inspecting the tongue, skin, and eyes, and looking at the eating and sleeping habits of the person as well as many other things.

History

Traces of therapeutic activities in China date from the Shang dynasty (14th–11th centuries BC). Though the Shang did not have a concept of "medicine" as distinct from other fields, their oracular inscriptions on bones and tortoise shells refer to illnesses that affected the Shang royal family: eye disorders, toothaches, bloated abdomen, etc., which Shang elites usually attributed to curses sent by their ancestors. There is no evidence that the Shang nobility used herbal remedies. According to a 2006 overview, the "Documentation of Chinese materia medica (CMM) dates back to around 1,100 BC when only dozens of drugs were first described. By the end of the 16th century, the number of drugs documented had reached close to 1,900. And by the end of the last century, published records of CMM have reached 12,800 drugs."

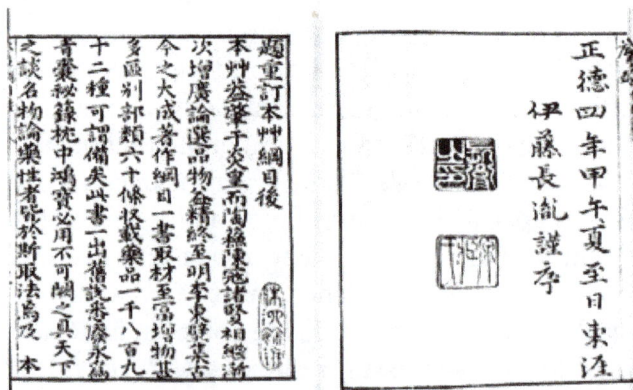

The Compendium of Materia Medica is a pharmaceutical text written by Li Shizhen (1518–1593 AD) during the Ming Dynasty of China. This edition was published in 1593.

Stone and bone needles found in ancient tombs led Joseph Needham to speculate that acupuncture might have been carried out in the Shang dynasty. But most historians now make a distinction between medical lancing (or bloodletting) and acupuncture in the narrower sense of using metal needles to treat illnesses by stimulating specific points along circulation channels ("meridians") in accordance with theories related to the circulation of Qi. The earliest evidence for acupuncture in this sense dates to the second or first century BC.

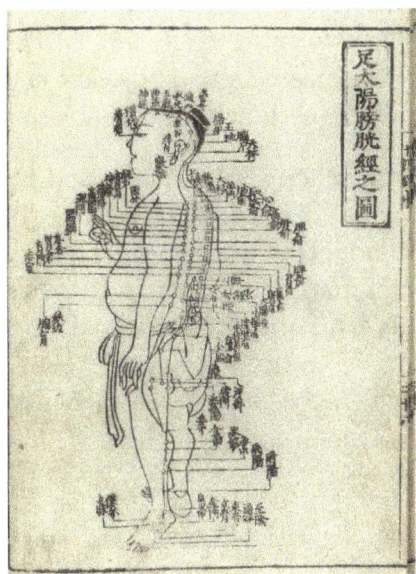

Acupuncture chart from Hua Shou (fl. 1340s, Yuan Dynasty). This image from *Shi si jing fa hui (Expression of the Fourteen Meridians)*. (Tokyo: Suharaya Heisuke kanko, Kyoho gan 1716).

The *Yellow Emperor's Inner Canon*, the oldest received work of Chinese medical theory, was compiled around the first century BC on the basis of shorter texts from different medical lineages. Written in the form of dialogues between the legendary Yellow Emperor and his ministers, it offers explanations on the relation between humans, their environment, and the cosmos, on the contents of the body, on human vitality and pathology, on the symptoms of illness, and on how to make diagnostic and therapeutic decisions in light of all these factors. Unlike earlier texts like *Recipes for Fifty-Two Ailments*, which was excavated in the 1970s from a tomb that had been sealed in 168 BC, the *Inner Canon* rejected the influence of spirits and the use of magic. It was also one of the first books in which the cosmological doctrines of Yinyang and the Five Phases were brought to a mature synthesis.

The *Treatise on Cold Damage Disorders and Miscellaneous Illnesses* was collated by Zhang Zhongjing sometime between 196 and 220 CE, at the end of the Han dynasty. Focusing on drug prescriptions rather than acupuncture, it was the first medical work to combine Yinyang and the Five Phases with drug therapy. This formulary was also the earliest public Chinese medical text to group symptoms into clinically useful "patterns" (*zheng* 證) that could serve as targets for therapy. Having gone through numerous changes over time, the formulary now circulates as two distinct books: the *Treatise on Cold Damage Disorders* and the *Essential Prescriptions of the Golden Casket*, which were edited separately in the eleventh century, under the Song dynasty.

In the centuries that followed the completion of the *Yellow Emperor's Inner Canon*, several shorter books tried to summarize or systematize its contents. The *Canon of Problems* (probably second century CE) tried to reconcile divergent doctrines from the *Inner Canon* and developed a complete medical system centered on needling therapy. The *AB Canon of Acupuncture and Moxibustion* (*Zhenjiu jiayi jing* 針灸甲乙經, compiled by Huangfu Mi sometime between 256 and 282 CE) assembled a consistent body of doctrines concerning acupuncture; whereas the *Canon of the Pulse* (*Maijing* 脈經; ca. 280) presented itself as a "comprehensive handbook of diagnostics and therapy."

In 1950, Chairman Mao Zedong made a speech in support of traditional Chinese medicine which was influenced by political necessity. Zedong believed he and the Chinese Communist Party should promote traditional Chinese medicine (TCM) but he did not personally believe in TCM and he didn't use it. In 1952, the president of the Chinese Medical Association said that, "This One Medicine, will possess a basis in modern natural sciences, will have absorbed the ancient and the new, the Chinese and the foreign, all medical achievements—and will be China's New Medicine!"

Historical Physicians

These include Zhang Zhongjing, Hua Tuo, Sun Simiao, Tao Hongjing, Zhang Jiegu, and Li Shizhen.

Philosophical Background

Traditional Chinese medicine (TCM) is a broad range of medicine practices sharing common concepts which have been developed in China and are based on a tradition of more than 2,000 years, including various forms of herbal medicine, acupuncture, massage (Tui na), exercise (qigong), and dietary therapy. It is primarily used as a complementary alternative medicine approach. TCM is widely used in China and it is also used in the West. Its philosophy is based on Yinyangism (i.e., the combination of Five Phases theory with Yin-yang theory), which was later absorbed by Daoism.

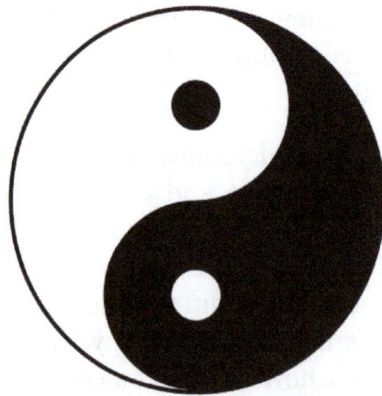

Yin and yang symbol for balance. In Traditional Chinese Medicine, good health is believed to be achieved by a balance between yin and yang.

Yin and Yang

Yin and yang are ancient Chinese concepts which can be traced back to the Shang dynasty (1600–1100 BC). They represent two abstract and complementary aspects that every phenomenon in the universe can be divided into. Primordial analogies for these aspects are the sun-facing (yang) and the shady (yin) side of a hill. Two other commonly used representational allegories of yin and yang are water and fire. In the yin-yang theory, detailed attributions are made regarding the yin or yang character of things:

Phenomenon	Yin	Yang
Celestial bodies	moon	sun
Gender	female	male
Location	inside	outside
Temperature	cold	hot
Direction	downward	upward
Degree of humidity	damp/moist	dry

The concept of yin and yang is also applicable to the human body; for example, the upper part of the body and the back are assigned to yang, while the lower part of the body are believed to have the yin character. Yin and yang characterization also extends to the various body functions, and – more importantly – to disease symptoms (e.g., cold and heat sensations are assumed to be yin and yang symptoms, respectively). Thus, yin and yang of the body are seen as phenomena whose lack (or over-abundance) comes with characteristic symptom combinations:

- Yin vacuity (also termed "vacuity-heat"): heat sensations, possible night sweats, insomnia, dry pharynx, dry mouth, dark urine, a red tongue with scant fur, and a "fine" and rapid pulse.

- Yang vacuity ("vacuity-cold"): aversion to cold, cold limbs, bright white complexion, long voidings of clear urine, diarrhea, pale and enlarged tongue, and a slightly weak, slow and fine pulse.

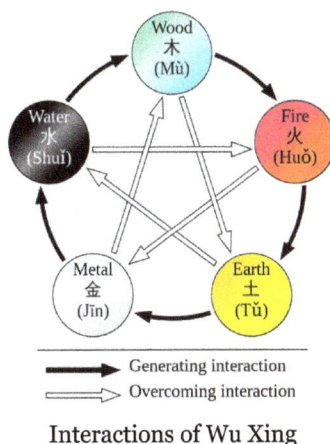

Interactions of Wu Xing

TCM also identifies drugs believed to treat these specific symptom combinations, i.e., to reinforce yin and yang.

Five Phases Theory

Five Phases (五行, pinyin: *wǔ xíng*), sometimes also translated as the "Five Elements" theory, presumes that all phenomena of the universe and nature can be broken down into five elemental qualities – represented by wood (木, pinyin: *mù*), fire (火pinyin: *huǒ*), earth (土, pinyin: *tǔ*), metal (金, pinyin: *jīn*), and water (水, pinyin: *shuǐ*). In this way, lines of correspondence can be drawn:

Phenomenon	Wood	Fire	Earth	Metal	Water
Direction	East	South	Centre	West	North
Colour	green/blue	red	yellow	white	black
Climate	wind	heat	damp	dryness	cold
Taste	sour	bitter	sweet	acrid	salty
Zang Organ	Liver	Heart	Spleen	Lung	Kidney
Fu Organ	Gallbladder	Small intestine	Stomach	Large intestine	Bladder
Sense organ	eye	tongue	mouth	nose	ears
Facial part	above bridge of nose	between eyes, lower part	bridge of nose	between eyes, middle part	cheeks (below cheekbone)
Eye part	iris	inner/outer corner of the eye	upper and lower lid	sclera	pupil

Strict rules are identified to apply to the relationships between the Five Phases in terms of sequence, of acting on each other, of counteraction, etc. All these aspects of Five Phases theory constitute the basis of the zàng-fǔ concept, and thus have great influence regarding the TCM model of the body. Five Phase theory is also applied in diagnosis and therapy.

Correspondences between the body and the universe have historically not only been seen in terms of the Five Elements, but also of the "Great Numbers" (大數, pinyin: *dà shū*) For example, the number of acu-points has at times been seen to be 365, corresponding with the number of days in a year; and the number of main meridians—12—has been seen as corresponding with the number of rivers flowing through the ancient Chinese empire.

Model of the Body

TCM "holds that the body's vital energy (*chi* or *qi*) circulates through channels, called *meridians*, that have branches connected to bodily organs and functions." Its view of the human body is only marginally concerned with anatomical structures, but focuses primarily on the body's *functions* (such as digestion, breathing, temperature maintenance, etc.):

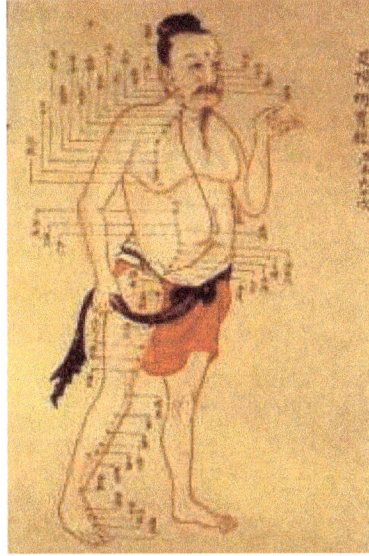

Old Chinese medical chart on acupuncture meridians

"The tendency of Chinese thought is to seek out dynamic functional activity rather than to look for the fixed somatic structures that perform the activities. Because of this, the Chinese have no system of anatomy comparable to that of the West."

— *Ted Kaptchuk, The Web That Has No Weaver*

These functions are aggregated and then associated with a primary functional entity – for instance, nourishment of the tissues and maintenance of their moisture are seen as connected functions, and the entity postulated to be responsible for these functions is xuě (blood). These functional entities thus constitute *concepts* rather than something with biochemical or anatomical properties.

The primary functional entities used by traditional Chinese medicine are qì, xuě, the five zàng organs, the six fǔ organs, and the meridians which extend through the organ systems. These are all theoretically interconnected: each zàng organ is paired with a fǔ organ, which are nourished by the blood and concentrate qi for a particular function, with meridians being extensions of those functional systems throughout the body.

Concepts of the body and of disease used in TCM have notions of a pre-scientific culture, similar to European humoral theory. – TCM is characterized as full of pseudoscience. Some practitioners no longer consider yin and yang and the idea of an energy flow to apply. Scientific investigation has not found any histological or physiological evidence for traditional Chinese concepts such as *qi*, meridians, and acupuncture points.[a] It is a generally held belief within the acupuncture community that acupuncture points and meridians structures are special conduits for electrical signals but no research has established any consistent anatomical structure or function for either acupuncture points or meridians. The scientific evidence for the anatomical existence of either meridians or acupuncture points is not compelling. Stephen Barrett of Quackwatch writes that, "TCM theory and practice are not based upon the body of knowledge related to health, disease, and health care that has been widely accepted by the scientific community. TCM practitioners disagree among themselves about how to diagnose patients and which treatments should go with which diagnoses. Even if they could agree, the TCM theories are so nebulous that no amount of scientific study will enable TCM to offer rational care."

TCM has been the subject of controversy within China. In 2006, the Chinese scholar Zhang Gongyao triggered a national debate when he published an article entitled "Farewell to Traditional Chinese Medicine," arguing that TCM was a pseudoscience that should be abolished in public healthcare and academia. The Chinese government however, interested in the opportunity of export revenues, took the stance that TCM is a science and continued to encourage its development.

Qi

TCM distinguishes many kinds of qi (simplified Chinese: 气; traditional Chinese: 氣; pinyin: *qì*). In a general sense, qi is something that is defined by five "cardinal functions":

1. Actuation (simplified Chinese: 推动; traditional Chinese: 推動; pinyin: *tuīdòng*) – of all physical processes in the body, especially the circulation of all body fluids such as blood in their vessels. This includes actuation of the functions of the zang-fu organs and meridians.

2. Warming (Chinese: 溫煦; pinyin: *wēnxù*) – the body, especially the limbs.

3. Defense (Chinese: 防御; pinyin: *fángyù*) – against Exogenous Pathogenic Factors

4. Containment (simplified Chinese: 固摄; traditional Chinese: 固攝; pinyin: *gùshè*) – of body fluids, i.e., keeping blood, sweat, urine, semen, etc. from leakage or excessive emission.

5. Transformation (simplified Chinese: 气化; traditional Chinese: 氣化; pinyin: *qìhuà*) – of food, drink, and breath into qi, xue (blood), and jinye ("fluids"), and/or transformation of all of the latter into each other.

Vacuity of qi will be characterized especially by pale complexion, lassitude of spirit, lack of strength, spontaneous sweating, laziness to speak, non-digestion of food, shortness of breath (especially on exertion), and a pale and enlarged tongue.

Qi is believed to be partially generated from food and drink, and partially from air (by breathing). Another considerable part of it is inherited from the parents and will be consumed in the course of life.

TCM uses special terms for qi running inside of the blood vessels and for qi that is distributed in the skin, muscles, and tissues between those. The former is called yíng-qì (simplified Chinese: 营气; traditional Chinese: 營氣); its function is to complement xuè and its nature has a strong yin aspect (although qi in general is considered to be yang). The latter is called weì-qì (simplified Chinese: 卫气; traditional Chinese: 衞氣); its main function is defence and it has pronounced yang nature.

Qi is said to circulate in the meridians. Just as the qi held by each of the zang-fu organs, this is considered to be part of the 'principal' qi (simplified Chinese: 元气; traditional Chinese: 元氣; pinyin: *yuánqì*) of the body (also called 真氣 Chinese: 真气; pinyin: *zhēn qì*, "true" qi, or 原氣 Chinese: 原气; pinyin: *yuán qì*, "original" qi).

Xue

In contrast to the majority of other functional entities, xuè (血, "blood") is correlated with a physical form – the red liquid running in the blood vessels. Its concept is, nevertheless, defined by its functions: nourishing all parts and tissues of the body, safeguarding an adequate degree of moisture, and sustaining and soothing both consciousness and sleep.

Typical symptoms of a lack of xuě (usually termed "blood vacuity" [血虚, pinyin: *xuě xū*]) are described as: Pale-white or withered-yellow complexion, dizziness, flowery vision, palpitations, insomnia, numbness of the extremities; pale tongue; "fine" pulse.

Jinye

Closely related to xuě are the jīnyè (津液, usually translated as "body fluids"), and just like xuě they are considered to be yin in nature, and defined first and foremost by the functions of nurturing and moisturizing the different structures of the body. Their other functions are to harmonize yin and yang, and to help with the secretion of waste products.

Jīnyè are ultimately extracted from food and drink, and constitute the raw material for the production of xuě; conversely, xuě can also be transformed into jīnyè. Their palpable manifestations are all bodily fluids: tears, sputum, saliva, gastric acid, joint fluid, sweat, urine, etc.

Zang-fu

The zàng-fǔ (simplified Chinese: 脏腑; traditional Chinese: 臟腑) constitute the centre piece of TCM's systematization of bodily functions. Bearing the names of organs, they are, however, only secondarily tied to (rudimentary) anatomical assumptions (the fǔ a little more, the zàng much less). As they are primarily defined by their functions, they are not equivalent to the anatomical organs–to highlight this fact, their names are usually capitalized.

The term zàng (臟) refers to the five entities considered to be yin in nature–Heart, Liver, Spleen, Lung, Kidney–, while fǔ (腑) refers to the six yang organs–Small Intestine, Large Intestine, Gallbladder, Urinary Bladder, Stomach and Sānjiaō.

The zàng's essential functions consist in production and storage of qì and xuě; they are said to regulate digestion, breathing, water metabolism, the musculoskeletal system, the skin, the sense organs, aging, emotional processes, and mental activity, among other structures and processes. The fǔ organs' main purpose is merely to transmit and digest (傳化, pinyin: *chuán-huà*) substances such as waste and food.

Since their concept was developed on the basis of Wǔ Xíng philosophy, each zàng is paired with a fǔ, and each zàng-fǔ pair is assigned to one of five elemental qualities (i.e., the Five Elements or Five Phases). These correspondences are stipulated as:

- Fire (火) = Heart (心, pinyin: *xīn*) and Small Intestine (小腸, pinyin: *xiaǒcháng*) (and, secondarily, Sānjiaō [三焦, "Triple Burner"] and Pericardium [心包, pinyin: *xīnbaò*])

- Earth (土) = Spleen (脾, pinyin: *pí*) and Stomach (胃, pinyin: *weì*)

- Metal (金) = Lung (肺, pinyin: *feì*) and Large Intestine (大腸, pinyin: *dàcháng*)

- Water (水) = Kidney (腎, pinyin: *shèn*) and Bladder (膀胱, pinyin: *pángguāng*)

- Wood (木) = Liver (肝, pinyin: *gān*) and Gallbladder (膽, pinyin: *dān*)

The zàng-fǔ are also connected to the twelve standard meridians–each yang meridian is attached to a fǔ organ, and five of the yin meridians are attached to a zàng. As there are only five zàng but six yin meridians, the sixth is assigned to the Pericardium, a peculiar entity almost similar to the Heart zàng.

Jing-luo

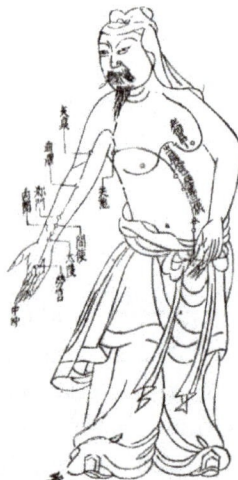

Acupuncture chart from the Ming Dynasty (c. 1368–1644)

The meridians (经络, pinyin: *jīng-luò*) are believed to be channels running from the zàng-fǔ in the interior (里, pinyin: *lǐ*) of the body to the limbs and joints ("the surface" [表, pinyin: *biǎo*]), transporting qi and xuě. TCM identifies 12 "regular" and 8 "extraordinary" meridians; the Chinese terms being 十二经脉 (pinyin: *shí-èr jīngmài*, lit. "the Twelve Vessels") and 奇经八脉 (pinyin: *qí jīng bā mài*) respectively. There's also a number of less customary channels branching from the "regular" meridians.

Concept of Disease

In general, disease is perceived as a disharmony (or imbalance) in the functions or interactions of yin, yang, qi, xuě, zàng-fǔ, meridians etc. and/or of the interaction between the human body and the environment. Therapy is based on which "pattern of disharmony" can be identified. Thus, "pattern discrimination" is the most important step in TCM diagnosis. It is also known to be the most difficult aspect of practicing TCM.

In order to determine which pattern is at hand, practitioners will examine things like the color and shape of the tongue, the relative strength of pulse-points, the smell of the breath, the quality of breathing or the sound of the voice. For example, depending on tongue and pulse conditions, a TCM practitioner might diagnose bleeding from the mouth and nose as: "Liver fire rushes upwards and scorches the Lung, injuring the blood vessels and giving rise to reckless pouring of blood from the mouth and nose.". He might then go on to prescribe treatments designed to clear heat or supplement the Lung.

Disease Entities

In TCM, a disease has two aspects: "bìng" and "zhèng". The former is often translated as "disease entity", "disease category", "illness", or simply "diagnosis". The latter, and more important one, is usually translated as "pattern" (or sometimes also as "syndrome"). For example, the disease entity of a common cold might present with a pattern of wind-cold in one person, and with the pattern of wind-heat in another.

From a scientific point of view, most of the disease entitites (病, pinyin: *bìng*) listed by TCM constitute mere symptoms. Examples include headache, cough, abdominal pain, constipation etc.

Since therapy will not be chosen according to the disease entity but according to the pattern, two people with the same disease entity but different patterns will receive different therapy. Vice versa, people with similar patterns might receive similar therapy even if their disease entities are different. This is called 异病同治，同病异治 (pinyin: *yì bìng tóng zhì, tóng bìng yì zhì*,"different diseases, same treatment; same disease, different treatments").

Patterns

In TCM, "pattern" (证, pinyin: *zhèng*) refers to a "pattern of disharmony" or "functional disturbance" within the functional entities the TCM model of the body is composed of. There are disharmony patterns of qi, xuě, the body fluids, the zàng-fǔ, and the meridians. They are ultimately defined by their symptoms and "signs" (i.e., for example, pulse and tongue findings).

In clinical practice, the identified pattern usually involves a combination of affected entities (compare with typical examples of patterns). The concrete pattern identified should account for *all* the symptoms a person has.

Six Excesses

The Six Excesses (六淫, pinyin: *liù yín*, sometimes also translated as "Pathogenic Factors", or "Six Pernicious Influences"; with the alternative term of 六邪, pinyin: *liù xié*, – "Six Evils" or "Six Devils") are allegorical terms used to describe disharmony patterns displaying certain typical symptoms. These symptoms resemble the effects of six climatic factors. In the allegory, these symptoms can occur because one or more of those climatic factors (called 六气, pinyin: *liù qì*, "the six qi") were able to invade the body surface and to proceed to the interior. This is sometimes used to draw causal relationships (i.e., prior exposure to wind/cold/etc. is identified as the cause of a disease), while other authors explicitly deny a direct cause-effect relationship between weather conditions and disease, pointing out that the Six Excesses are primarily descriptions of a certain combination of symptoms translated into a pattern of disharmony. It is undisputed, though, that the Six Excesses can manifest inside the body without an external cause. In this case, they might be denoted "internal", e.g., "internal wind" or "internal fire (or heat)".

The Six Excesses and their characteristic clinical signs are:

1. Wind (风, pinyin: *fēng*): rapid onset of symptoms, wandering location of symptoms, itching, nasal congestion, "floating" pulse; tremor, paralysis, convulsion.

2. Cold (寒, pinyin: *hán*): cold sensations, aversion to cold, relief of symptoms by warmth, watery/clear excreta, severe pain, abdominal pain, contracture/hypertonicity of muscles, (slimy) white tongue fur, "deep"/"hidden" or "string-like" pulse, or slow pulse.

3. Fire/Heat (火, pinyin: *huǒ*): aversion to heat, high fever, thirst, concentrated urine, red face, red tongue, yellow tongue fur, rapid pulse. (Fire and heat are basically seen to be the same)

4. Dampness (湿, pinyin: *shī*): sensation of heaviness, sensation of fullness, symptoms of Spleen dysfunction, greasy tongue fur, "slippery" pulse.

5. Dryness (燥, pinyin: *zào*): dry cough, dry mouth, dry throat, dry lips, nosebleeds, dry skin, dry stools.

6. Summerheat (暑, pinyin: *shǔ*): either heat or mixed damp-heat symptoms.

Six-Excesses-patterns can consist of only one or a combination of Excesses (e.g., wind-cold, wind-damp-heat). They can also transform from one into another.

Typical Examples of Patterns

For each of the functional entities (qi, xuě, zàng-fǔ, meridians etc.), typical disharmony patterns are recognized; for example: qi vacuity and qi stagnation in the case of qi; blood vacuity, blood stasis, and blood heat in the case of xuě; Spleen qi vacuity, Spleen yang vacuity, Spleen qi vacuity with down-bearing qi, Spleen qi vacuity with lack of blood containment, cold-damp invasion of the Spleen, damp-heat invasion of Spleen and Stomach in case of the Spleen zàng; wind/cold/damp invasion in the case of the meridians.

TCM gives detailed prescriptions of these patterns regarding their typical symptoms, mostly including characteristic tongue and/or pulse findings. For example:

- "Upflaming Liver fire" (肝火上炎, pinyin: *gānhuǒ shàng yán*): Headache, red face, reddened eyes, dry mouth, nosebleeds, constipation, dry or hard stools, profuse menstruation, sudden tinnitus or deafness, vomiting of sour or bitter fluids, expectoration of blood, irascibility, impatience; red tongue with dry yellow fur; slippery and string-like pulse.

Eight Principles of Diagnosis

The process of determining which actual pattern is on hand is called 辩证 (pinyin: *biàn zhèng*, usually translated as "pattern diagnosis", "pattern identification" or "pattern discrimination"). Generally, the first and most important step in pattern diagnosis is an evaluation of the present signs and symptoms on the basis of the "Eight Principles" (八纲, pinyin: *bā gāng*). These eight principles refer to four pairs of fundamental qualities of a disease: exterior/interior, heat/cold, vacuity/repletion, and yin/yang. Out of these, heat/cold and vacuity/repletion have the biggest clinical importance. The yin/yang quality, on the other side, has the smallest importance and is somewhat seen aside from the other three pairs, since it merely presents a general and vague conclusion regarding what other qualities are found. In detail, the Eight Principles refer to the following:

- *Yin and yang* are universal aspects all things can be classified under, this includes diseases in general as well as the Eight Principles' first three couples. For example, cold is identified to be a yin aspect, while heat is attributed to yang. Since descriptions of patterns in terms of yin and yang lack complexity and clinical practicality, though, patterns are usually not labelled this way anymore. Exceptions are vacuity-cold and repletion-heat patterns, who are sometimes referred to as "yin patterns" and "yang patterns" respectively.

- *Exterior* (表, pinyin: *biǎo*) refers to a disease manifesting in the superficial layers of the body – skin, hair, flesh, and meridians. It is characterized by aversion to cold and/or wind, headache, muscle ache, mild fever, a "floating" pulse, and a normal tongue appearance.

- *Interior* (里, pinyin: *lǐ*) refers to disease manifestation in the zàng-fǔ, or (in a wider sense) to any disease that can not be counted as exterior. There are no generalized characteristic symptoms of interior patterns, since they'll be determined by the affected zàng or fǔ entity.

- *Cold* (寒, pinyin: *hán*) is generally characterized by aversion to cold, absence of thirst, and a white tongue fur. More detailed characterization depends on whether cold is coupled with vacuity or repletion.

- *Heat* (热, pinyin: *rè*) is characterized by absence of aversion to cold, a red and painful throat, a dry tongue fur and a rapid and floating pulse, if it falls together with an exterior pattern. In all other cases, symptoms depend on whether heat is coupled with vacuity or repletion.

- *Deficiency* (虚, pinyin: *xū*), can be further differentiated into deficiency of qi, xuě, yin and yang, with all their respective characteristic symptoms. Yin deficiency can also cause "empty-heat".

- *Excess* (实, pinyin: *shí*) generally refers to any disease that can't be identified as a deficient pattern, and usually indicates the presence of one of the Six Excesses, or a pattern of stagnation (of qi, xuě, etc.). In a concurrent exterior pattern, excess is characterized by the absence of sweating.

After the fundamental nature of a disease in terms of the Eight Principles is determined, the investigation focuses on more specific aspects. By evaluating the present signs and symptoms against the background of typical disharmony patterns of the various entities, evidence is collected whether or how specific entities are affected. This evaluation can be done

1. in respect of the meridians (经络辩证, pinyin: *jīng-luò biàn zhèng*)

2. in respect of qi (气血辩证, pinyin: *qì xuě biàn zhèng*)

3. in respect of xuě (气血辩证, pinyin: *qì xuě biàn zhèng*)

4. in respect of the body fluids (津液辩证, pinyin: *jīn-yè biàn zhèng*)

5. in respect of the zàng-fǔ (脏腑辩证, pinyin: *zàng-fǔ biàn zhèng*) – very similar to this, though less specific, is disharmony pattern description in terms of the Five Elements [五行辩证, pinyin: *wǔ xíng biàn zhèng*])

There are also three special pattern diagnosis systems used in case of febrile and infectious diseases only ("Six Channel system" or "six division pattern" [六经辩证, pinyin: *liù jīng biàn zhèng*]; "Wei Qi Ying Xue system" or "four division pattern" [卫气营血辩证, pinyin: *wei qì yíng xuě biàn zhèng*]; "San Jiao system" or "three burners pattern" [三角辩证, pinyin: *sānjiaō biàn zhèng*]).

Considerations of Disease Causes

Although TCM and its concept of disease do not strongly differentiate between cause and effect, pattern discrimination can include considerations regarding the disease cause; this is called 病因辩证 (pinyin: *bìngyīn biàn zhèng*, "disease-cause pattern discrimination").

There are three fundamental categories of disease causes (三因, pinyin: *sān yīn*) recognized:

1. external causes: these include the Six Excesses and "Pestilential Qi".

2. internal causes: the "Seven Affects" (七情, pinyin: *qì qíng*, sometimes also translated as "Seven Emotions") – joy, anger, brooding, sorrow, fear, fright and grief. These are believed to be able to cause damage to the functions of the zàng-fú, especially of the Liver.

3. non-external-non-internal causes: dietary irregularities (especially: too much raw, cold, spicy, fatty or sweet food; voracious eating; too much alcohol), fatigue, sexual intemperance, trauma, and parasites (虫, pinyin: *chóng*).

Diagnostics

In TCM, there are five diagnostic methods: inspection, auscultation, olfaction, inquiry, and palpation.

*   Inspection focuses on the face and particularly on the tongue, including analysis of the tongue size, shape, tension, color and coating, and the absence or presence of teeth marks around the edge.

*   Auscultation refers to listening for particular sounds (such as wheezing).

*   Olfaction refers to attending to body odor.

*   Inquiry focuses on the "seven inquiries", which involve asking the person about the regularity, severity, or other characteristics of: chills, fever, perspiration, appetite, thirst, taste, defecation, urination, pain, sleep, menses, leukorrhea.

*   Palpation which includes feeling the body for tender A-shi points, and the palpation of the wrist pulses as well as various other pulses, and palpation of the abdomen.

Tongue and Pulse

Examination of the tongue and the pulse are among the principal diagnostic methods in TCM. Certain sectors of the tongue's surface are believed to correspond to the zàng-fǔ. For example, teeth marks on one part of the tongue might indicate a problem with the Heart, while teeth marks on another part of the tongue might indicate a problem with the Liver.

Pulse palpation involves measuring the pulse both at a superficial and at a deep level at three different locations on the radial artery (*Cun, Guan, Chi*, located two finger-breadths from the wrist crease, one fingerbreadth from the wrist crease, and right at the wrist crease, respectively, usually palpated with the index, middle and ring finger) of each arm, for a total of twelve pulses, all of which are thought to correspond with certain zàng-fǔ. The pulse is examined for several characteristics including rhythm, strength and volume, and described with qualities like "floating, slippery, bolstering-like, feeble, thready and quick"; each of these qualities indicate certain disease patterns. Learning TCM pulse diagnosis can take several years.

Herbal Medicine

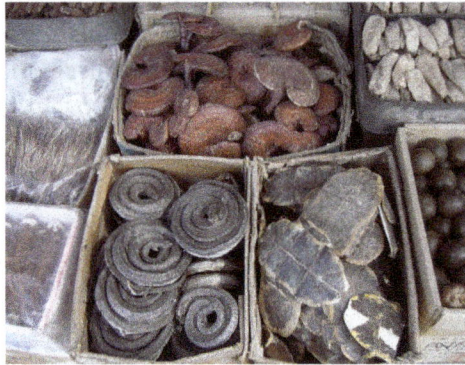

Assorted dried plant and animal parts used in traditional Chinese medicines, clockwise from top left corner: dried Lingzhi (lit. "spirit mushrooms"), ginseng, Luo Han Guo, turtle shell underbelly (plastron), and dried curled snakes.

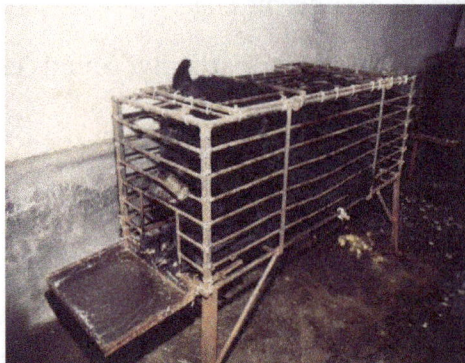

A bile bear in a "crush cage" on Huizhou Farm, China.

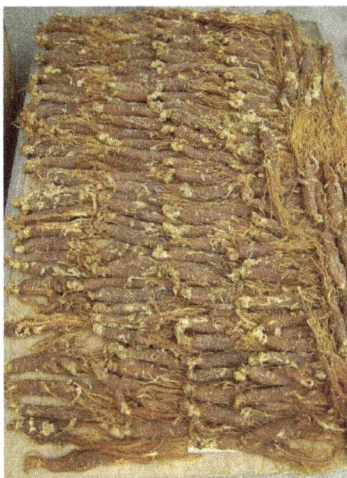
Chinese red ginseng roots

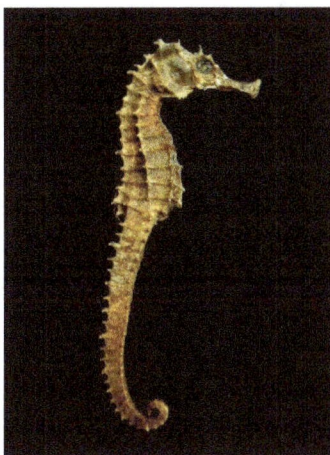
Dried seahorses are extensively used in traditional medicine in China and elsewhere.

The term "herbal medicine" is somewhat misleading in that, while plant elements are by far the most commonly used substances in TCM, other, non-botanic substances are used as well: animal, human, and mineral products are also utilized. Thus, the term "medicinal" (instead of herb) is usually preferred.

Prescriptions

Typically, one batch of medicinals is prepared as a decoction of about 9 to 18 substances. Some of these are considered as main herbs, some as ancillary herbs; within the ancillary herbs, up to three categories can be distinguished.

Raw Materials

There are roughly 13,000 medicinals used in China and over 100,000 medicinal recipes recorded in the ancient literature. Plant elements and extracts are by far the most common elements used. In the classic *Handbook of Traditional Drugs* from 1941, 517 drugs were listed – out of these, 45 were animal parts, and 30 were minerals.

Animal Substances

Some animal parts used as medicinals can be considered rather strange such as cows' gallstones, hornet's nest, leech, and scorpion. Other examples of animal parts include horn of the antelope or buffalo, deer antlers, testicles and penis bone of the dog, and snake bile. Some TCM textbooks still recommend preparations containing animal tissues, but there has been little research to justify the claimed clinical efficacy of many TCM animal products.

Some medicinals can include the parts of endangered species, including tiger bones and rhinoceros horn which is used for many ailments (though not as an aphrodisiac as is commonly misunderstood by the West). The black market in rhinoceros horn (driven not just by TMC but also unrelated status-seeking) has reduced the world's rhino population by more than 90 percent over the past 40 years. Concerns have also arisen over the use of pangolin scales, turtle plastron, seahorses, and the gill plates of mobula and manta rays. Poachers hunt restricted or endangered species animals to supply the black market with TCM products. There is no scientific evidence of efficacy for tiger medicines. Concern over China considering to legalize the trade in tiger parts prompted the 171-nation Convention on International Trade in Endangered Species (CITES) to endorse a decision opposing the resurgence of trade in tigers. Fewer than 30,000 saiga antelopes remain, which are exported to China for use in traditional fever therapies. Organized gangs illegally export the horn of the antelopes to China. The pressures on seahorses (Hippocampus spp.) used in traditional medicine is large; tens of millions of animals are unsustainably caught annually. Many species of syngnathid are currently part of the IUCN Red List of Threatened Species or national equivalents.

Since TCM recognizes bear bile as a medicinal, more than 12,000 asiatic black bears are held in bear farms. The bile is extracted through a permanent hole in the abdomen leading to the gall bladder, which can cause severe pain. This can lead to bears trying to kill themselves. As of 2012, approximately 10,000 bears are farmed in China for their bile. This practice has spurred public outcry across the country. The bile is collected from live bears via a surgical procedure. The deer penis is believed to have therapeutic benefits according to traditional Chinese medicine. It is typically very big and, proponents believe, in order to preserve its properties, it should be extracted from a living deer. Medicinal tiger parts from poached animals include tiger penis, believed to improve virility, and tiger eyes. The illegal trade for tiger parts in China has driven the species to near-extinction because of its popularity in traditional medicine. Laws protecting even critically endangered species such as the Sumatran tiger fail to stop the display and sale of these items in open markets. Shark fin soup is traditionally regarded in Chinese medicine as beneficial for health in East Asia, and its status as an elite dish has led to huge demand with the increase of affluence in China, devastating shark populations. The shark fins have been a part of traditional Chinese medicine for centuries. Shark finning is banned in many countries, but the trade is thriving in Hong Kong and China, where the fins are part of shark fin soup, a dish considered a delicacy, and used in some types of traditional Chinese medicine.

The tortoise (guiban) and the turtle (biejia) species used in traditional Chinese medicine are raised on farms, while restrictions are made on the accumulation and export of other endangered species. However, issues concerning the overexploitation of Asian turtles in China have not been completely solved. Australian scientists have developed methods to identify medicines containing DNA traces of endangered species. Finally, although not an endangered species, sharp rises in exports of donkeys and donkey hide from Africa to China to make the traditional remedy ejiao have prompted export restrictions by some African countries.

Human Body Parts

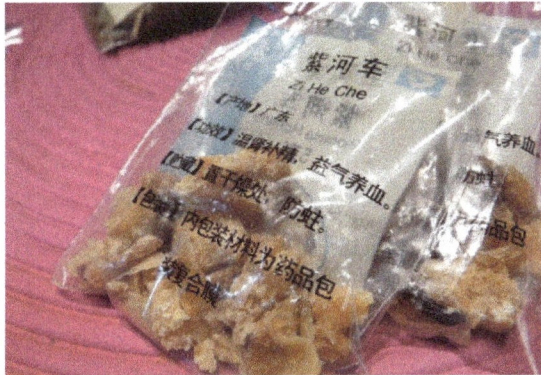

Dried human placenta (Ziheche (紫河车) is used in traditional Chinese medicine.

Traditional Chinese Medicine also includes some human parts: the classic Materia medica (Bencao Gangmu) describes the use of 35 human body parts and excreta in medicines, including bones, fingernail, hairs, dandruff, earwax, impurities on the teeth, feces, urine, sweat, organs, but most are no longer in use.

Human placenta has been used an ingredient in certain traditional Chinese medicines, including using dried human placenta, known as "Ziheche", to treat infertility, impotence and other conditions. The consumption of the human placenta is a potential source of infection.

Traditional Categorization

The traditional categorizations and classifications that can still be found today are:

The classification according to the Four Natures (四气, pinyin: *sì qì*): hot, warm, cool, or cold (or, neutral in terms of temperature) and hot and warm herbs are used to treat cold diseases, while cool and cold herbs are used to treat heat diseases.

The classification according to the Five Flavors, (五味, pinyin: *wǔ wèi*, sometimes also translated as Five Tastes): acrid, sweet, bitter, sour, and salty. Substances may also have more than one flavor, or none (i.e., a "bland" flavor). Each of the Five Flavors corresponds to one of zàng organs, which in turn corresponds to one of the Five Phases. A flavor implies certain properties and therapeutic actions of a substance; e.g., saltiness drains downward and softens hard masses, while sweetness is supplementing, harmonizing, and moistening.

The classification according to the meridian – more precise, the zàng-organ including its associated meridian – which can be expected to be primarily affected by a given medicinal.

The categorization according to the specific function mainly include: exterior-releasing or exterior-resolving, heat-clearing, downward-draining, or precipitating wind-damp-dispelling, dampness-transforming, promoting the movement of water and percolating dampness or dampness-percolating, interior-warming, qi-regulating or qi-rectifying, dispersing food accumulation or food-dispersing, worm-expelling, stopping bleeding or blood-stanching, quickening the Blood and dispelling stasis or blood-quickening, transforming phlegm, stopping coughing and calming wheezing or phlegm-transforming and cough- and panting-suppressing, Spirit-quieting, calming the liver and expelling wind or liver-calming and wind-extinguishingl orifice-openingl supplementing which includes qi-supplementing, blood-nourishing, yin-enriching, and yang-fortifying, astriction-promoting or securing and astringing, vomiting-inducing, and substances for external application.

Efficacy

As of 2007 there were not enough good-quality trials of herbal therapies to allow their effectiveness to be determined. A high percentage of relevant studies on traditional Chinese medicine are in Chinese databases. Fifty percent of systematic reviews on TCM did not search Chinese databases, which could lead to a bias in the results. Many systematic reviews of TCM interventions published in Chinese journals are incomplete, some contained errors or were misleading. The herbs recommended by traditional Chinese practitioners in the US are unregulated.

A 2013 review found the data too weak to support use of Chinese herbal medicine (CHM) for benign prostatic hyperplasia. A 2013 review found the research on the benefit and safety of CHM for idiopathic sudden sensorineural hearing loss is of poor quality and cannot be relied upon to support their use. A 2013 Cochrane review found inconclusive evidence that CHM reduces the severity of eczema. The traditional medicine ginger, which has shown anti-inflammatory properties in laboratory experiments, has been used to treat rheumatism, headache and digestive and respiratory issues, though there is no firm evidence supporting these uses. A 2012 Cochrane review found no difference in decreased mortality when Chinese herbs were used alongside Western medicine versus Western medicine exclusively. A 2012 Cochrane review found insufficient evidence to support the use of TCM for people with adhesive small bowel obstruction. A 2011 review found low quality evidence that suggests CHM improves the symptoms of Sjogren's syndrome. A 2010 review found TCM seems to be effective for the treatment of fibromyalgia but the findings were of insufficient methodological rigor. A 2009 Cochrane review found insufficient evidence to recommend the use of TCM for the treatment of epilepsy. A 2008 Cochrane review found promising evidence for the use of Chinese herbal medicine in relieving painful menstruation, but the trials assessed were of such low methodological quality that no conclusion could be drawn about the remedies' suitability as a recommendable treatment option. Turmeric has been used in traditional Chinese medicine for centuries to treat various conditions. This includes jaundice and hepatic disorders, rheumatism, anorexia, diabetic wounds, and menstrual complications. Most of its effects have been attributed to curcumin. Research that curcumin shows strong anti-inflammatory and antioxidant activities have instigated mechanism of action studies on the possibility for cancer and inflammatory diseases prevention and treatment. It also exhibits immunomodulatory effects. A 2005 Cochrane review found insufficient evidence for the use of CHM in HIV-infected people and people with AIDS.

Drug Research

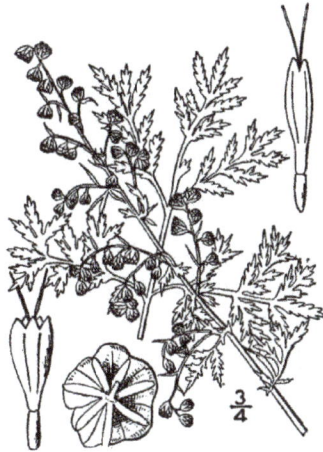

Artemisia annua is traditionally used to treat fever. It has been found to have antimalarial properties.

With an eye to the enormous Chinese market, pharmaceutical companies have explored the potential for creating new drugs from traditional remedies. A *Nature* editorial described TCM as "fraught with pseudoscience", and stated that having "no rational mechanism of action for most of its therapies" is the "most obvious answer" to why its study didn't provide a "flood of cures", while advocates responded that "researchers are missing aspects of the art, notably the interactions between different ingredients in traditional therapies."

One of the few successes was the development in the 1970s of the antimalarial drug artemisinin, which is a processed extract of *Artemisia annua*, a herb traditionally used as a fever treatment. Researcher Tu Youyou discovered that a low-temperature extraction process could isolate an effective antimalarial substance from the plant. She says she was influenced by a traditional source saying that this herb should be steeped in cold water, after initially finding high-temperature extraction unsatisfactory. The extracted substance, once subject to detoxification and purification processes, is a usable antimalarial drug – a 2012 review found that artemisinin-based remedies were the most effective drugs for the treatment of malaria. For her work on malaria, Tu received the 2015 Nobel Prize in Physiology or Medicine. Despite global efforts in combating malaria, it remains a large burden for the population. Although WHO recommends artemisinin-based remedies for treating uncomplicated malaria, artemisinin resistance can no longer be ignored.

Also in the 1970s Chinese researcher Zhang TingDong and colleagues investigated the potential use of the traditionally used substance arsenic trioxide to treat acute promyelocytic leukemia (APL). Building on his work, research both in China and the West eventually led to the development of the drug Trisenox, which was approved for leukemia treatment by the FDA in 2000.

Huperzine A, which is extracted from traditional herb *Huperzia serrata*, has attracted the interest of medical science because of alleged neuroprotective properties. Despite earlier promising results, a 2013 systematic review and meta-analysis found "Huperzine A appears to have beneficial effects on improvement of cognitive function, daily living activity, and global clinical assessment in participants with Alzheimer's disease. However, the findings should be interpreted with caution due to the poor methodological quality of the included trials."

Ephedrine in its natural form, known as *má huáng* (麻黄) in traditional Chinese medicine, has been documented in China since the Han dynasty (206 BC – 220 AD) as an antiasthmatic and stimulant. In 1885, the chemical synthesis of ephedrine was first accomplished by Japanese organic chemist Nagai Nagayoshi based on his research on Japanese and Chinese traditional herbal medicines

Cost-effectiveness

A 2012 systematic review found there is a lack of available cost-effectiveness evidence in TCM.

Safety

From the earliest records regarding the use of medicinals to today, the toxicity of certain substances has been described in all Chinese materiae medicae. Since TCM has become more popular in the Western world, there are increasing concerns about the potential toxicity of many traditional Chinese medicinals including plants, animal parts and minerals. Traditional Chinese herbal remedies are conveniently available from grocery stores in most Chinese neighborhoods; some of these items may contain toxic ingredients, are imported into the U.S. illegally, and are associated with claims of therapeutic benefit without evidence. For most medicinals, efficacy and toxicity testing are based on traditional knowledge rather than laboratory analysis. The toxicity in some cases could be confirmed by modern research (i.e., in scorpion); in some cases it couldn't (i.e., in *Curculigo*). Traditional herbal medicines can contain extremely toxic chemicals and heavy metals, and naturally occurring toxins, which can cause illness, exacerbate pre-existing poor health or result in death. Botanical misidentification of plants can cause toxic reactions in humans. The description on some plants used in traditional Chinese medicine have changed, leading to unintended intoxication of the wrong plants. A concern is also contaminated herbal medicines with microorganisms and fungal toxins, including aflatoxin. Traditional herbal medicines are sometimes contaminated with toxic heavy metals, including lead, arsenic, mercury and cadmium, which inflict serious health risks to consumers.

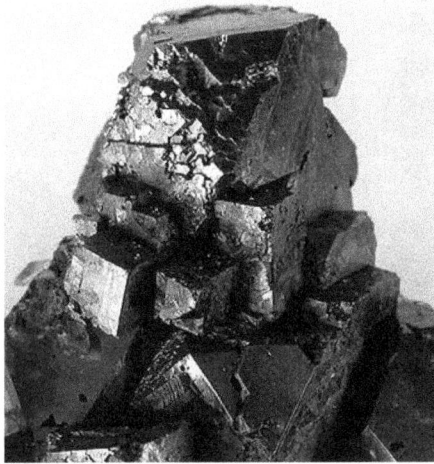

Galena (lead ore) is part of TCM.

Substances known to be potentially dangerous include *Aconitum*, secretions from the Asiatic toad, powdered centipede, the Chinese beetle (*Mylabris phalerata*), certain fungi, *Aristolochia*, *Aconitum*, Arsenic sulfide (Realgar), mercury sulfide, and cinnabar. Asbestos ore (Actinolite, Yang Qi Shi, 阳起石) is used to treat impotence in TCM. Due to galena's (litharge, lead(II) oxide) high lead content, it is known to be toxic. Lead, mercury, arsenic, copper, cadmium, and thallium have been detected in TCM products sold in the U.S. and China.

To avoid its toxic adverse effects *Xanthium sibiricum* must be processed. Hepatotoxicity has been reported with products containing *Polygonum multiflorum*, glycyrrhizin, *Senecio* and *Symphytum*. The herbs indicated as being hepatotoxic included *Dict-*

amnus dasycarpus, *Astragalus membranaceous*, and *Paeonia lactiflora*. Contrary to popular belief, *Ganoderma lucidum* mushroom extract, as an adjuvant for cancer immunotherapy, appears to have the potential for toxicity. A 2013 review suggested that although the antimalarial herb *Artemisia annua* may not cause hepatotoxicity, haematotoxicity, or hyperlipidemia, it should be used cautiously during pregnancy due to a potential risk of embryotoxicity at a high dose.

However, many adverse reactions are due to misuse or abuse of Chinese medicine. For example, the misuse of the dietary supplement *Ephedra* (containing ephedrine) can lead to adverse events including gastrointestinal problems as well as sudden death from cardiomyopathy. Products adulterated with pharmaceuticals for weight loss or erectile dysfunction are one of the main concerns. Chinese herbal medicine has been a major cause of acute liver failure in China.

Acupuncture and Moxibustion

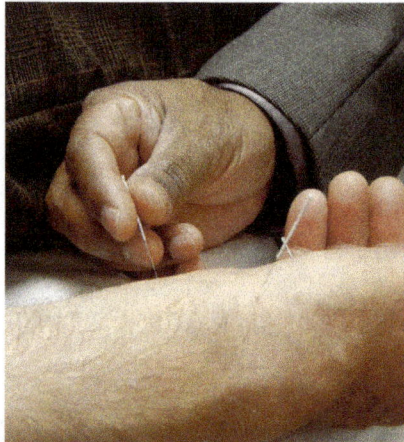

Needles being inserted into the skin.

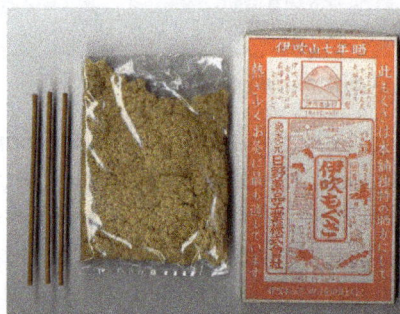

Traditional moxibustion set from Ibuki (Japan)

Acupuncture is the insertion of needles into superficial structures of the body (skin, subcutaneous tissue, muscles) – usually at acupuncture points (acupoints) – and their subsequent manipulation; this aims at influencing the flow of qi. According to TCM it relieves pain and treats (and prevents) various diseases.

Acupuncture is often accompanied by moxibustion – the Chinese characters for acupuncture (simplified Chinese: 针灸; traditional Chinese: 針灸; pinyin: *zhēnjiǔ*) literally meaning "acupuncture-moxibustion" – which involves burning mugwort on or near the skin at an acupuncture point. According to the American Cancer Society, "available scientific evidence does not support claims that moxibustion is effective in preventing or treating cancer or any other disease".

In electroacupuncture, an electric current is applied to the needles once they are inserted, in order to further stimulate the respective acupuncture points.

Efficacy

A 2013 editorial by Steven P. Novella and David Colquhoun found that the inconsistency of results of acupuncture studies (i.e. acupuncture relieved pain in some conditions but had no effect in other very similar conditions) suggests false positive results, which may be caused by factors like biased study designs, poor blinding, and the classification of electrified needles (a type of TENS) as a form of acupuncture. The same editorial suggested that given the inability to find consistent results despite more than 3,000 studies of acupuncture, the treatment seems to be a placebo effect and the existing equivocal positive results are noise one expects to see after a large number of studies are performed on an inert therapy. The editorial concluded that the best controlled studies showed a clear pattern, in which the outcome does not rely upon needle location or even needle insertion, and since "these variables are those that define acupuncture, the only sensible conclusion is that acupuncture does not work."

A 2012 meta-analysis concluded that the mechanisms of acupuncture "are clinically relevant, but that an important part of these total effects is not due to issues considered to be crucial by most acupuncturists, such as the correct location of points and depth of needling ... [but are] ... associated with more potent placebo or context effects". Commenting on this meta-analysis, both Edzard Ernst and David Colquhoun said the results were of negligible clinical significance.

A 2011 overview of Cochrane reviews found high quality evidence that suggests acupuncture is effective for some but not all kinds of pain. A 2010 systematic review found that there is evidence "that acupuncture provides a short-term clinically relevant effect when compared with a waiting list control or when acupuncture is added to another intervention" in the treatment of chronic low back pain. Two review articles discussing the effectiveness of acupuncture, from 2008 and 2009, have concluded that there is not enough evidence to conclude that it is effective beyond the placebo effect.

Acupuncture is generally safe when administered using Clean Needle Technique (CNT). Although serious adverse effects are rare, acupuncture is not without risk. Severe adverse effects, including death, have continued to be reported.

Tui Na

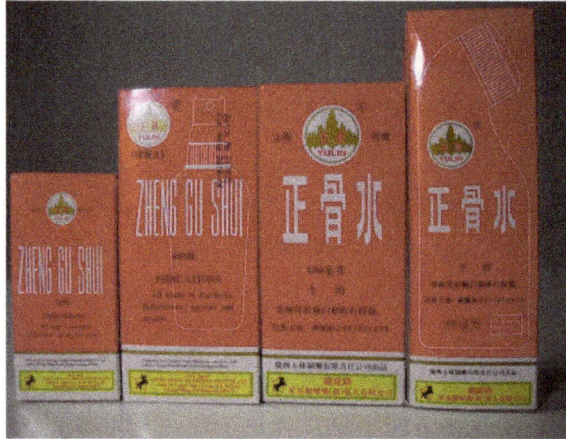

An example of a Traditional Chinese medicine used in Tui Na

Tui na (推拿) is a form of massage akin to acupressure (from which shiatsu evolved). Asian massage is typically administered with the person fully clothed, without the application of grease or oils. Techniques employed may include thumb presses, rubbing, percussion, and assisted stretching.

Qigong

Qìgōng (气功 or 氣功) is a TCM system of exercise and meditation that combines regulated breathing, slow movement, and focused awareness, purportedly to cultivate and balance qi. One branch of qigong is qigong massage, in which the practitioner combines massage techniques with awareness of the acupuncture channels and points.

Other Therapies

Cupping

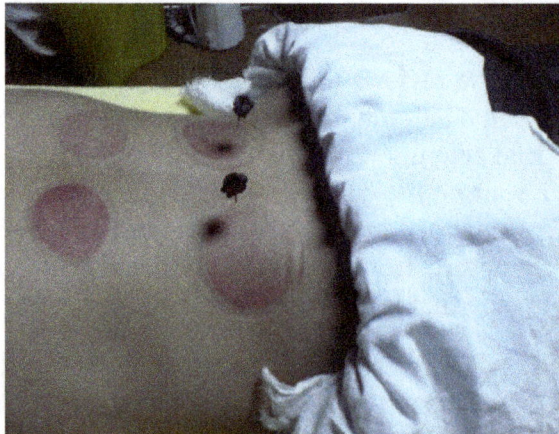

Acupuncture and moxibustion after cupping in Japan

Cupping (Chinese: 拔罐; pinyin: báguàn) is a type of Chinese massage, consisting of placing several glass "cups" (open spheres) on the body. A match is lit and placed inside the cup and then removed before placing the cup against the skin. As the air in the cup is heated, it expands, and after placing in the skin, cools, creating lower pressure inside the cup that allows the cup to stick to the skin via suction. When combined with massage oil, the cups can be slid around the back, offering "reverse-pressure massage".

It has not been found to be effective for the treatment of any disease. The 2008 *Trick or Treatment* book said that no evidence exists of any beneficial effects of cupping for any medical condition.

Gua Sha

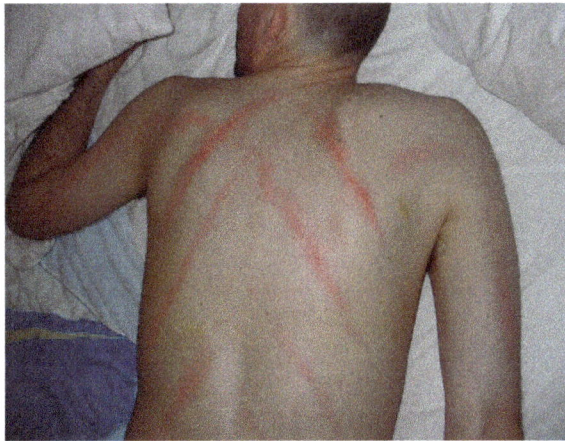

Gua Sha

Gua Sha (Chinese: 刮痧； pinyin: guāshā) is abrading the skin with pieces of smooth jade, bone, animal tusks or horns or smooth stones; until red spots then bruising cover the area to which it is done. It is believed that this treatment is for almost any ailment including cholera. The red spots and bruising take 3 to 10 days to heal, there is often some soreness in the area that has been treated.

Die-da

Diē-dá (跌打) or bone-setting is usually practiced by martial artists who know aspects of Chinese medicine that apply to the treatment of trauma and injuries such as bone fractures, sprains, and bruises. Some of these specialists may also use or recommend other disciplines of Chinese medical therapies (or Western medicine in modern times) if serious injury is involved. Such practice of bone-setting (整骨 or 正骨) is not common in the West.

Chinese Food Therapy

Traditional Chinese characters 陰 and 陽 for the words *yin* and *yang* denote different classes of foods, and it is important to consume them in a balanced fashion. The meal sequence should also observe these classes:

> In the Orient, it is traditional to eat yang before yin. Miso soup (yang — fermented soybean protein) for breakfast; raw fish (more yang protein); and then the vegetables which are yin.

Regulations

Many governments have enacted laws to regulate TCM practice.

Australia

From 1 July 2012 Chinese medicine practitioners must be registered under the national registration and accreditation scheme with the Chinese Medicine Board of Australia and meet the Board's Registration Standards, in order to practice in Australia.

Canada

TCM is regulated in five provinces in Canada: Alberta, British Columbia, Ontario, Quebec, and Newfoundland.

Hong Kong

The Chinese Medicine Council of Hong Kong was established in 1999. It regulates the medicinals and professional standards for TCM practitioners. All TCM practitioners in Hong Kong are required to register with the Council. The eligibility for registration includes a recognised 5-year university degree of TCM, a 30-week minimum supervised clinical internship, and passing the licensing exam.

Malaysia

The Traditional and Complementary Medicine Bill was passed by Parliament in 2012 establishing the Traditional and Complementary Medicine Council to register and regulate traditional and complementary medicine practitioners, including traditional Chinese medicine practitioners as well as other traditional and complementary medicine practitioners such as those in traditional Malay medicine and traditional Indian medicine.

Singapore

The TCM Practitioners Act was passed by Parliament in 2000 and the TCM Practitioners Board was established in 2001 as a statutory board under the Ministry of Health, to register and regulate TCM practitioners. The requirements for registration include possession of a diploma or degree from a TCM educational institution/university on a gazetted list, either structured TCM clinical training at an approved local TCM educational institution or foreign TCM registration together with supervised TCM clinical attachment/practice at an approved local TCM clinic, and upon meeting these requirements, passing the Singapore TCM Physicians Registration Examination (STRE) conducted by the TCM Practitioners Board.

United States

As of July 2012, only six states do not have existing legislation to regulate the professional practice of TCM. These six states are Alabama, Kansas, North Dakota, South Dakota, Oklahoma, and Wyoming. In 1976, California established an Acupuncture Board and became the first state licensing professional acupuncturists.

Indonesia

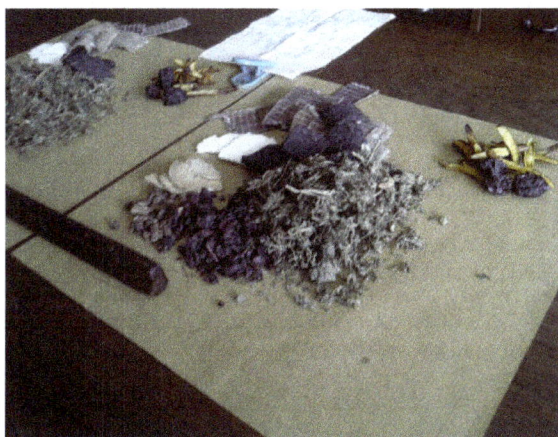

The Chinese traditional medicine at one of Chinese traditional medicine shop at Jagalan Road, Surabaya, Indonesia.

All traditional medicines, including TCM, are regulated on Indonesian Minister of Health Regulation in 2013 about Traditional Medicine. Traditional Medicine License (*Surat Izin Pengobatan Tradisional* -SIPT) will be granted to the practitioners whose methods are scientifically recognized as safe and bring the benefit for health. The TCM clinics are registered but there is no explicit regulation for it. The only TCM method which is accepted by medical logic and is empirically proofed is acupuncture. The acupuncturists can get SIPT and participate on health care facilities.

References

- Sivin, Nathan (1987). Traditional Medicine in Contemporary China. Ann Arbor: Center for Chinese Studies, University of Michigan. ISBN 978-0-89264-074-4.

- Goldschmidt, Asaf (2009). The Evolution of Chinese Medicine: Song Dynasty, 960–1200. London and New York: Routledge. ISBN 978-0-415-42655-8.

- Lu, Gwei-djen; Needham, Joseph (2002). Celestial Lancets: A History and Rationale of Acupuncture and Moxa. Routledge. ISBN 978-0-700-71458-2.

- Harper, Donald (1998). Early Chinese Medical Literature: The Mawangdui Medical Manuscripts. London and New York: Kegan Paul International. ISBN 978-0-7103-0582-4.

- Unschuld, Paul U. (1985). Medicine in China: A History of Ideas. Berkeley, California: University of California Press. ISBN 978-0-520-05023-5.

- Liu, Zheng-Cai (1999): "A Study of Daoist Acupuncture & Moxibustion" Blue Poppy Press, first edition. ISBN 978-1-891845-08-6

- Men, J. & Guo, L. (2010) "A General Introduction to Traditional Chinese Medicine" Science Press. ISBN 978-1-4200-9173-1

- Deng, T. (1999): "Practical diagnosis in traditional Chinese medicine". Elsevier. 5th reprint, 2005. ISBN 978-0-443-04582-0

- Maciocia, Giovanni, (1989): The Foundations of Chinese Medicine: A Comprehensive Text for Acupuncturists and Herbalists; Churchill Livingstone; ISBN 978-0-443-03980-5, p. 26

- Ross, Jeremy (1984) "Zang Fu, the organ systems of traditional Chinese medicine" Elsevier. First edition 1984. ISBN 978-0-443-03482-4

- Aung, S.K.H. & Chen, W.P.D. (2007): Clinical introduction to medical acupuncture. Thieme Mecial Publishers. ISBN 978-1-58890-221-4, p. 19

- Williams, WF (2013). Encyclopedia of Pseudoscience: From Alien Abductions to Zone Therapy. Encyclopedia of Pseudoscience. Routledge. pp. 3–4. ISBN 1135955220.

- Aung, S.K.H. & Chen, W.P.D. (2007): Clinical introduction to medical acupuncture. Thieme Mecial Publishers. ISBN 978-1-58890-221-4, p. 20

- Flaws, B., & Finney, D., (1996): "A handbook of TCM patterns & their treatments" Blue Poppy Press. 6th Printing 2007. ISBN 978-0-936185-70-5

- Clavey, Steven (1995): "Fluid physiology and pathology in traditional Chinese medicine". Elsevier. 2nd edition, 2003. ISBN 978-0-443-07194-2

- Marcus & Kuchera (2004). Foundations for integrative musculoskeletal medicine: an east-west approach. North Atlantic Books. ISBN 978-1-55643-540-9. Retrieved 22 March 2011. p. 159

2

Chinese Herbology: An Integrated Study

Chinese herbology or herbal therapy are an undocumented school of alternate medicine that uses ancient and modern medicinal recipes, derived from plant extracts, animal parts and other elements. Different regions of China have different approaches to Chinese herbology. The chapter strategically encompasses and incorporates the major components and key concepts of Chinese herbology, providing a complete understanding.

Chinese herbology

Chinese herbology (simplified Chinese: 中药学; traditional Chinese: 中藥學; pinyin: *zhōngyào xué*) is the theory of traditional Chinese herbal therapy, which accounts for the majority of treatments in traditional Chinese medicine (TCM). A *Nature* editorial described TCM as "fraught with pseudoscience", and said that the most obvious reason why it has not delivered many cures is that the majority of its treatments have no logical mechanism of action.

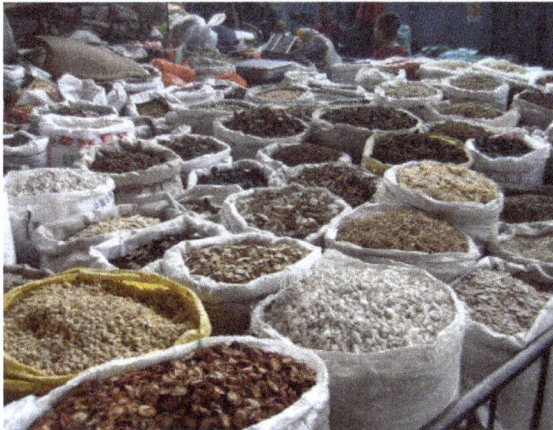

Dried herbs and plant portions for Chinese herbology at a Xi'an market

The term herbology is misleading in the sense that, while plant elements are by far the most commonly used substances, animal, human, and mineral products are also utilized. In the Neijing they are referred to as 毒藥 [duyao] which means toxin, poison or medicine. Unschuld points out that this is similar etymology to the Greek *pharmakon* and so he uses the term 'pharmaceutic'. Thus, the term "medicinal" (instead of herb) is usually preferred as a translation for 药 (pinyin: *yào*).

The effectiveness of traditional Chinese herbal therapy remains poorly documented. There are concerns over a number of potentially toxic Chinese herbs.

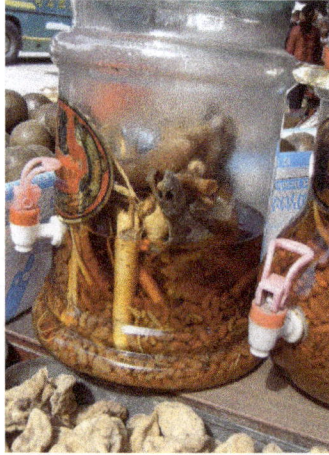

Ready-to-drink macerated medicinal liquor with goji berry, tokay gecko, and ginseng, for sale at a traditional medicine market in Xi'an, China

History

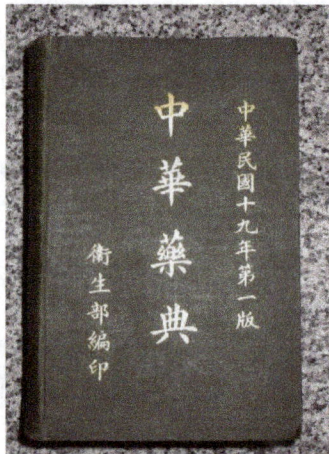

Chinese pharmacopoeia

Chinese herbs have been used for centuries. Among the earliest literature are lists of prescriptions for specific ailments, exemplified by the manuscript "Recipes for 52 Ailments", found in the Mawangdui which were sealed in 168 BC.

The first traditionally recognized herbalist is Shénnóng (神农, lit. "Divine Farmer"), a mythical god-like figure, who is said to have lived around 2800 BC. He allegedly tasted hundreds of herbs and imparted his knowledge of medicinal and poisonous plants to farmers. His *Shénnóng Běn Cǎo Jīng* (神农本草经, *Shennong's Materia Medica*) is considered as the oldest book on Chinese herbal medicine. It classifies 365 species of roots, grass, woods, furs, animals and stones into three categories of herbal medicine:

1. The "superior" category, which includes herbs effective for multiple diseases and are mostly responsible for maintaining and restoring the body balance. They have almost no unfavorable side-effects.

2. A category comprising tonics and boosters, whose consumption must not be prolonged.

3. A category of substances which must usually be taken in small doses, and for the treatment of specific diseases only.

The original text of Shennong's Materia Medica has been lost; however, there are extant translations. The true date of origin is believed to fall into the late Western Han dynasty (i.e., the first century BC).

The *Treatise on Cold Damage Disorders and Miscellaneous Illnesses* was collated by Zhang Zhongjing, also sometime at the end of the Han dynasty, between 196 and 220 CE. Focusing on drug prescriptions, it was the first medical work to combine Yinyang and the Five Phases with drug therapy. This formulary was also the earliest Chinese medical text to group symptoms into clinically useful "patterns" (*zheng* □) that could serve as targets for therapy. Having gone through numerous changes over time, it now circulates as two distinct books: the *Treatise on Cold Damage Disorders* and the *Essential Prescriptions of the Golden Casket*, which were edited separately in the eleventh century, under the Song dynasty.

Succeeding generations augmented these works, as in the *Yaoxing Lun* (simplified Chinese: 药性论; traditional Chinese: 藥性論; literally "Treatise on the Nature of Medicinal Herbs"), a 7th-century Tang Dynasty Chinese treatise on herbal medicine.

There was a shift in emphasis in treatment over several centuries. A section of the Neijing Suwen including Chapter 74 was added by Wang Bing [王冰 Wáng Bīng] in his 765 edition. In which it says: 主病之謂君，佐君之謂臣，應臣之謂使，非上下三品之謂也。 "Ruler of disease it called Sovereign, aid to Sovereign it called Minister, comply with Minister it called Envoy (Assistant), not upper lower three classes (qualities) it called." The last part is interpreted as stating that these three rulers are not the three classes of Shénnóng mentioned previously. This chapter in particular outlines a more forceful approach. Later on Zhang Zihe [張子和 Zháng Zǐ-hè (or hē?), aka Zhang Cong-zhen] (1156-1228) is credited with founding the 'Attacking School' which criticized the overus of tonics.

Arguably the most important of these later works is the *Compendium of Materia Medica* (*Bencao Gangmu*:本草綱目) compiled during the Ming dynasty by Li Shizhen, which is still used today for consultation and reference.

The use of Chinese herbs was popular during the medieval age in western Asian and Islamic countries. They were traded through the Silk Road from the East to the West.

Cinnamon, ginger, rhubarb, nutmeg and cubeb are mentioned as Chinese herbs by medieval Islamic medical scholars Such as Rhazes (854– 925 CE), Haly Abbas (930-994 CE) and Avicenna (980-1037 CE). There were also multiple similarities between the clinical uses of these herbs in Chinese and Islamic medicine.

Raw Materials

There are roughly 13,000 medicinals used in China and over 100,000 medicinal recipes recorded in the ancient literature. Plant elements and extracts are by far the most common elements used. In the classic *Handbook of Traditional Drugs* from 1941, 517 drugs were listed – out of these, only 45 were animal parts, and 30 were minerals. For many plants used as medicinals, detailed instructions have been handed down not only regarding the locations and areas where they grow best, but also regarding the best timing of planting and harvesting them.

Some animal parts used as medicinals can be considered rather strange such as cows' gallstones.

Furthermore, the classic materia medica *Bencao Gangmu* describes the use of 35 traditional Chinese medicines derived from the human body, including bones, fingernail, hairs, dandruff, earwax, impurities on the teeth, feces, urine, sweat, and organs, but most are no longer in use.

Preparation

Each herbal medicine prescription is a cocktail of many substances, usually tailored to the individual patient.

Decoction

Typically, one batch of medicinals is prepared as a decoction of about 9 to 18 substances. Some of these are considered as main herbs, some as ancillary herbs; within the ancillary herbs, up to three categories can be distinguished. Some ingredients are added in order to cancel out toxicity or side-effects of the main ingredients; on top of that, some medicinals require the use of other substances as catalysts.

Chinese Patent Medicine

Chinese patent medicine (traditional Chinese: 中成藥, Simplified Chinese: 中成药, pinyin: zhōngchéng yào) is a kind of traditional Chinese medicine. They are standardized herbal formulas. From ancient times, pills were formed by combining several herbs and other ingredients, which were dried and ground into a powder. They were then mixed with a binder and formed into pills by hand. The binder was traditionally honey. Modern teapills, however, are extracted in stainless steel extractors to create either a water decoction or water-alcohol decoction, depending on the herbs used.

They are extracted at a low temperature (below 100 degrees Celsius) to preserve essential ingredients. The extracted liquid is then further condensed, and some raw herb powder from one of the herbal ingredients is mixed in to form an herbal dough. This dough is then machine cut into tiny pieces, a small amount of excipients are added for a smooth and consistent exterior, and they are spun into pills. Teapills are characteristically little round black pills.

Chinese patent medicines are easy and convenient. They are not easy to customize on a patient-by-patient basis, however. They are often used when a patient's condition is not severe and the medicine can be taken as a long-term treatment.

These medicines are not patented in the traditional sense of the word. No one has exclusive rights to the formula. Instead, "patent" refers to the standardization of the formula. In China, all Chinese patent medicines of the same name will have the same proportions of ingredients, and manufactured in accordance with the PRC Pharmacopoeia, which is mandated by law. However, in western countries there may be variations in the proportions of ingredients in patent medicines of the same name, and even different ingredients altogether.

Several producers of Chinese herbal medicines are pursuing FDA clinical trials to market their products as drugs in U.S. and European markets.

Chinese Herbal Extracts

Chinese herbal extracts are herbal decoctions that have been condensed into a granular or powdered form. Herbal extracts, similar to patent medicines, are easier and more convenient for patients to take. The industry extraction standard is 5:1, meaning for every five pounds of raw materials, one pound of herbal extract is derived.

Categorization

There are several different methods to classify traditional Chinese medicinals:

- The Four Natures (simplified Chinese: 四气; traditional Chinese: 四氣; pinyin: *sìqì*)

- The Five Flavors (Chinese: 五味; pinyin: *wǔwèi*)

- The meridians (simplified Chinese: 经络; traditional Chinese: 經絡; pinyin: *jīngluò*)

- The specific function.

Four Natures

The Four Natures are: hot (热), warm (温), cool (凉), cold (寒) or neutral (平), in terms of temperature. Hot and warm herbs are used to treat cold diseases, while cool and cold herbs are used to treat heat diseases.

Five Flavors

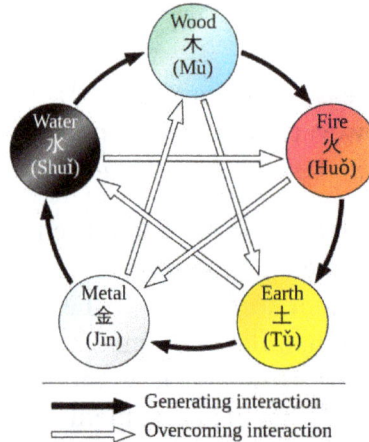

The Five Phases, which correspond to the Five Flavors

The Five Flavors, sometimes also translated as *Five Tastes*, are: acrid/pungent (辛), sweet (甘), bitter (苦), sour (酸), and salty (咸). Substances may also have more than one flavor, or none (i.e., a bland (淡) flavor). Each of the Five Flavors corresponds to one of the zàng organs, which in turn corresponds to one of the Five Phases: A flavor implies certain properties and therapeutic actions of a substance: saltiness "drains downward and softens hard masses"; sweetness is "supplementing, harmonizing, and moistening"; pungent substances are thought to induce sweat and act on qi and blood; sourness tends to be astringent (涩) in nature; bitterness "drains heat, purges the bowels, and eliminates dampness".

Meridians

This classification refers not just to the meridian, but also to the meridian-associated zàng-organ, which can be expected to be primarily affected by a given medicinal (there are 12 standard meridians in the body a medicinal can act upon). For example, traditional beliefs hold that menthol is pungent and cool and goes to the lung and the liver channels. The traditional Chinese concept of the lungs includes the function of protecting the body from colds, and menthol is thought to cool the lungs and purge heat toxins caused by wind-heat invasion (one of the patterns of common cold).

Specific Function

These categories mainly include:

- exterior-releasing or exterior-resolving
- heat-clearing

- downward-draining or precipitating

- wind-damp-dispelling

- dampness-transforming

- promoting the movement of water and percolating dampness or dampness-per-colating

- interior-warming

- qi-regulating or qi-rectifying

- dispersing food accumulation or food-dispersing

- worm-expelling

- stopping bleeding or blood-stanching

- quickening the Blood and dispelling stasis or blood-quickening or Blood-moving.

- transforming phlegm, stopping coughing and calming wheezing or phlegm-transforming and cough- and panting-suppressing

- Spirit-quieting or Shen-calming.

- calming the Liver and expelling wind or Liver-calming and wind-extinguishing

- orifice-opening

- supplementing or tonifying: this includes qi-supplementing, blood-nourishing, yin-enriching, and yang-fortifying.

- astriction-promoting or securing and astringing

- vomiting-inducing

- substances for external application

Nomenclature

Many herbs earn their names from their unique physical appearance. Examples of such names include *Niu Xi* (Radix cyathulae seu achyranthis), "cow's knees," which has big joints that might look like cow knees; *Bai Mu Er* (Fructificatio tremellae fuciformis), white wood ear,' which is white and resembles an ear; *Gou Ji* (Rhizoma cibotii), 'dog spine,' which resembles the spine of a dog.

Color

Color is not only a valuable means of identifying herbs, but in many cases also provides information about the therapeutic attributes of the herb. For example, yellow herbs are referred to as *huang* (yellow) or *jin* (gold). Huang Bai (Cortex Phellodendri) means 'yellow fir," and *Jin Yin Hua* (Flos Lonicerae) has the label 'golden silver flower."

Smell and Taste

Unique flavors define specific names for some substances. *Gan* means 'sweet,' so *Gan Cao* (Radix glycyrrhizae) is 'sweet herb," an adequate description for the licorice root. "Ku" means bitter, thus Ku Shen (Sophorae flavescentis) translates as 'bitter herb.'

Geographic Location

The locations or provinces in which herbs are grown often figure into herb names. For example, *Bei Sha Shen* (Radix glehniae) is grown and harvested in northern China, whereas *Nan Sha Shen* (Radix adenophorae) originated in southern China. And the Chinese words for north and south are respectively *bei* and *nan*.

Chuan Bei Mu (Bulbus fritillariae cirrhosae) and *Chuan Niu Xi* (Radix cyathulae) are both found in Sichuan province, as the character "chuan" indicates in their names.

Function

Some herbs, like Fang Feng (Radix Saposhnikoviae), literally 'prevent wind," prevents or treats wind-related illnesses. Xu Duan (Radix Dipsaci), literally 'restore the broken,' effectively treats torn soft tissues and broken bones.

Country of Origin

Many herbs indigenous to other countries have been incorporated into the Chinese materia medica. *Xi Yang Shen* (Radix panacis quinquefolii), imported from North American crops, translates as 'western ginseng," while *Dong Yang Shen* (Radix ginseng Japonica), grown in and imported from North Asian countries, is 'eastern ginseng.' Similar examples are noted in the text whenever geography matters in herb selection.

Toxicity

From the earliest records regarding the use of medicinals to today, the toxicity of certain substances has been described in all Chinese materia medica. Since TCM has become more popular in the Western world, there are increasing concerns about the potential toxicity of many traditional Chinese medicinals including plants, animal parts and minerals. For most medicinals, efficacy and toxicity testing are based on traditional knowledge rather than laboratory analysis. The toxicity in some cases could be confirmed by modern research (i.e., in scorpion); in some cases it could not (i.e., in *Curculigo*). Further, ingredients may have different names in different locales or in historical texts, and different preparations may have similar names for the same reason, which can create inconsistencies and confusion in the creation of medicinals, with the possible danger of poisoning. Edzard Ernst "concluded that adverse effects of herbal medicines are an important albeit neglected subject in dermatology, which deserves further systematic investigation." Research suggests that the toxic heavy metals and undeclared drugs found in Chinese herbal medicines might be a serious health issue.

Substances known to be potentially dangerous include aconite, secretions from the Asiatic toad, powdered centipede, the Chinese beetle (*Mylabris phalerata*, Ban mao), and certain fungi. There are health problems associated with *Aristolochia*. Toxic effects are also frequent with *Aconitum*. To avoid its toxic adverse effects *Xanthium sibiricum* must be processed. Hepatotoxicity has been reported with products containing *Polygonum multiflorum*, glycyrrhizin, *Senecio* and *Symphytum*. The evidence suggests that hepatotoxic herbs also include *Dictamnus dasycarpus*, *Astragalus membranaceous*, and *Paeonia lactiflora*; although there is no evidence that they cause liver damage. Contrary to popular belief, *Ganoderma lucidum* mushroom extract, as an adjuvant for cancer immunotherapy, appears to have the potential for toxicity.

A 2013 review suggested that although the antimalarial herb *Artemisia annua* may not cause hepatotoxicity, haematotoxicity, or hyperlipidemia, it should be used cautiously during pregnancy due to a potential risk of embryotoxicity at a high dose.

However, many adverse reactions are due to misuse or abuse of Chinese medicine. For example, the misuse of the dietary supplement *Ephedra* (containing ephedrine) can lead to adverse events including gastrointestinal problems as well as sudden death from cardiomyopathy. Products adulterated with pharmaceuticals for weight loss or erectile dysfunction are one of the main concerns. Chinese herbal medicine has been a major cause of acute liver failure in China.

Efficacy

Regarding Traditional Chinese herbal therapy, only few trials exist that are considered to be of adequate methodology by modern western medical researchers, and its effectiveness therefore is considered poorly documented. A 2016 Cochrane review found "insufficient evidence that Chinese Herbal Medicines were any more or less effective than placebo or Hormonal Therapy" for the relief of menopause related symptoms. A 2012 Cochrane review found no difference in decreased mortality when Chinese herbs were used alongside Western medicine versus Western medicine exclusively. A 2010 Cochrane review found there is not enough robust evidence to support the effectiveness of traditional Chinese medicine herbs to stop the bleeding from haemorrhoids. A 2008 Cochrane review found promising evidence for the use of Chinese herbal medicine in relieving painful menstruation, compared to conventional medicine such as NSAIDs and the oral contraceptive pill, but the findings are of low methodological quality. A 2007 Cochrane review found there is not enough evidence to support or dismiss the use of Chinese medicinal herbs for the treatment of influenza. A 2005 Cochrane review found that although the evidence was weak for the use of any single herb, there was low quality evidence that some Chinese medicinal herbs may be effective for the treatment of acute pancreatitis.

Successful results have however been scarce: artemisinin, for example, which is an effective treatment for malaria, was discovered from an herb traditionally used to treat fever. Although advocates have argued that research had missed some key features of TCM, such as the subtle interrelationships between ingredients, it is largely pseudoscience, with no valid mechanism of action for the majority of its treatments.

Ecological Impacts

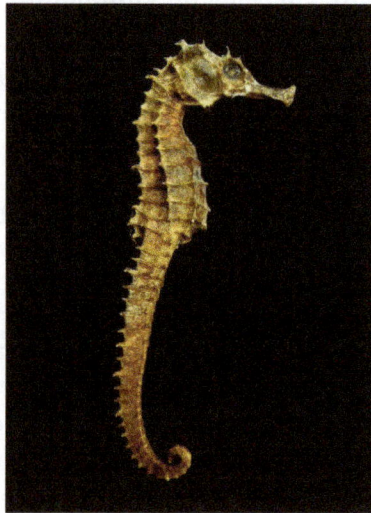

Dried seahorses like these are extensively used in traditional medicine in China and elsewhere.

The traditional practice of using (by now) endangered species is controversial within TCM. Modern Materia Medicas such as Bensky, Clavey and Stoger's comprehensive Chinese herbal text discuss substances derived from endangered species in an appendix, emphasizing alternatives.

Parts of endangered species used as TCM drugs include tiger bones and rhinoceros horn. Poachers supply the black market with such substances, and the black market in rhinoceros horn, for example, has reduced the world's rhino population by more than 90 percent over the past 40 years. Concerns have also arisen over the use of turtle plastron and seahorses.

TCM recognizes bear bile as a medicinal. In 1988, the Chinese Ministry of Health started controlling bile production, which previously used bears killed before winter. Now bears are fitted with a sort of permanent catheter, which is more profitable than killing the bears. More than 12,000 asiatic black bears are held in "bear farms", where they suffer cruel conditions while being held in tiny cages. The catheter leads through a permanent hole in the abdomen directly to the gall bladder, which can cause severe pain.

Increased international attention has mostly stopped the use of bile outside of China; gallbladders from butchered cattle (niú dǎn / 牛膽 / 牛胆) are recommended as a substitute for this ingredient.

Collecting American ginseng to assist the Asian traditional medicine trade has made ginseng the most harvested wild plant in North America for the last two centuries, which eventually led to a listing on CITES Appendix II.

Herbs in Use

There are over three hundred herbs that are commonly being used today. Some of the most commonly used herbs are Ginseng (人参, 人參, *rénshēn*), wolfberry (枸杞子), *dong quai* (*Angelica sinensis*, 当归, 當歸, *dāngguī*), astragalus (黄耆, 黃耆, *huángqí*), atractylodes (白术, 白朮, *báizhú*), bupleurum (柴胡, *cháihú*), cinnamon (cinnamon twigs (桂枝, *guìzhī*) and cinnamon bark (肉桂, *ròuguì*)), coptis (黄莲, 黃蓮, *huánglián*), ginger (姜, 薑, *jiāng*), hoelen (茯苓, *fúlíng*), licorice (甘草, *gāncǎo*), *ephedra sinica* (麻黄, 麻黃, *máhuáng*), peony (white: 白芍, *báisháo* and reddish: 赤芍, *chìsháo*), rehmannia (地黄, 地黃, *dìhuáng*), rhubarb (大黄, 大黃, *dàhuáng*), and salvia (丹参, 丹參, *dānshēn*).

Ginseng

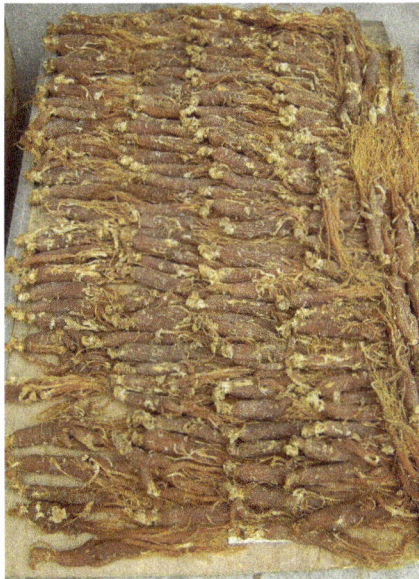

Chinese red ginseng roots

The use of ginseng (人参) is well over 2,000 years old in Chinese medicine. Ginseng contains ginsenosides. The amount of ginsenosides in ginseng depends on how the plant was cultivated and the age of the root. Wild ginseng is rare and commands the highest prices on the market. Red Panax ginseng is the most popular form of ginseng and it is usually packaged as a liquid or tea. Ginseng comes in two kinds, red and white. The color of the ginseng depends on how it is processed. White ginseng is unprocessed and dries naturally. Red ginseng is processed with steam and is believed to be more effective. Native Americans have used American ginseng for dry coughs, constipation, and fevers.

TCM Information: Species: Panax ginseng. Pinyin: Ren Shen. Common Name: Chinese Ginseng. Quality: Sweet, Bitter, Warm. Meridians: Lung, Spleen, Heart. Actions: Tonifies yuan qi to treat collapse of qi, tonifies spleen and lung, generates fluids, mildly tonifies heart qi.

Species: Elutherococcus senticosus. Pinyin: Ci Wu Jia. Common Name: Siberian Ginseng. Quality: Pungent (Acrid), Slightly bitter, Warm. Meridians: Spleen, Heart, Kidney. Actions: Tonifies spleen and kidney, mildly tonifies heart qi, promotes blood circulation, calms shen.

Species: Panax quinquefolius. Pinyin: Xi Yang Shen. Common Name: American Ginseng. Quality: Sweet, Slightly bitter, Cold. Meridians: Heart, Kidney, Lung. Actions: Tonifies lung and spleen qi, tonifies lung yin, cools fire from lung yin deficiency, generates fluids.

Ginkgo

Mushrooms

Mushrooms have long been used as a medicinal food and as a tea in Chinese herbology. Clinical, animal, and cellular research has shown some mushrooms may be able to up-regulate aspects of the immune system. Notable mushrooms used in Chinese herbology include Reishi and Shiitake.

Wolfberry

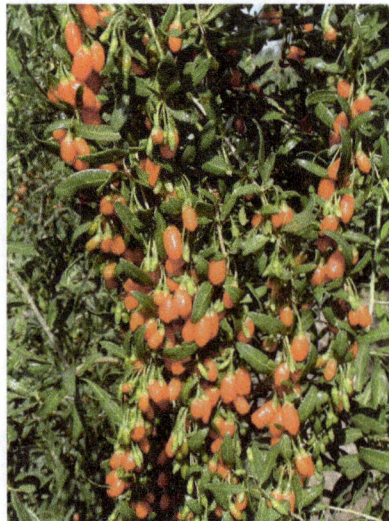

Lycium barbarum, Wolfberry (枸杞子)

Wolfberry (枸杞子) is grown in the Far East and is grown from shrubs with long vines. The shrubs are covered with small trumpet-shaped flowers, which turn into small, bright red berries. The berries are usually fresh and sometimes used when dried.

TCM Information: Species: *Lycium barbarum*. Pinyin: Gou Qi Zi. Common Name: Chinese Wolfberry. Quality: Sweet, Neutral. Meridians: Liver, Lung, Kidney. Actions: Tonifies kidney and lung yin, tonifies liver blood, tonifies jing, improves vision.

Dang Gui

Dang Gui (当归, *Angelica sinensis* or "female ginseng") is an aromatic herb that grows in China, Korea, and Japan.

TCM Information: Species: Angelica sinensis. Pinyin: Dang Gui. Common Name: Chinese Angelica Root. Quality: Sweet, Pungent(Acrid), Warm. Meridians: Liver, Heart, Spleen. Actions: Tonifies blood, invigorates blood, regulates menstruation, relieves pain, unblocks bowels by moistening intestine.

Astragalus

Astragalus (黄芪) is a root used for immune deficiencies and allergies.

TCM Information: Species: Astragalus membranaceus. Pinyin: Huang Qi. Common Name: Astragalus Root, Milkvetch Root. Quality: Sweet, Slightly warm. Meridians: Lung, Spleen. Actions: Raises yang qi to treat prolapse, tonifies spleen and lung qi, tonifies wei qi, increases urination, promotes drainage of pus, generates flesh.

Atractylodes

Atractylodes (白术) is believed to be important in the treatment of digestive disorders and problems of moisture accumulation.

TCM Information: Species: Atractylodes lancea. Pinyin: Cang Zhu. Common Name: Atractylodes Rhizome. Quality: Pungent(Acrid), Bitter, Warm. Meridians: Spleen, Stomach. Actions: Strong to dry dampness, strengthens the spleen, induce sweating, expels wind-cold, clears damp-heat from lower jiao, improves vision.

Bupleurum

Bupleurum (柴胡) is believed to be useful for the treatment of liver diseases, skin ailments, arthritis, menopausal syndrome, withdrawal from corticosteroid use, nephritis, stress-induced ulcers, and mental disorders.

TCM Information: Species: Bupleurnum chinense. Pinyin: Chai Hu. Common Name: Hare's Ear Root. Quality: Bitter, Pungent(Acrid), Cool. Meridians: Gallbladder, Liver, Pericardium, San Jiao. Actions: Treats alternating chills and fever, clears lesser yang disorders, relieves liver qi stagnation, raises yang qi to treat prolapse, treats certain menstrual disorders.

Cinnamon

Cinnamon (桂枝, 肉桂), mostly *gui zhi* and *rou gui*, is the twigs and bark from large tropical trees.

Studies show that cinnamon reduces serum glucose, triglyceride, LDL cholesterol, and total cholesterol in people with type 2 diabetes, and the findings suggest that the inclusion of cinnamon in the diet of people with type 2 diabetes will reduce risk factors associated with diabetes and cardiovascular diseases.

TCM Information: Species: Cinnamomum cassia. Pinyin: Gui Zhi. Common Name: Cinnamon Twig. Quality: Pungent (Acrid), Sweet, Warm. Meridians: Heart, Lung, Bladder. Actions: Induces sweating, warms and unblocks channels, unblocks yang qi of the chest, treats dysmenorrhea.

Species: Cinnamomum cassia. Pinyin: Rou Gui. Common Name: Cinnamon Bark. Quality: Pungent (Acrid), Sweet, Hot. Meridians: Heart, Kidney, Liver, Spleen. Actions: Tonifies kidney yang, leads fire back to its source, disperses cold, encourages generation of qi and blood, promotes blood circulation, alleviates pain due to cold, dysmenorrhea.

Coptis Chinensis

Coptis chinensis (黄莲) is a rhizome that is one of the bitterest herbs used in Chinese medicine.

TCM Information: Species: Coptis chinensis. Pinyin: Huang Lian. Common Name: Coptis Rhizome. Qualities: Bitter, Cold. Meridians: Heart, Large Intestine, Liver, Stomach. Actions: Clears heat and drains damp, drains fire(especially from heart and stomach), eliminates toxicity.

Ginger

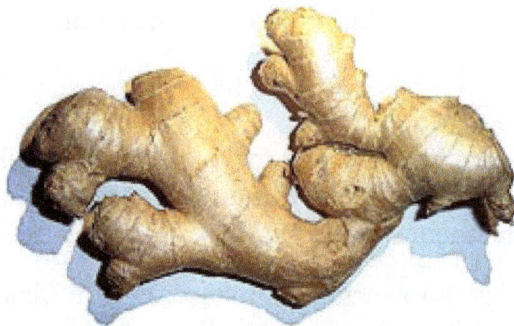

Ginger is consumed in China as food and as medicine.

Ginger (姜, 薑) is a herb and a spice that is used in Chinese cuisine. There are four main kinds of preparations in Chinese herbology: fresh ginger, dried ginger, roasted ginger, and ginger charcoal, all made of the rhizomes.

TCM Information:

Species: Zingiber officinalis.

Pinyin: Sheng Jiang (生姜, 生薑).

Common Name: Fresh Ginger Rhizome.

Quality: Pungent(Acrid), Slightly warm.

Meridians: Lung, Spleen, Stomach.

Actions: Releases the exterior, expels cold, warms the middle *jiao*, relieves nausea, transforms phlegm, warms lung to stop coughing, treats toxicity, and moderates the toxicity of other herbs.

Species: Zingiber officinalis.

Pinyin: Gan Jiang (干姜, 乾薑).

Common Name: Dried Ginger Rhizome.

Quality: Pungent(Acrid), Hot.

Meridians: Heart, Lung, Spleen, Stomach.

Actions: Warms the spleen and stomach, restores devastated yang, warms the lung to transform thin mucus, warms and unblocks channels.

Licorice

The use of the licorice plant (甘草) *Glycyrrhiza glabra* L. is thought to help treat hepatitis, sore throat, and muscle spasms.

TCM Information:

Species: *Glycyrrhiza inflata* or *Glycyrrhiza glabra*.

Pinyin: Gan Cao.

Common Name: Licorice Root.

Quality: Sweet, Neutral.

Meridians: All 12 channels, but mainly Heart, Lung, Spleen, Stomach.

Actions: Tonify spleen qi, moisten lung for dry cough, clears heat and fire toxicity, tonifies heart qi to regulate pulse, alleviates spasmodic pain, antidote for toxicity, moderates the effects of harsh herbs.

Ephedra

Ephedra (麻黄)

TCM Information: Species: Ephedra sinica or Ephedra intermedia. Pinyin: Ma Huang. Common Name: Ephedra Stem. Quality: Pungent(Acrid), Slightly Bitter, Warm. Meridians: Lung, Bladder. Actions: Induce sweating and release exterior for wind-cold invasion with no sweating, promotes urination, move lung qi for wheezing, cough or asthma.

Peony

Peony (白芍, 赤芍) comes in two varieties: bai shao (white) and chi shao (red), the root of the plant is used in both varieties.

TCM Information: Species: Paeonia lactiflora. Pinyin: Bai Shao. Common Name: White Peony Root. Quality: Bitter, Sour, Cool. Meridians: Liver, Spleen. Actions: Tonify liver blood, calms liver yang, alleviates flank/abdominal pain from liver qi stagnation or liver and spleen disharmony, preserves yin and adjusts nutritive and protective levels, regulates menses for blood deficiency problem.

Species: Paeonia lactiflora or Paeonia veitchii. Pinyin: Chi Shao. Common Name: Red Peony Root. Quality: Sour, Bitter, Cool. Meridians: Liver, Spleen. Actions: Clears heat, cools blood, invigorates blood and dispel stasis to treat irregular menses, dysmenorrhoea, amenorrhea, abdominal pain, and fixed abdominal masses.

Rehmannia

Rehmannia (地黄) is a root where the dark, moist part of the herb is used.

TCM Information: Species: Rehmannia glucinosa. Pinyin: Sheng Di Huang. Common Name: Chinese Foxglove Root. Qualities: Sweet, Bitter, Cold. Meridians: Heart, Kidney, Liver. Actions: Clears heat, cools blood, nourishes yin, generates fluids, treats wasting and thirsting disorder.

Species: Rehmannia glucinosa. Pinyin: Shu Di Huang. Common Name: Chinese Foxglove Root Prepared with Wine. Qualities: Sweet, Slightly warm. Meridians: Heart, Kidney, Liver. Actions: Tonifies blood, tonifies liver and kidney yin, treats wasting and thirsting disorder, nourishes jing.

Rhubarb

Rhubarb (大黄), used medicinally for its root, was one of the first herbs to be imported from China.

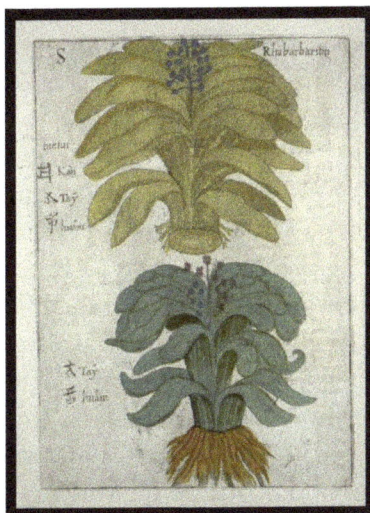

Chinese rhubarb depicted by Michał Boym (1655)

TCM Information: Species: Rheum palmatum, Rheum ranguticum, or Rheum officinale. Pinyin: Da Huang. Common Name: Rhubarb Root and Rhizome. Quality: Bitter, Cold. Meridians: Heart, Large Intestine, Liver, Stomach. Actions: Purge accumulation, cool blood, invigorate blood, drain damp-heat.

Salvia

Salvia (丹参) are the deep roots of the Chinese sage plant.

TCM Information: Species: Salvia miltiorrhiza. Pinyin: Dan Shen. Common Name: Salvia Root. Qualities: Bitter, Cool. Meridians: Heart, Pericardium, Liver. Actions: Invigorate blood, tonify blood, regulate menstruation, clear heat and soothe irritability.

Herbalism

Herbalism (also herbology or herbal medicine) is the use of plants for medicinal purposes, and the study of botany for such use. Plants have been the basis for medical treatments through much of human history, and such traditional medicine is still widely practiced today. Modern medicine recognizes herbalism as a form of alternative medicine, as the practice of herbalism is not strictly based on evidence gathered using the scientific method. Modern medicine, does, however, make use of many plant-derived compounds as the basis for evidence-tested pharmaceutical drugs. Phytotherapy, and phytochemistry work to apply modern standards of effectiveness testing to herbs and medicines that are derived from natural sources. The scope of herbal medicine is sometimes extended to include fungal and bee products, as well as minerals, shells and certain animal parts.

History

Archaeological evidence indicates that the use of medicinal plants dates at least to the Paleolithic age, approximately 60,000 years ago. Written evidence of herbal remedies dates back over 5,000 years, to the Sumerians, who compiled lists of plants. A number of ancient cultures wrote about plants and their medical uses in books called *herbals*. In ancient Egypt, herbs are mentioned in Egyptian medical papyri, depicted in tomb illustrations, or on rare occasions found in medical jars containing trace amounts of herbs. Among the oldest, lengthiest, and most important medical papyri of ancient Egypt, the Ebers Papyrus dates from about 1550 BC, and covers more than 700 drugs, mainly of plant origin. The earliest known Greek herbals come from Theophrastus of Eresos who in the 4th c. B.C. wrote in Greek *Historia Plantarum*, from Diocles of Carystus who wrote during the 3rd century B.C, and from Krateuas who wrote in the 1st century B.C. Only a few fragments of these works have survived intact, but from what remains scholars have noted a large amount of overlap with the Egyptian herbals. Seeds likely used for herbalism have been found in archaeological sites of Bronze Age China dating from the Shang Dynasty (c. 1600 BC–c. 1046 BC). Over a hundred of the 224 drugs mentioned in the *Huangdi Neijing*, an early Chinese medical text, are herbs. Herbs also commonly featured in the medicine of ancient India, where the principal treatment for diseases was diet. *De Materia Medica*, originally written in Greek by Pedanius Dioscorides (c. 40 – 90 AD) of Anazarbus, Cilicia, a Greek physician, pharmacologist and botanist, is a particularly important example of such[which?] writings. The documentation of herbs and their uses was a central part of both Western and Eastern medical scholarship through to the 1600s, and these works played an important role in the development of the science of botany.

Modern Herbal Medicine

The World Health Organization (WHO) estimates that 80 percent of the population of some Asian and African countries presently use herbal medicine for some aspect of primary health care. Pharmaceuticals are prohibitively expensive for most of the world's population, half of whom lived on less than $2 U.S. per day in 2002. In comparison, herbal medicines can be grown from seed or gathered from nature for little or no cost.

Many of the pharmaceuticals currently available to physicians have a long history of use as herbal remedies, including opium, aspirin, digitalis, and quinine. According to the World Health Organization, approximately 25% of modern drugs used in the United States have been derived from plants. At least 7,000 medical compounds in the modern pharmacopoeia are derived from plants. Among the 120 active compounds currently isolated from the higher plants and widely used in modern medicine today, 80% show a positive correlation between their modern therapeutic use and the traditional use of the plants from which they are derived.

Clinical Tests

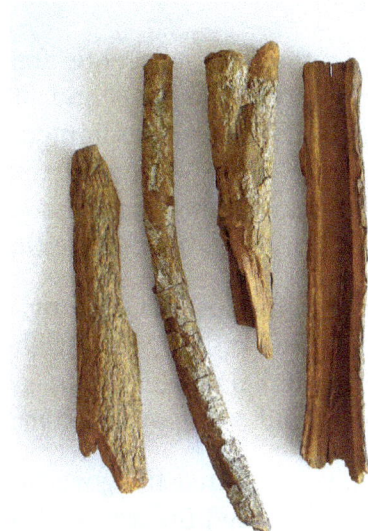

The bark of the cinchona tree contains quinine, which today is a widely prescribed treatment for malaria, especially in countries that cannot afford to purchase the more expensive anti-malarial drugs produced by the pharmaceutical industry.

In 2015 the Australian Government's Department of Health published the results of a review of alternative therapies that sought to determine if any were suitable for being covered by health insurance; Herbalism was one of 17 topics evaluated for which no clear evidence of effectiveness was found.

In a 2010 survey of the most common 1000 plant-derived compounds, only 156 had clinical trials published. Preclinical studies (tissue-culture and animal studies) were reported for about one-half of the plant products, while 12% of the plants, although available in the Western market, had "no substantial studies" of their properties. Strong evidence was found that 5 were toxic or allergenic, so that their use ought to be discouraged or forbidden. Nine plants had considerable evidence of therapeutic effect.

According to Cancer Research UK, "there is currently no strong evidence from studies in people that herbal remedies can treat, prevent or cure cancer".

The U.S. National Center for Complementary and Integrative Health of the National Institutes of Health funds clinical trials of the effectiveness of herbal medicines and provides "fact sheets" summarizing the effectiveness and side effects of many plant-derived preparations.

Prevalence of Use

The use of herbal remedies is more prevalent in patients with chronic diseases such as cancer, diabetes, asthma and end-stage renal disease. Multiple factors such as gender, age, ethnicity, education and social class are also shown to have association with prevalence of herbal remedies use.

A survey released in May 2004 by the National Center for Complementary and Integrative Health focused on who used complementary and alternative medicines (CAM), what was used, and why it was used. The survey was limited to adults, aged 18 years and over during 2002, living in the United States. According to this survey, herbal therapy, or use of natural products other than vitamins and minerals, was the most commonly used CAM therapy (18.9%) when all use of prayer was excluded.

Herbal remedies are very common in Europe. In Germany, herbal medications are dispensed by apothecaries (e.g., Apotheke). Prescription drugs are sold alongside essential oils, herbal extracts, or herbal teas. Herbal remedies are seen by some as a treatment to be preferred to pure medical compounds that have been industrially produced.

In India the herbal remedy is so popular that the government of India has created a separate department—AYUSH—under the Ministry of Health & Family Welfare. The National Medicinal Plants Board was also established in 2000 by the Indian government in order to deal with the herbal medical system.

Herbal Preparations

There are many forms in which herbs can be administered, the most common of which is in the form of a liquid that is drunk by the patient—either an herbal tea or a (possibly diluted) plant extract. Whole herb consumption is also practiced either fresh, in dried form or as fresh juice.

Several methods of standardization may be determining the amount of herbs used. One is the ratio of raw materials to solvent. However different specimens of even the same plant species may vary in chemical content. For this reason, thin layer chromatography is sometimes used by growers to assess the content of their products before use. Another method is standardization on a signal chemical.

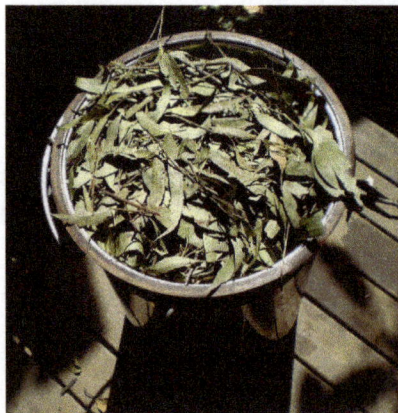

Leaves of *Eucalyptus olida* being packed into a steam distillation unit to gather its essential oil.

Herbal teas, or tisanes, are the resultant liquid of extracting herbs into water, though they are made in a few different ways. Infusions are hot water extracts of herbs, such as chamomile or mint, through steeping. Decoctions are the long-term boiled extracts, usually of harder substances like roots or bark. Maceration is the old infusion of plants with high mucilage-content, such as sage, thyme, etc. To make macerates, plants are chopped and added to cold water. They are then left to stand for 7 to 12 hours (depending on herb used). For most macerates 10 hours is used.

Tinctures are alcoholic extracts of herbs, which are generally stronger than herbal teas. Tinctures are usually obtained by combining 100% pure ethanol (or a mixture of 100% ethanol with water) with the herb. A completed tincture has an ethanol percentage of at least 25% (sometimes up to 90%). Herbal wine and elixirs are alcoholic extract of herbs, usually with an ethanol percentage of 12-38%. Herbal wine is a maceration of herbs in wine, while an elixir is a maceration of herbs in spirits (e.g., vodka, grappa, etc.). Extracts include liquid extracts, dry extracts, and nebulisates. Liquid extracts are liquids with a lower ethanol percentage than tinctures. They are usually made by vacuum distilling tinctures. Dry extracts are extracts of plant material that are evaporated into a dry mass. They can then be further refined to a capsule or tablet. A nebulisate is a dry extract created by freeze-drying. Vinegars are prepared in the same way as tinctures, except using a solution of acetic acid as the solvent. Syrups are extracts of herbs made with syrup or honey. Sixty-five parts of sugar are mixed with thirty-five parts of water and herb. The whole is then boiled and macerated for three weeks.

The exact composition of an herbal product is influenced by the method of extraction. A tea will be rich in polar components because water is a polar solvent. Oil on the other hand is a non-polar solvent and it will absorb non-polar compounds. Alcohol lies somewhere in between.

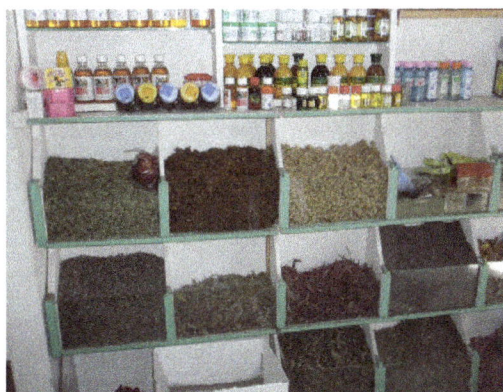

A herb shop in the souk of Marrakesh, Morocco

Many herbs are applied topically to the skin in a variety of forms. Essential oil extracts can be applied to the skin, usually diluted in a carrier oil. Many essential oils can burn the skin or are simply too high dose used straight; diluting them in olive oil or another food grade oil such as almond oil can allow these to be used safely as a topical.Salves, oils, balms, creams and lotions are other forms of topical delivery mechanisms. Most topical applications are oil extractions of herbs. Taking a food grade oil and soaking herbs in it for anywhere from weeks to months allows certain phytochemicals to be extracted into the oil. This oil can then be made into salves, creams, lotions, or simply used as an oil for topical application. Many massage oils, antibacterial salves, and wound healing compounds are made this way. One can also make a poultice or compress using the whole herb or the appropriate part of the plant, which is usually crushed or dried and re-hydrated with a small amount of water and then applied directly in a bandage, cloth, or just as is.

Inhalation, as in aromatherapy, can be used as a mood changing treatment to fight a sinus infection or cough , or to cleanse the skin on a deeper level (steam rather than direct inhalation here)

Safety

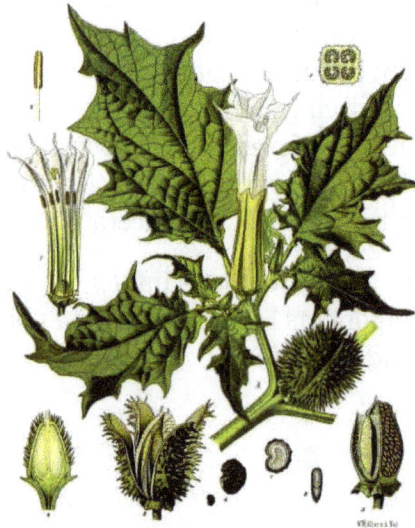

Datura stramonium is a highly effective treatment for asthma symptoms when smoked, because it contains atropine, which acts as an antispasmodic in the lungs. However, datura is also an extremely powerful hallucinogen and overdoses of the tropane alkaloids in it can result in hospitalization or death.

A number of herbs are thought to be likely to cause adverse effects. Furthermore, "adulteration, inappropriate formulation, or lack of understanding of plant and drug interactions have led to adverse reactions that are sometimes life threatening or lethal." Proper double-blind clinical trials are needed to determine the safety and efficacy of each plant before they can be recommended for medical use. Although many consumers believe that herbal medicines are safe because they are "natural", herbal medicines and synthetic drugs may interact, causing toxicity to the patient. Herbal remedies can also be dangerously contaminated, and herbal medicines without established efficacy, may unknowingly be used to replace medicines that do have corroborated efficacy.

Standardization of purity and dosage is not mandated in the United States, but even products made to the same specification may differ as a result of biochemical variations within a species of plant. Plants have chemical defense mechanisms against predators that can have adverse or lethal effects on humans. Examples of highly toxic herbs include poison hemlock and nightshade. They are not marketed to the public as herbs, because the risks are well known, partly due to a long and colorful history in Europe, associated with "sorcery", "magic" and intrigue. Although not frequent, adverse reactions have been reported for herbs in widespread use. On occasion serious untoward outcomes have been linked to herb consumption. A case of major potassium depletion has been attributed to chronic licorice ingestion., and consequently professional herbalists avoid the use of licorice where they recognize that this may be a risk. Black cohosh has been implicated in a case of liver failure. Few studies are available on the safety of herbs for pregnant women, and one study found that use of complementary and alternative medicines are associated with a 30% lower ongoing pregnancy and live birth rate during fertility treatment. Examples of herbal treatments with likely cause-effect relationships with adverse events include aconite, which is often a legally restricted herb, ayurvedic remedies, broom, chaparral, Chinese herb mixtures, comfrey, herbs containing certain flavonoids, germander, guar gum, liquorice root, and pennyroyal. Examples of herbs where a high degree of confidence of a risk long term adverse effects can be asserted include ginseng, which is unpopular among herbalists for this reason, the endangered herb goldenseal, milk thistle, senna, against which herbalists generally advise and rarely use, aloe vera juice, buckthorn bark and berry, cascara sagrada bark, saw palmetto, valerian, kava, which is banned in the European Union, St. John's wort, Khat, Betel nut, the restricted herb Ephedra, and Guarana.

There is also concern with respect to the numerous well-established interactions of herbs and drugs. In consultation with a physician, usage of herbal remedies should be clarified, as some herbal remedies have the potential to cause adverse drug interactions when used in combination with various prescription and over-the-counter pharmaceuticals, just as a patient should inform a herbalist of their consumption of orthodox prescription and other medication.

For example, dangerously low blood pressure may result from the combination of an herbal remedy that lowers blood pressure together with prescription medicine that has the same effect. Some herbs may amplify the effects of anticoagulants. Certain herbs as well as common fruit interfere with cytochrome P450, an enzyme critical to much drug metabolism.

Labeling Accuracy

A 2013 study published in the journal BMC Medicine found that one-third of herbal supplements sampled contained no trace of the herb listed on the label. The study found products adulterated with filler including allergens such as soy, wheat, and black walnut. One bottle labeled as St. John's Wort was found to actually contain Alexandrian senna, a laxative.

Researchers at the University of Adelaide found in 2014 that almost 20 per cent of herbal remedies surveyed were not registered with the Therapeutic Goods Administration, despite this being a condition for their sale. They also found that nearly 60 per cent of products surveyed had ingredients that did not match what was on the label. Out of 121 products, only 15 had ingredients that matched their TGA listing and packaging.

In 2015 the New York Attorney General issued cease and desist letters to four major U.S. retailers (GNC, Target, Walgreens, and Walmart) who are accused of selling herbal supplements that were mislabeled and potentially dangerous. 24 products were tested by DNA barcoding as part of the investigation, all but five contained DNA that did not match the products' labels. The investigation was prompted by the 2013 BMC study.

Practitioners of Herbalism

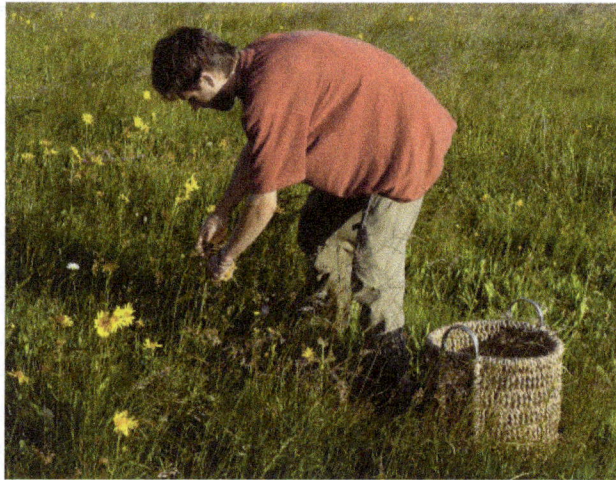

A herbalist gathers the flower heads of *Arnica montana*.

A herbalist is:

1. A person whose life is dedicated to the economic or medicinal uses of plants.

2. One skilled in the harvesting and collection of medicinal plants.

3. Traditional Chinese herbalist: one who is trained or skilled in the dispensing of herbal prescriptions; traditional Chinese herb doctor. Similarly, traditional Ayurvedic herbalist: one who is trained or skilled in the dispensing of herbal prescriptions in the Ayurvedic tradition.

4. One trained or skilled in the therapeutic use of medicinal plants.

5. One who is skilled in the preparation/manufacture of dried and/or liquid herbal products who possesses a pharmacognostic, formulary and/or clinical understanding of the products being prepared/manufactured.

Herbalists must learn many skills, including the wildcrafting or cultivation of herbs, diagnosis and treatment of conditions or dispensing herbal medication, and preparations of herbal medications. Education of herbalists varies considerably in different areas of the world. Lay herbalists and traditional indigenous medicine people generally rely upon apprenticeship and recognition from their communities in lieu of formal schooling.

In some countries formalized training and minimum education standards exist, although these are not necessarily uniform within or between countries. For example, in Australia the currently self-regulated status of the profession (as of April 2008) results in different associations setting different educational standards, and subsequently recognising an educational institution or course of training. The National Herbalists Association of Australia is generally recognised as having the most rigorous professional standard within Australia. In the United Kingdom, the training of medical herbalists is done by state funded Universities. For example, Bachelor of Science degrees in herbal medicine are offered at Universities such as University of East London, Middlesex University, University of Central Lancashire, University of Westminster, University of Lincoln and Napier University in Edinburgh at the present.

Government Regulations

The World Health Organization (WHO), the specialized agency of the United Nations (UN) that is concerned with international public health, published *Quality control methods for medicinal plant materials* in 1998 in order to support WHO Member States in establishing quality standards and specifications for herbal materials, within the overall context of quality assurance and control of herbal medicines.

In the European Union (EU), herbal medicines are now regulated under the European Directive on Traditional Herbal Medicinal Products.

In the United States, herbal remedies are regulated dietary supplements by the Food and Drug Administration under current good manufacturing practice (cGMP) policy for dietary supplements. Manufacturers of products falling into this category are not required to prove the safety or efficacy of their product so long as they don't make 'medical' claims or imply being other than for 'dietary supplement' use, though the FDA may withdraw a product from sale should it prove harmful.

The National Nutritional Foods Association, the industry's largest trade association, has run a program since 2002, examining the products and factory conditions of member companies, giving them the right to display the GMP (Good Manufacturing Practices) seal of approval on their products.

Some herbs, such as cannabis and coca, are outright banned in most countries though coca is legal in most of the South American countries where it is grown. The *Cannabis* plant is used as an herbal medicine, and as such is legal in some parts of the world.

Since 2004, the sales of ephedra as a dietary supplement is prohibited in the United States by the Food and Drug Administration., and subject to Schedule III restrictions in the United Kingdom.

Traditional Herbal Medicine Systems

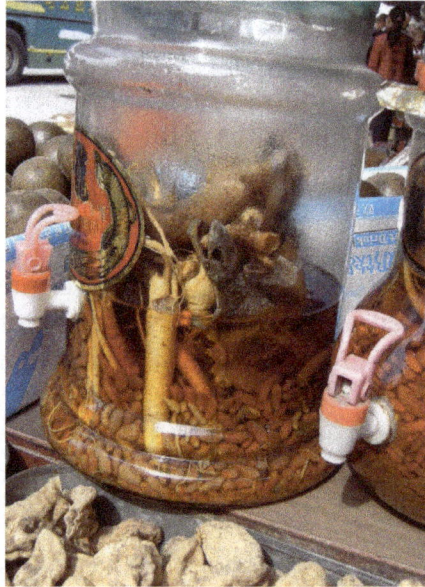

Ready to drink macerated medicinal liquor with goji berry, tokay gecko, and ginseng, for sale at a traditional medicine market in Xi'an, China.

Africa

Americas

Native Americans medicinally used about 2,500 of the approximately 20,000 plant species that are native to North America.

China

Some researchers trained in both western and traditional Chinese medicine have attempted to deconstruct ancient medical texts in the light of modern science. One idea is that the yin-yang balance, at least with regard to herbs, corresponds to the pro-oxidant and anti-oxidant balance. This interpretation is supported by several investigations of the ORAC ratings of various yin and yang herbs.

India

In India, Ayurvedic medicine has quite complex formulas with 30 or more ingredients, including a sizable number of ingredients that have undergone "alchemical processing", chosen to balance "Vata", "Pitta" or "Kapha".

In Ladakh, Lahul-Spiti and Tibet, the Tibetan Medical System is prevalent, also called the 'Amichi Medical System'. Over 337 species of medicinal plants have been documented by C.P. Kala. Those are used by Amchis, the practitioners of this medical system.

In Tamil Nadu, Tamils have their own medicinal system now popularly called Siddha medicine. The Siddha system is entirely in the Tamil language. It contains roughly 300,000 verses covering diverse aspects of medicine. This work includes herbal, mineral and metallic compositions used as medicine. Ayurveda is in Sanskrit, but Sanskrit was not generally used as a mother tongue and hence its medicines are mostly taken from Siddha and other local traditions.

Indonesia

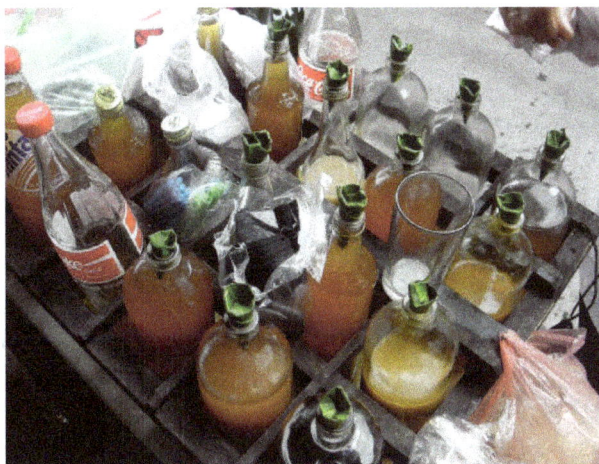

Different types of Indonesian jamu herbal medicines held in bottles.

In Indonesia, especially among the Javanese, the jamu traditional herbal medicine is an age old tradition preserved for centuries. Jamu is thought to have originated in the Mataram Kingdom era, some 1300 years ago. The bas-reliefs on Borobudur depicts the image of people ground herbs with stone mortar and pestle, drink seller, physician and masseuse treating their clients. All of these scenes might be interpreted as a traditional herbal medicine and health-related treatments in ancient Java. The Madhawapura inscription from Majapahit period mentioned a specific profession of herbs mixer and combiner (herbalist), called *Acaraki*. The medicine book from Mataram dated from circa 1700 contains 3,000 entries of jamu herbal recipes, while Javanese classical literature Serat Centhini (1814) describes some jamu herbal concoction recipes.

Though highly possible influenced by Indian Ayurveda system, Indonesia is a vast archipelago with numerous indigenous plants not to be found in India, which include plants similar to Australia beyond the Wallace Line. Indonesians might experimented and figure out the medicinal uses of these native herbal plants. Jamu may vary from region to region, and often not written down, especially in remote areas of the country.

Although primarily herbal, materials acquired from animals, such as honey, royal jelly, milk and *ayam kampung* eggs are also often used in jamu.

Herbal Philosophy and Spiritual Practices

According to Eisenburg: "The Chinese and Western medical models are like two frames of reference in which identical phenomena are studied. Neither frame of reference provides an unobstructed view of health and illness. Each is incomplete and in need of refinement." Specifically, the traditional Chinese medical model could effect change on the recognized, and expected, phenomena of detachment to patients as people and estrangement unique to the clinical and impersonal relationships between patient and physician of the Western school of medicine.

Four approaches to the use of plants as medicine include:

1. The magical/shamanic—Almost all societies, with the exception of cultures influenced by Western-style industrialization, recognize this kind of use. The practitioner is regarded as endowed with gifts or powers that allow him/her to use herbs in a way that is hidden from the average person, and the herbs are said to affect the spirit or soul of the person.

2. The energetic—This approach includes the major systems of Traditional Chinese Medicine, Ayurveda, and Unani. Herbs are regarded as having actions in terms of their energies and affecting the energies of the body. The practitioner may have extensive training, and ideally be sensitive to energy, but need not have supernatural powers.

3. The functional dynamic—This approach was used by early physiomedical practitioners, whose doctrine forms the basis of contemporary practice in the UK. Herbs have a functional action, which is not necessarily linked to a physical compound, although often to a physiological function, but there is no explicit recourse to concepts involving energy.

4. The chemical—Modern practitioners - called Phytotherapists - attempt to explain herb actions in terms of their chemical constituents. It is generally assumed that the specific combination of secondary metabolites in the plant are responsible for the activity claimed or demonstrated, a concept called synergy.

Herbalists tend to use extracts from parts of plants, such as the roots or leaves but not isolate particular phytochemicals. Pharmaceutical medicine prefers single ingredients on the grounds that dosage can be more easily quantified. It is also possible to patent single compounds, and therefore generate income. Herbalists often reject the notion of a single active ingredient, arguing that the different phytochemicals present in many herbs will interact to enhance the therapeutic effects of the herb and dilute toxicity. Furthermore, they argue that a single ingredient may contribute to multiple effects.

Herbalists deny that herbal synergism can be duplicated with synthetic chemicals They argue that phytochemical interactions and trace components may alter the drug response in ways that cannot currently be replicated with a combination of a few potentially active ingredients. Pharmaceutical researchers recognize the concept of drug synergism but note that clinical trials may be used to investigate the efficacy of a particular herbal preparation, provided the formulation of that herb is consistent.

In specific cases the claims of synergy and multifunctionality have been supported by science. The open question is how widely both can be generalized. Herbalists would argue that cases of synergy can be widely generalized, on the basis of their interpretation of evolutionary history, not necessarily shared by the pharmaceutical community. Plants are subject to similar selection pressures as humans and therefore they must develop resistance to threats such as radiation, reactive oxygen species and microbial attack in order to survive. Optimal chemical defenses have been selected for and have thus developed over millions of years. Human diseases are multifactorial and may be treated by consuming the chemical defences that they believe to be present in herbs. Bacteria, inflammation, nutrition and ROS (reactive oxygen species) may all play a role in arterial disease. Herbalists claim a single herb may simultaneously address several of these factors. Likewise a factor such as ROS may underlie more than one condition. In short herbalists view their field as the study of a web of relationships rather than a quest for single cause and a single cure for a single condition.

In selecting herbal treatments herbalists may use forms of information that are not applicable to pharmacists. Because herbs can moonlight as vegetables, teas or spices they have a huge consumer base and large-scale epidemiological studies become feasible. Ethnobotanical studies are another source of information. For example, when indigenous peoples from geographically dispersed areas use closely related herbs for the same purpose that is taken as supporting evidence for its efficacy. Herbalists contend that historical medical records and herbals are underutilized resources. They favor the use of convergent information in assessing the medical value of plants. An example would be when in-vitro activity is consistent with traditional use.

Uses of Herbal Medicines by Animals

Indigenous healers often claim to have learned by observing that sick animals change their food preferences to nibble at bitter herbs they would normally reject. Field biologists have provided corroborating evidence based on observation of diverse species, such as chickens, sheep, butterflies, and chimpanzee.The habit has been shown to be a physical means of purging intestinal parasites. Lowland gorillas take 90% of their diet from the fruits of *Aframomum melegueta*, a relative of the ginger plant, that is a potent antimicrobial and apparently keeps shigellosis and similar infections at bay. Current research focuses on the possibility that this plants also protects gorillas from fibrosing cardiomyopathy which has a devastating effect on captive animals.

Sick animals tend to forage plants rich in secondary metabolites, such as tannins and alkaloids. Since these phytochemicals often have antiviral, antibacterial, antifungal and antihelminthic properties, a plausible case can be made for self-medication by animals in the wild.

Chinese Patent Medicine

Chinese patent medicine (simplified Chinese: 提取中药; traditional Chinese: 科學中藥; pinyin: *zhōngyào*) are herbal medicines in Traditional Chinese medicine. Many kinds of Chinese patent medicines are still sold today.

Description

Chinese patent medicines generally consist of extracted condensed pills called teapills, which are usually small, spherical, and black, appearing like black pearls. They are called teapills because the herbs are cooked into an herbal tea to make the pills. Honey or water pills made from ground raw herbs are also a popular format in China, and tend to be bigger and slightly to significantly softer than teapills.

Modern teapills are created from herbs extracted in stainless steel extractors to create either a water decoction or water-alcohol decoction, depending on the herbs used. They are extracted at a low temperature (below 100 degrees Celsius) to preserve essential ingredients. The extracted liquid is then further condensed and a bit of raw herb powder from one of the herbal ingredients is mixed in to form an herbal dough. This dough is then machine cut into tiny pieces, a small amount of excipients are added for a smooth and consistent exterior, and they are spun into pills.

Honey pills and water pills have been made since ancient times by combining several dried herbs and other ingredients, which are ground into a powder, mixed with a binder and traditionally formed into pills by hand. Modern honey or water pills are formed into pills by machine. The binder is traditionally honey for honey pills. For water pills the binder may simply be water, or may include another binder, such as molasses. Modern manufacturers still produce many patent formulas as honey or water pills, such as Wuji Baifeng Wan, a popular honey pill formula to "nourish qi and blood", to strengthen the body.

Patents may come in other forms such as dripping pills, liquids, syrups, powders, granules, instant teas, and capsules. Companies make Chinese patent medicines both within and outside China.

Like other patent medicines, they are not patented in the traditional sense of the word. No one has exclusive rights to the formula. Instead, "patent" refers to the standardization of the formula.

In China, all Chinese patent medicines of the same name have the same proportions of ingredients, and are manufactured in accordance with the PRC Pharmacopoeia's monograph on that particular formula, which is mandated by Chinese law. Each monograph details the exact herbal ingredients that make up the patent formula, usually accompanied by the specific tests that should be used for correct herb identification, such as thin layer chromatography (TLC) or high performance liquid chromatography (HPLC), the percentage of each ingredient, and specific cautions and contraindications. The monograph also details the manufacturing methods that must be followed, how to process and cook the herbs, often including specific requirements for finished product testing including authenticating and assessing the potency of the formula with active ingredient markers where known, as well as testing for dissolution time and content uniformity. All good manufacturing practice (GMP) certified factories must also test for heavy metal levels and microbials for all patent medicines they produce.

However, many patents do not list all ingredients, presumably to protect the secrecy of the formula. An example of this is Yunnan Baiyao, a popular formula used to stop bleeding, whose ingredients have never been revealed. This is an acceptable practice in China, where no other protection exists to protect family or "secret" Chinese herbal formulas.

In western countries, there is considerable variation of ingredients and in the proportions of ingredients in products sharing the same name. This is because the Chinese government allows foreign companies to apply for modifications of patent formulas to be sold outside of China. For example, Hebei brand Lifei pills contain Kadsura (feng sha teng) and Morus (sang ye), whereas Plum Flower brand Li Fei Pian contains Schizandra (we wei zi) and Gecko (ge jie) instead. Another example is Qing Qi Hua Tan Wan. The Lanzou brand uses Citrus (ju hong). The Lanzhou Foci Min Shan brand and the Plum Flower brand do not, but use Ginger (sheng jiang).

Herbal Formulas

Chinese classic herbal formulas form the basis of Chinese patent medicine. These are the basic herbal formulas that students of traditional Chinese medicine learn. Many of these formulas are quite old. For example, "Liu Wei Di Huang Wan" (六味地黄丸 liù wèi dì huáng wán) was developed by Qian Yi (钱乙 Qián Yǐ) (c. 1032–1113 CE). It was published in the "Xiao'er Yao Zheng Zhi Jue" (also known as "Key to Therapeutics of Children's Diseases" 小儿药证直诀 xiǎoér yào zhèng zhí jué) in 1119 by Qian Yi's student. Interestingly, although Liu Wei Di Huang Wan can be prepared as a raw herb decoction (or herbal tea), it was originally created to be made into honey pills. The last word in Liu Wei Di Huang Wan, "Wan" (丸) means "pill".

Criticisms

Heavy Metal Contamination

Some Chinese patent medicines were tested and found to contain high to dangerous levels of heavy metals. The most common heavy metals found were mercury, lead, and arsenic. These ingredients can cause serious medical problems.

Pharmaceutical Adulterants

Some Chinese patent medicines were found to contain pharmaceutical drugs such as decongestants, analgesics or antihistamines. The most common Chinese patent medicines found to carry pharmaceutical drugs were for the treatment of asthma, pain, and arthritis.

Prohibited Ingredients

Some Chinese patent medicines contain ingredients which are banned in other countries. The two most common prohibited herbs are Ma Huang (麻黃 má huáng) (Ephedra) and Ban Xia (半夏 bàn xià) (Pinellia). On 30 December 2003, the FDA in the US announced a ban (effective 12 April 2004), on these herbs from all dietary supplements. Traditional Chinese herbal remedies are exempt from this law.

Development

Problems Conquered

In modern-day Taiwan, due to Chinese patent medicines are prescription drugs since the 1970s, and also adopted in public health system since 1995.

Heavy Metal Contamination and Pesticide Residue

All Chinese patent medicine products sold in Taiwan must pass a heavy metal limitation test and pesticide residue test according to Taiwan Herbal Pharmacopeia. There are several manufacturers in Taiwan certified ISO 17025 Lab, for example: Sun-Ten (Chinese: 順天堂), Chuang Song Zong Pharmaceutical Co., Ltd. (Chinese: 莊松榮)

NPharmaceutical Adulterants

According to Taiwanese government law, products licenses will be suspended if there exists pharmaceutical adulterants. Furthermore, it could cause GMP certificate to be cancelled. In Taiwan, those main manufacturer in order to export products abroad, few of them has passed PIC/S GMP audition. For example: Sun-Ten (Chinese: 順天堂), Chuang Song Zong Pharmaceutical Co., Ltd. (Chinese: 莊松榮).

List of Traditional Chinese Medicines

In traditional Chinese medicine, there are roughly 13,000 medicinals used in China and over 100,000 medicinal prescriptions recorded in the ancient literature. Plant elements and extracts are the most common elements used in medicines. In the classic *Handbook of Traditional Drugs* from 1941, 517 drugs were listed - 442 were plant parts, 45 were animal parts, and 30 were minerals.

Herbal medicine, as used in traditional Chinese medicine (TCM), came to widespread attention in the United States in the 1970s. At least 40 states in the United States license practitioners of Oriental medicine, and there are about 50 colleges of Oriental medicine in the United States today.

In Japan, the use of TCM herbs and herbal formulas is traditionally known as Kampo, literally "Han Chinese Medical Formulas". Many Kampo combinations are manufactured in Japan on a large scale by reputable manufacturers.

In Korea, more than 5000 herbs and 7000 herbal formulas are used in Traditional Korean Medicine for the prevention and treatment of ailments. These are herbs and formulas that are traditionally Korean or derived from, or are used in TCM.

In Vietnam, traditional medicine comprises Thuoc Bac (Northern Medicine) and Thuoc Nam (Southern Medicine). Only those who can understand Chinese characters could diagnose and prescribe remedies in Northern Medicine. The theory of Northern Medicine is based on the Yin-Yang interactions and the eight trigrams, as used in Chinese Medicine. Herbs such as Gleditsia sinensis are used in both Traditional Vietnamese Medicine and TCM.

Ginseng is the most broadly used substance for the most broad set of alleged cures. Powdered antlers, horns, teeth, and bones are second in importance to ginseng, with claims ranging from curing cancer to curing impotence.

Mammals

Human Parts and Excreta

Human body parts and excreta are currently used in TCM medicines and are included in its new textbooks and handbooks, such as licorice in human feces, dried human placenta, finger nails, child's urine, hair, and urinary sediments (*Hominis Urinae Sedimentum*, Ren Zhong Bai). The current consumption of human parts is considered cannibalism by some. Other parts include pubic hair, flesh, blood, bone, semen, and menstrual blood. The Bencao Gangmu describes the use of 35 human waste products and body parts as medicines, such as bones, fingernail, hairs, dandruff, earwax, impurities on the teeth, feces, urine, sweat, and organs. - Also listed are human breath and the "soul of criminals that were hanged", which is considered under TCM to be a material object resembling charcoal that is dug out of the ground beneath the body shortly after a hanged criminal died, but very few human or allegedly human products remain in use today.

There is considerable controversy about the ethics of use of criminals for body parts, using humans as commodities, and consumption of human body parts which some consider to be cannibalism.

Dried Human Placenta

Dried human placenta is believed to treat male impotence, male and female infertility, chronic cough, asthma, and insomnia.

Human Feces and Urine

The contemporary use of licorice in prepared human feces is known as Ren Zhong Huang Human urine sediment is called Ren Zhong Bai. Both Ren Zhong Huang and Ren Zhong Bai are used to treat inflammatory conditions and fungal infections of the skin and mouth.

In Traditional Chinese medicine, human feces is used in a decoction of licorice. These feces-licorice decoctions have been found to have profound differences in pharmacokinetics as compared to pure glycyrrhizin. Initial studies investigating traditional Chinese Medicine indicate that taking the fecal bacteria alongside the licorice may improve the pharmacokinetics of glycyrrhizin, and certain strains of gut bacteria may produce an anti-tumor effect and an immune boosting effect. Human gut flora may protect against cell damage caused by hydrogen peroxide.

Human Penis

The human penis is not a drug

— Li Shizhen

Human penis is believed under TCM to stop bleeding, and as with other TCM medicines, the basis for belief in its therapeutic effects is anecdotal and not based on the scientific method; Li Shizhen, author of the greatest pharmacological work in pre-modern China, the Bencao Gangmu, objected to use of human penis, but cited the anecdotal evidence and included it in the Bencao Gangmu, which is still a standard reference today.

Human Pubic Hair

Human pubic hair ("shady hair") was claimed to cure snakebite, difficult birth, abnormal urination, and "yin and yang disorder" (A disease unique to TCM based on its views of sexual behavior).

Donkey-hide Gelatin

Gelatin made from the hide of donkeys (ejiao) is made into pellets for use in making teas.

Deer Penis

Deer penis is commonly sold in Chinese pharmacies. and served in specialized restaurants such as the Guo Li Zhuang restaurant in Beijing. The deer penis is typically very large and, under TCM it must be extracted from the deer whilst still alive. Often it is then sliced into small pieces, typically by women and then roasted and dried in the sun and then preserved while the deer looks on. China banned deer penis wine during the 2008 Summer Olympics, as it is believed that the wine is an effective treatment for athletic injuries.

Flying Squirrel Feces

Flying squirrel feces is used to stop bleeding.

The text *Chinese Medical Herbology and Pharmacology* notes that flying squirrel feces has a *"distinct odor"* that *"may decrease patient compliance"* with ingesting it.

It is believed to have uses for amenorrhea, menses pain, postpartum abdominal pain, epigastric pain, and chest pain. It is boiled in a decoction with other herbs prior to ingestion. If it is to be used in a formula to stop heavy bleeding; it is dry fried prior to making the decoction. Use of flying squirrel feces as medicine has been associated with *Rickettsia* infections.

Rhinoceros Horn

The horn of a rhinoceros is used as an antipyretic - because it is believed to "cool the blood" - however several scientific studies failed to find any active antipyretic molecule in rhinoceros horn. The illegal trade in rhinoceros horns has decimated the world's rhino population by more than 90 percent over the past 40 years.

Tiger Penis

The penis and testicles of male tigers is used by some to treat erectile dysfunction and to improve sexual performance, despite tiger penis being a placebo. Critically endangered species such as the Sumatran tiger are often being hunted to keep up with the illegal demand for tiger parts.

Reptiles and Amphibians

Snake Oil

Snake oil is the most widely known Chinese medicine in the west, due to extensive marketing in the west in the late 1800s and early 1900s, and wild claims of its efficacy to treat many maladies. Snake oil is a traditional Chinese medicine used to treat joint pain by rubbing it on joints as a liniment.

This is theoretically possible because snake oil is higher in eicosapentaenoic acid than most other oils. But there are no scientific studies showing that rubbing it on joints has any positive effect, or that snake oil is safe for daily consumption.

Toad Secretions

The secretions of various species of toads are an ingredient in certain traditional Chinese teas. However, these teas may contain deadly amounts of cardiac glycosides and thus should be avoided

Toad-headed Gecko

Toad-head geckos are gutted, beheaded, dried and then crushed, and are used to treat asthma, male impotence and the common cold.

Turtle Shell

Widespread medicinal use of turtle shells is of concern to conservationists.

Marine Life

Seahorse

Seahorse (*Hai Ma*) is a fundamental ingredient in therapies for a variety of disorders, including asthma, arteriosclerosis, incontinence, impotence, insomnia, thyroid disorders, skin ailments, broken bones, heart disease, throat infections, abdominal pain, sores, skin infections; it is also used as an aphrodisiac and to facilitate childbirth. As many as 20 million seahorses per year may be used for TCM purposes. In one study, 58 seahorse samples were collected from various TCM vendors in Taiwan, and of all the eight species identified from the fifty-eight samples, seven were vulnerable, and one was endangered.

Shark Fin Soup

Shark fin soup is traditionally regarded as beneficial for health in East Asia, and its status as an elite dish has led to huge demand with the increase of affluence in China, devastating shark populations.

Insects

Blister Beetle

Blister beetles (Ban mao) are believed under TCM to treat skin lesions, because they cause them. They contain the blister agent cantharidin.

Centipede

Powdered centipede (wu gong) is believed under TCM to treat tetanus, seizures, convulsions, skin lesions, and pain. It is toxic.

Hornets Nest

Hornets nest (lu feng fang) is used to treat skin disorders and ringworm. It may be toxic.

Leech

Hirudo medicinalis is used in TCM to treat amenorrhea, abdominal and chest pain, and constipation.

Scorpion

Dried scorpions (Chinese: 全蝎, Pinyin:*quan xie*) may be ground into a powder and mixed with water. In TCM, powdered scorpion is toxic and is therefore used to treat poisoning. A scorpion venom peptide was found to help with arthritis in vitro.

Fungi

Various fungi are used in TCM. Some may have scientifically proven medicinal value, while others may be extremely toxic.

Supernatural Mushroom

The supernatural mushroom (lingzhi mushroom, Chinese "linh chi" = "supernatural mushroom", "reishi mushroom" in Japan) encompasses several fungal species of the genus *Ganoderma*, and most commonly refers to the closely related species, *Ganoderma lucidum* and *Ganoderma tsugae*. *G. lucidum* enjoys special veneration in East Asia, where it has been used as a medicinal mushroom in traditional Chinese medicine for more than 2,000 years, making it one of the oldest mushrooms known to have been used medicinally. Today, the ling zhi mushroom is used in a herbal formula designed to minimize the side effects of chemotherapy.

Extracts of the mushroom are used as a commercial pharmaceutical to suppress cancer cell proliferation and migration, although the mechanisms by which this is achieved are currently unknown.

Tremella Fuciformis

Tremella fuciformis is used as a beauty product by women in China and Japan as it reportedly increases moisture retention in the skin and prevents senile degradation of micro-blood vessels in the skin, reducing wrinkles and smoothing fine lines. Other beneficial effects come from its ability to increase the activity of SOD in the brain and liver.

Plants

There are thousands of plants that are used as medicines. The following list represents a very small portion of the pharmacopoeia.

Aconite

Monkshood root is commonly used in TCM. It was once so commonly used it was called "the king of the 100 herbs".

The monkshood plant contains what is called "the queen of poisons", the highly toxic alkaloid aconitine. Aconitine is easily absorbed through the skin, eyes and through the lining of the nose; Death may occur through respiratory paralysis. A few minutes after exposure, paresthesia starts at the mouth and slowly beings to cover the whole body, Anesthesia, hot and cold flashes, nausea and vomiting and other similar symptoms follow. Sometimes there is strong pain, accompanied by cramps, or diarrhea.

When a person has a negative reaction to the alkaloid, some practitioners of classical Chinese medicine think that this is because it was that the monkshood plant was processed incorrectly or planted on the wrong place or on the wrong day of the year; Not because of an overdose

The Chinese also used aconitine both for hunting and for warfare.

Birthworts

Birthworts (family Aristolochiaceae) are often used to treat many aliments, including hypertension, hemorrhoids, and colic. However - they are of little medicinal value and contain the carcinogen aristolochic acid. The over-use of this plant family in TCM is thought be a significant cause of upper urinary tract cancer and kidney failure in Taiwan; in 2012, approximately a third of all herbal prescriptions in Taiwan contained birthworts. Supplements containing birthwort may be responsible for BEN.

Camellia Sinensis

Tea from India, Sri Lanka, Java and Japan is used in TCM for aches and pains, digestion, depression, detoxification, as an energizer and, to prolong life.

Cayenne Pepper

Cayenne pepper is believed under TCM to be a prophylactic medicine.

Chinese Cucumber

The fruit of *Trichosanthes kirilowii* is believed to treat tumors, reduce fevers, swelling and coughing, abscesses, amenorrhea, jaundice, and polyuria. The plant is deadly if improperly prepared; causing pulmonary edema, cerebral hemorrhage, seizures, and high fever.

Chrysanthemum Flowers

Chrysanthemum flowers (Ju Hua) are used in TCM to treat headaches, fever, dizziness and dry eyes. They are also used to make certain beverages. Chrysanthemum flowers are believed to "brighten the eyes, pacify the liver, break blood, clear heat, stop dysentery, disperse wind, relieve toxicity, and regulate the center".

Cocklebur Fruit

Cocklebur fruit (*Xanthium*, cang er zi) is one of the most important herbs in TCM, and is commonly to treat sinus congestion, chronic nasal obstructions and discharges, and respiratory allergies.

The plant is mildly toxic and can cause gastrointestinal upset

Crow Dipper

Pinellia ternata is believed under TCM to be the strongest of all TCM herbs for removing phlegm.

Active ingredinets of this herb include: methionine, glycine, β-aminobutyric acid, γ-aminobutyric acid, ephedrine, trigonelline, phytosterols and glucoronic acid.

Care should be taken as crow dipper is toxic.

Croton Seed

Seeds of *Croton tiglium* are used in TCM to treat gastrointestinal disorders, convulsions, and skin lesions. They are often used with rhubarb, dried ginger and apricot seed. Care should be taken as the seeds are toxic and carcinogenic.

Dioscorea Root

In TCM, Dioscorea Root (Radix Dioscorea, *Huai Shan Yao* or *Shan Yao* in Chinese), benefits both the *Yin* and *Yang*, and is used to *tonify* the lungs, spleen and kidney. It can "be used in large amounts and 30g is suggested when treating diabetes". If taken habitually, it "brightens the intellect and prolongs life".

Ginger

Ginger root, *Zingiber officinale*, has been used in China for over 2,000 years to treat indigestion, upset stomach, diarrhea, and nausea. It is also used in TCM to treat arthritis, colic, diarrhea, heart conditions, the common cold, flu-like symptoms, headaches, and menstrual cramps. Today, health care professionals worldwide commonly recommend ginger to help prevent or treat nausea and vomiting associated with motion sickness, pregnancy, and cancer chemotherapy. It is also used as a treatment for minor stomach upset, as a supplement for arthritis, and may even help prevent heart disease and cancer.

Ginkgo

Ginkgo biloba seeds are crushed and believed under TCM to treat asthma. *G. biloba* has been used by humans for nearly 5,000 years. However, further scientific studies are needed to establish the efficacy of *G. biloba* as a medicine.

Ginseng

Ginseng root is the most widely sold traditional Chinese medicine. The name "ginseng" is used to refer to both American (*Panax quinquefolius*) and Asian or Korean ginseng (*P. ginseng*), which belong to the species Panax and have a similar chemical makeup. Siberian ginseng or Eleuthero (*Eleutherococcus senticosus*) is another type of plant. Asian ginseng has a light tan, gnarled root that often looks like a human body with stringy shoots for arms and legs. In ancient times, herbalists thought that because of the way ginseng looks it could treat many different kinds of syndromes, from fatigue and stress to asthma and cancer. In traditional Chinese medicine, ginseng was often combined with other herbs and used often to bring longevity, strength, and mental alacrity to its users. Asian ginseng is believed to enhance the immune system in preventing and treating infection and disease. Several clinical studies report that Asian ginseng can improve immune function. Studies have found that ginseng seems to increase the number of immune cells in the blood, and improve the immune system's response to a flu vaccine. In one study, 227 participants received either ginseng or placebo for 12 weeks, with a flu shot administered after 4 weeks. The number of colds and flu were two-thirds lower in the group that took ginseng.

Ginseng contains stimulants, but may produce side effect including high blood pressure, low blood pressure, and mastalgia. Ginseng may also lead to induction of mania in depressed patients who mix it with antidepressants. One of the most common and characteristic symptoms of acute overdose of ginseng from the genus *Panax* is bleeding. Symptoms of mild overdose with *Panax* ginseng may include dry mouth and lips, excitation, fidgeting, irritability, tremor, palpitations, blurred vision, headache, insomnia, increased body temperature, increased blood pressure, edema, decreased appetite, increased sexual desire, dizziness, itching, eczema, early morning diarrhea, bleeding, and fatigue. Symptoms of gross overdose with *Panax* ginseng may include nausea, vomiting, irritability, restlessness, urinary and bowel incontinence, fever, increased blood pressure, increased respiration, decreased sensitivity and reaction to light, decreased heart rate, cyanotic facial complexion, red face, seizures, convulsions, and delirium.

The constituents of ginseng include triterpene saponins, aglycone protopanaxadiol, aglycone protopanaxytriol, aglycone oleanolic acid and water-soluble polysaccharides.

Goji Berry

Marketing literature for goji berry (wolfberry) products including several "goji juices" suggest that wolfberry polysaccharides have extensive biological effects and health benefits, although none of these claims have been supported by peer-reviewed research.

A May 2008 clinical study published by the peer-reviewed Journal of Alternative and Complementary Medicine indicated that parametric data, including body weight, did not show significant differences between subjects receiving *Lycium barbarum* berry juice and subjects receiving the placebo; the study concluded that subjective measures of health were improved and suggested further research in humans was necessary. This study, however, was subject to a variety of criticisms concerning its experimental design and interpretations.

Published studies have also reported possible medicinal benefits of *Lycium barbarum*, especially due to its antioxidant properties, including potential benefits against cardiovascular and inflammatory diseases, vision-related diseases (such as age-related macular degeneration and glaucoma), having neuroprotective properties or as an anticancer and immunomodulatory agent.

Wolfberry leaves may be used to make tea, together with *Lycium* root bark (called *dìgǔpí*; 地骨皮 in Chinese), for traditional Chinese medicine (TCM). A glucopyranoside isolated from wolfberry root bark have inhibitory activity in vitro against human pathogenic bacteria and fungi.

Horny Goat Weed

Horny goat weed (Yin Yang Huo, 淫羊藿) may have use in treating erectile dysfunction. Exploitation of wild populations may have a serious impact on the surrounding environment.

Lily Bulb

Lily bulbs (Bai He) are used in TCM to treat dry cough, dry and sore throat, and wheezing.

Chinese Rhubarb

The root of "Chinese rhubarb," or "da huang," (大黄) either *Rheum palmatum*, or *Rheum officinale*, is an important herb that is used primarily as a laxative in Chinese Traditional Medicine. The degree of potency depends on how long the root is cooked during preparation after harvesting.

Round Cardamon Fruit

Round cardamon fruit (Bai Dou Kou) is used in TCM to treat poor appetite, breathing problems, vomiting and diarreahea

Thunder God Vine

Thunder god vine is used in TCM to treat arthritis, relieve pain and reduce joint swelling. It can be extremely toxic, if not processed properly If used inappropriately, within two to three hours after ingestion, a patient may begin to have diarrhea, headache, dizziness, severe vomiting (sometimes with blood), chills, high fever, and irregular heart beat. Long term inproper use may result in nervous system damage.

Trichosanthis Root

In TCM, Trichosanthis Root (Radix Trichosanthis or *Tian Hua Fen* in Chinese), is used to clear *heat*, generate *fluids* when *heat* injures *fluids* causing thirst, in the *wasting and thirsting* syndrome. The pairing of *Tian Hua Fen* and *Zhi Mu* had a faster, stronger and longer effect in reducing blood sugar levels than either herb alone.

Strychnine Tree Seed

The seeds of the Strychnine tree, *Strychnos nux-vomica*, are sometimes used to treat diseases of the respiratory tract, anemia, and geriatric complaints. The active molecule is strychnine, a compound often used as a pesticide. Strychnine can also be used as a medication - however it has an extremely low therapeutic index and better, less toxic replacements are available.

Sweet Wormwood

Sweet wormwood (*Artemisia annua*, Qing Hao) is believed under TCM to treat fever, headache, dizziness, stopping bleeding, and alternating fever and chills.

Sweet wormwood had fallen out of common use under TCM until it was rediscovered in the 1970s when the *Chinese Handbook of Prescriptions for Emergency Treatments* (340 AD) was found. This pharmacopeia contained recipes for a tea from dried leaves, prescribed for fevers (not specifically malaria). The plant extracts often used in TCM are antimalarial, due to the presence of artemisinin.

However, it has been questioned as to whether tea made from *A. annua* is effective against malaria, since artemesinin is not soluble in water and the resulting tea would not be expected to contain any significant amount of artemesinin.

Willow Bark

Plants of the genus *Salix* have been used since the time of Hippocrates (400 BC) when patients were advised to chew on the bark to reduce fever and inflammation. Willow bark has been used throughout the centuries in China and Europe to the present for the treatment of pain (particularly low back pain and osteoarthritis), headache, and inflammatory conditions such as bursitis and tendinitis. The bark of white willow contains salicin, which is a chemical similar to aspirin (acetylsalicylic acid). It is thought to be responsible for the pain-relieving and anti-inflammatory effects of the herb. In 1829, salicin was used to develop aspirin. White willow appears to be slower than aspirin to bring pain relief, but its effects may last longer.

Minerals

Arsenic

Arsenic sulfide (Xiong Huang) is a toxic mineral used in TCM to kill parasitic worms and treat sore throats, swellings, abscesses, itching, rashes, and malaria.

Arsenic, while possibly essential for life in tiny amounts, is extremely toxic in the amounts used and arsenic poisoning may result from improper use of arsenic containing remedies. They are most commonly given as a pill or capsule, although are sometimes incorporated into a mixture with other substances.

Lead

Galena is used in TCM to treat ringworm, skin disorders and ulcers, and is thought to "detoxify" the body. It is crushed and taken orally or used on the skin. Lead tetroxide (Qian Dan) is used to treat anxiety, itching, and malaria. It is important to note that most lead compounds are extremely toxic.

Mercury

Cinnabar

Despite its toxicity, mercury sulfide (cinnabar) has historically been used in Chinese medicine, where it is called *zhūshā* (朱砂), and was highly valued in Chinese Alchemy. It was also referred to as *dān* (丹), meaning all of Chinese alchemy, cinnabar, and the "elixir of immortality". Cinnabar has been used in Traditional Chinese medicine as a sedative for more than 2000 years, and has been shown to have sedative and toxic effects in mice. In addition to being used for insomnia, cinnabar is thought to be effective for cold sores, sore throat, and some skin infections.

Corrosive Sublimate

Mercury(II) chloride (*Qing Fen*) is used in TCM to "detoxify" the body, kill intestinal parasites, and as a mild tranquilizer.

Traditional Chinese Medicines Derived from the Human Body

Li Shizhen's (1597) *Bencao gangmu*, the classic materia medica of traditional Chinese medicine (TCM), included 35 human drugs, including organs, bodily fluids, and excreta. Crude drugs derived from the human body were commonplace in the early history of medicine. Some of these TCM human drug usages are familiar from alternative medicine, such as medicinal breast milk and urine therapy. Others are uncommon, such as the "mellified man", which was a foreign nostrum allegedly prepared from the mummy of a holy man who only ate honey during his last days and whose corpse had been immersed in honey for 100 years.

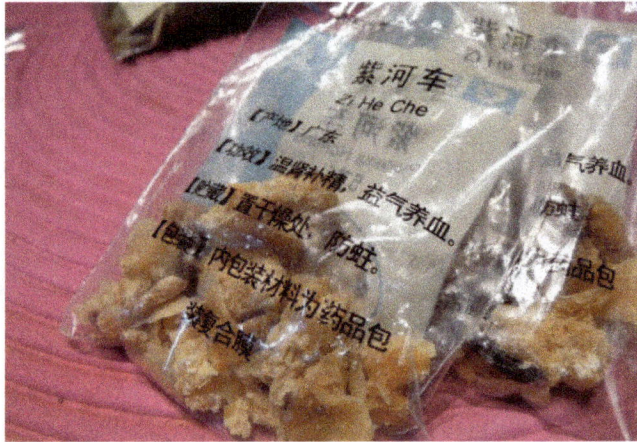

Modern Chinese medicinal *zǐhéchē* 紫河车 "dried human placenta"

Contents

Li Shizhen's (1518-1593) magnum opus, the *Bencao gangmu* or "Compendium of Materia Medica" is still one of the traditional Chinese physician's standard reference books.

Chapter 52 *Renbu* 人部 "human section" is classified under the fourth category of animals (兽之四), and is the last chapter in the *Bencao gangmu*. Li's preface explains this internal ordering (tr. Unschuld 1986: 151), "At the beginning, I have placed the waters and fires, followed by the soils. ... They are followed by the worms, scaly animals and crustaceans, fowl and quadruped; and man concludes the list. From the low I have ascended to the noble."

The human-drug chapter contains 37 entries (*zhǒng* 種 "kind; type"). Unlike the first 35 that discuss human pharmaceuticals and drug prescriptions, the last two are only recorded "for doctors as a reference" (tr. Luo 2003: 4190). Number 36 "Human beings from different locations" discusses personal influences from astrology, environment, geography, and climate (perhaps historical climatology in modern terms). Number 37

"Human beings in extraordinary conditions and of odd forms" ranges across cosmology, male and female sterility, pregnancy, hermaphroditism, metamorphosis, evolution, and monsters.

Some of these *Bencao gangmu* human drug names use obscure classical Chinese terms. *Chǐyìn* 齒垽 "tartar; dental calculus; plaque" (52.20) uses the rare name *yìn* 垽 "sediment: dregs" instead of *gòu* 垢 "filth" in the common *yágòu* 牙垢. *Renshi* 人勢 "penis" (52.32) uses *shì* 勢 "power; circumstance" in the archaic sense of "male genitals" seen in *qùshì* 去勢 "castrate; emasculate".

While most names of these 35 Chinese "human drugs" (translated as hair, dandruff, and earwax) are understandable, several culture-specific terms need explanation.

Li Shizhen distinguishes drugs from four types of human hair: 52.1 *fàbèi* "(esp. boy's) hair cut from the head", 52.2 *luànfà* 亂髮 "hair left on a comb after using it", 52.25 *zīxū* 髭鬚 "facial hair", and 52.26 *yīnmáo* 陰毛 "pubic hair". Li details additional names and their corresponding pulse diagnosis acupuncture channels.

Hair from different positions is given different names: Hair on the head, called Fa [髮] (hair), pertains to Kidney Channel of Foot Lesser Yin and Stomach Channel of Foot Greater Yang. Hair in front of the ears, called Bin [鬢] (temples), pertains to Sanjiao Channel of Hand Lesser Yang and Gall Bladder Channel of Foot Lesser Yang. Hair above the eyes, called Mei [眉] (eyebrow), pertains to Large Intestine Channel of Hand Greater Yang and Stomach Channel of Foot Greater Yang. Hair on the upper lip, called Zi [髭] (moustache), pertains to Large Intestine Channel of Hand Greater Yang. Hair under the chin, called Xu [鬚] (beard), pertains to Gall Bladder Channel of Foot Lesser Yang and Stomach Channel of Foot Greater Yang. Hair on the cheeks, called Ran [髯] (whiskers), pertains to Gall Bladder Channel of Foot Lesser Yang. (52.2, tr. Luo 2003: 4138)

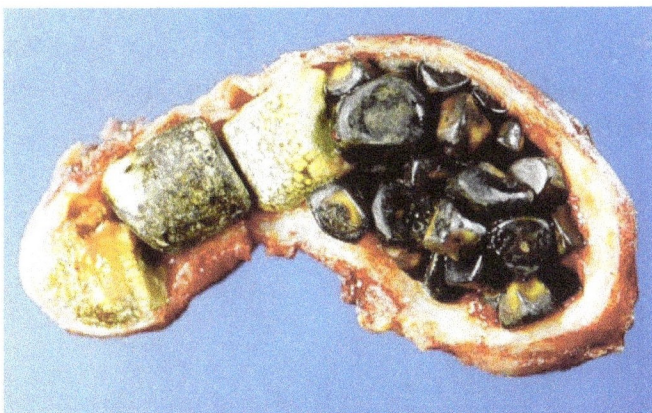

Gallstones in a gall bladder

The obscure drug 52.14 *pǐshí* 癖石, translated as "gall-stones" (Read), "gallstones" (Cooper & Sivin), and described as "hard masses formed from extraordinary addiction or devotion" (Luo), combines words meaning "craving; addiction; extreme devotion; idiosyncrasy; indigestion" and "stone; rock". Li Shizhen (tr. Luo 2003: 4165) explains, "If a person is especially devoted to a certain habit or thing, or when a person is suffering from the formation of hard masses, a strange thing will take shape." Li gives examples of similar things "formed due to congelation of a kind of essence substance": *niúhuáng* 牛黄 "ox bezoar; calculus bovis", *gǒubǎo* 狗寶 "stone in a dog's kidney/gall bladder", *zhǎdá* 鮓答 "white stone that forms between the liver and gall of livestock, used for rain prayers", and *shèlìzi* 舍利子 "śarīra; a Buddhist relic supposedly found in cremated ashes".

Medicinal 52.18 *rénjīng* 人精 "human semen" includes both male and female *jīngyè* 精液, meaning male "seminal fluid; semen" and female "vaginal lubrication". Read (1941: no. 425) notes the (c. 1550 BCE) Ebers Papyrus refers to both male and female semen. Li Shizhen says,

The essence substance of Ying (nutrient essence in blood) can be transformed into semen and gathered at the Mingmen (Gate of Life), which is the house of Jing (Vital Essence) and blood. When a boy is 16 years old, the volume of his semen is one *sheng* and six *ge* [over 1.5 liters]. If it is well protected, it will accumulate to three *sheng* [nearly 5 liters]. If it is not protected and is exhausted too quickly, less than a *sheng* of it can be retained. Without blood, semen cannot form. Semen is a treasured thing within the body and is well nourished by qi (Vital Energy). Therefore, when blood is at its full capacity, the amount of semen will be increased. When qi (Vital Energy) accumulates, semen becomes overfilled. Evil alchemists [邪術家] fool stupid maidens and mate with them. Then they drink the vaginal secretions of the girls. Or they blend their own semen with the menstrual blood of a maiden and eat it. This mixture is called Qiangong [鉛汞] (lead and mercury). They consider this a treasured drug and indulge in sex excessively, eating such a foul thing. This practice will shorten their lifespans greatly. What a stupid thing! (tr. Luo 2003: 4173)

Both 52.12 *qiūshí* 秋石 "processed white sediment of human urine with salt" and 52.30 *bāoyīshuǐ* 胞衣水 "processed fluid of human placenta" specify particular methods of iatrochemical or medical-chemical preparation.

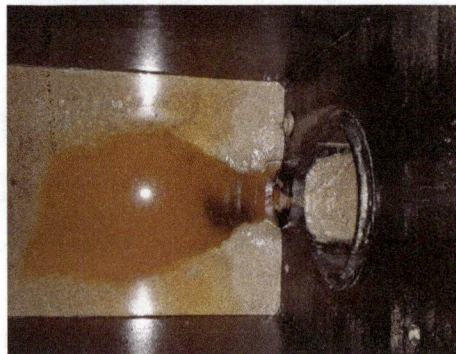

Urine precipitate in a tank collecting urine from urine diversion flush toilets in Germany

Qiūshí 秋石 (lit. "autumn mineral"), translated as "urea" (Read) and "processed white sediment of human urine with salt" (Luo), was prepared from 52.11 *nibaiyin* "white urinary sediment" from the urine of either Yin girls or Yang boys. The *qiushi* drug was called *qiūbīng* 秋冰 (lit. "autumn ice") after recrystallization, similar to boiling seawater to get salt. Li Shenzhen (tr. Luo 2003: 4161) warns that, "Some alchemists fake the product by calcining salt in a furnace. Any substance alleged to be Qiubing should be examined carefully to make sure it is genuine." Li Shizhen (tr. Lu & Needham1964: 109) outlines historical changes in the use of steroid-rich urine drugs. In ancient times, doctors used urinary precipitates to "keep the blood in motion, greatly help sexual debility, bring down heat, kill parasites, and disperse poisons; but the princes and wealthy patricians disliked using it because they considered it unhygienic. So the iatro-chemists ([*fangshi*]) began to purify the sediment, making first [*qiushi*] and later on [*qiubing*]", which licentious people used as aphrodisiacs. The *Bencao gangmu* lists six methods of processing *qiushi* through techniques including dilution, precipitation, filtration, evaporation, calcination, and sublimation.

Bāoyīshuǐ 胞衣水, translated as "old liquefied placenta" (Read) and "fluid of human placenta" (Luo), was traditionally processed in two ways (tr. Luo 2003: 4186). In north China, people bury a human placenta in the ground for 7 to 8 years, and it dissolves into a fluid that is as clean as ice. In south China, people blend human placenta with *gāncǎo* 甘草 "*Glycyrrhiza uralensis*; Chinese licorice root", *shēngmá* 升麻 "*Cimicifuga simplex*; bugbane", and other drugs, which they store in a bottle, and bury in the ground for 3 to 5 years. Then they dig it up and use it medicinally.

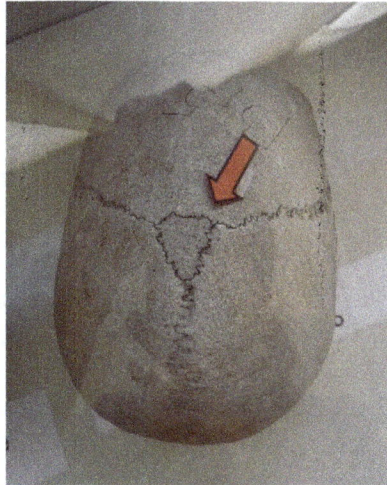

Human skull showing bregma

The 52.24 *rénpò* 人魄 "Human ghost (of a hanged person)" medicine refers to Chinese hun and po soul dualism between the *hun* 魂 "spiritual, ethereal, yang soul" that leaves the body after death and the *po* 魄 "corporeal, substantive, yin soul" that remains with the corpse. Li Shizhen (tr. Luo 2003: 4177) explains, "Renpo is found in the soil under a person who has hanged himself or herself. It resembles soft charcoal. If the Renpo is not dug out in time, it will penetrate deep into the earth where it cannot be traced." The *Bencao gangmu* compares a hanged person's soul with similar phenomena, "When a star descends to the earth it turns into a stone. When a tiger dies, his eyesight descends and turns into a white stone. Human blood will turn into phosphorus or jade when it drops to the ground." Li only gives one prescription, "Renpo pacifies the Heart and tranquilizes the soul and boldness. It treats convulsions, fright, and manic-depressive psychosis. Grind Renpo with water and take it by mouth."

52.28 *Tiānlínggài* 天靈蓋 "bregma; skullcap; calvaria" is translated as "human skull" (Read), "human skull top" (Luo), and "bregma" (Cooper & Sivin). In Daoist meditation and *qigong* breathing practices, the bregma is considered the locus of the upper *dantian* "elixir field". Li Shizhen (tr. Luo 2003: 4179) says, "The skull of a human looks like a round cover. It is shaped like the sky. It is the palace of Niwan" – *níwán* 泥丸 "clay pellet" is a Chinese transcription of "nirvana". Furthermore, "It is a place where ancestral wisdom is stored. Taoist alchemists stimulate the Li (Fire) by Kan (Water) so as to restore its condition of pure Qian (Yang). In this way, a sacred fetus will form. Then it may go out and come back in as it wishes. So the top of the skull is called Tianlinggai (meaning "cover of the Heavenly wisdom")." This *shèngtāi* 聖胎 "sacred embryo/fetus; Embryo of Sainthood" denotes achieving *xian* immortality through *neidan* "internal alchemy". Cooper & Sivin (1973: 249) say drilling the skull in order to provide a passage is still part of the initiation ritual for members of the esoteric Shingon sect in Taiwan today.

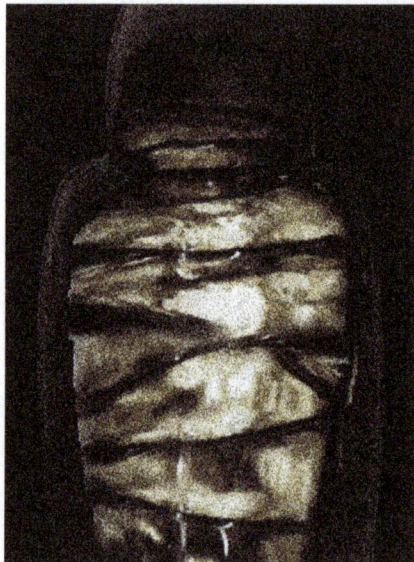

Mellified man (artistic impression)

The 52.35 *mùnǎiyī* 木乃伊 "mummy; mellified man" drug was not a Chinese drug and came from *Tianfangguo* (lit. 天方國 "Kaaba countries"), which was an archaic name for "Arabia; Middle East". Li Shizhen recounts this foreign legend and expresses skepticism,

The book *Chuogeng Lu* by Tao Jiucheng: It is recorded that in the Tianfang country there was an old man 70 or 80 years old was willing to sacrifice his body for the general public. So he stopped taking any food except for drinking honey daily. He washed himself repeatedly. After a month, his stools and urine all turned into honey. After his death, people in the country kept him in a stone coffin filled with honey. The date was inscribed on the stone coffin and it was buried in the ground. After 100 years, the body became a kind of honey-preserved thing that was used as a drug. When someone was suffering from an injury to his body, including bone fractures, a little of the "honey man" could be taken as a drug. It worked right away. Even in that country, this was something very precious. It was called "honey man. The above is quoted from Tao Jiucheng's book. It is not known whether this is true or not. So it is recorded at the end of this section for further study. (tr. Luo 2003:4189)

Read (1931: no. 442) says Burmese priests have the custom of preserving their chief abbots in coffins full of honey.

Among this total content of 35 entries with 287 prescriptions, 13 human drugs with 217 prescriptions first appeared in the *Bencao gangmu* while 22 types with 67 prescriptions came from earlier Chinese materia medica: 1 from the Eastern Han dynasty (25-220) *Shennong bencaojing*; 5 from the Liang dynasty (502-557) *Mingyi bielu*; 9 from the Tang dynasty (618-907) *Xinxiu bencao* and *Bencao shiyi*; 8 from Song dynasty (960-1279) texts *Da Ming rihua bencao*, *Kaibao bencao*, *Jiayou bencao*, and *Zhenglei bencao*; and 1 other from the Ming dynasty (1368-1644) *Bencao mengquan*. A few *Bencao gangmu* prescriptions are cited from non-medical literature, such as Zhang Hua's (c. 290) *Bowuzhi* "Record of Wide Knowledge" collection of wonders (but this magical marital formula is not found in the current reconstituted version). Prescription 52.16.5 (tr. Cooper & Sivin 1973: 236), "To keep one's wife from being jealous. Wrap a toad in the cloth the wife uses to absorb her menses 婦人月水布 and bury it five [*cun*] (15 cm) deep, one [*chi*] (31 cm) in front of the privy."

Since more than one-third of the human drugs were first added in Li Shizhen's time, Read (1931) suggested that "research into the origin of these relatively recent remedies which may reveal a new interchange of thought and practice between China and other civilizations. It may have been that the Arabs were in this matter a common source of both Chinese and European medicine."

Sample Entry

Bencao gangmu drug entries typically give the name used in the earliest materia medica reference, synonyms, explanations from earlier authors, information about preparing the drug, indications, effects, and prescriptions. As an example of these human drug entries, compare Read's partial summary and Luo's full translation of 52.26.

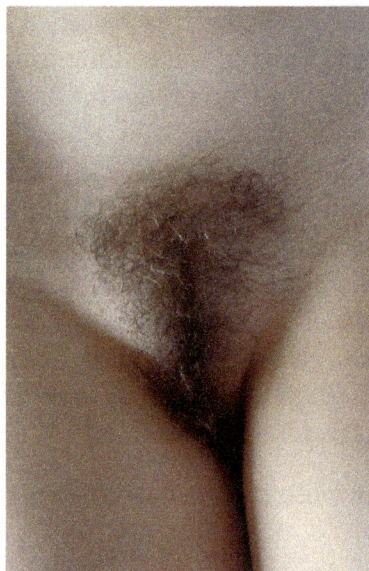

Female pubic hair

433. 陰毛 *YIN MAO*. PUBIC HAIR (M & F).

Shih-Yi: Pubic hair of the male is used for snake bite. Twelve [*sic*] hairs held in the mouth and sucked will keep the poison from entering the viscera.

For difficult labour, 14 hairs from the husband ashed and taken with lard in the form of a pill.

Pubic hair from the female is used to treat gonorrhea and sexual diseases. Also for swollen belly in the cow. (tr. Read 1931: no. 433)

This "Shih-Yi" abbreviates Chen Cangqi's (c. 720) *Bencao Shiyi* 本草拾遺 "Supplement to Materia Medica". Read translates *yinyangyibing* 陰陽易病 (lit. "yin-yang exchange disorders") as "gonorrhea and sexual diseases", compare Luo's "febrile disease transmitted by sex" below. According to Cooper & Sivin (1973: 220-221), *yinyangyi* is a general name for "illnesses contracted through sexual intercourse with someone who has just recovered from them", which are diagnosed by the appearance of a yang pulse on the wrist under conditions in which a yin pulse is normally read, and vice versa.

CLAUSE 52-26 YINMAO

Human pubic hair – *Bencao Shiyi* (*Supplement to Materia Medica* by Chen Cangqi).

[Indications]

Chen Cangqi: Male pubic hair is a good antidote for snake bite. Hold 20 strands of pubic hair in the mouth, and swallow the juice. This will prevent the snake's toxin from entering the abdomen.

Human pubic hair is good for treating dystocia with transverse or footling presentation. Burn l4 pieces of pubic hair of the patient's husband, blend the residue with pig lard, and make into pills the size of soy beans. Swallow the pills. – *Qiaijin Yaofang* (*Essential Prescriptions worth a Thousand Gold*).

Li Shizhen: Female pubic hair is good for treating stranguria of five types and the Yinyangyi syndrome (febrile disease transmitted by sex).

[Prescriptions] Two prescriptions collected recently.

Prescription 52.26.1: To treat the Yinyangyi syndrome (febrile disease transmitted by sex): After a man has just recovered from a serious disease, and he has sex too soon, his scrotum will become swollen and will shrink into his abdomen. This will be accompanied by severe colic. Burn female pubic hair into ash and take it by mouth right away. Also drink water in which female genitalia have been washed. – *Puji Fang* (*Prescriptions for Universal Relief*).

Prescription 52.26.2: To treat an ox that is dying from the effects of a distended abdomen: Wrap female pubic hair in straw and feed it to the ox. This will work. – *Waitai Miyao* (*Medical Secrets of an Official*). (tr. Luo 2003: 4178)

Luo (2003: 4133) explains translating "Clause" instead of "Drug" in chapter 52: "As most of the "drugs" from human being are no more used medically, it seems rude to list them as drugs." Note the medical terms *dystocia* "A slow or difficult labor or delivery" and *stranguria* (i.e., *strangury* "A painful, frequent need to urinate, when the bladder is largely empty or with little urine production").

Moral Aspects

Reflecting the well-known Confucianist inhibition against mutilating one's body (Cooper & Sivin 1973: 212), Li Shizhen's preface to chapter 52 ethically condemns the use of some human drugs.

The human is a different species from all the other organisms used as sources of drugs. In later times, Taoist alchemists [方伎之士] considered that many parts of the human body should be used as drugs, such as bone, flesh, and gall. This is really very rude and inhuman. In the present category, all parts of the human body that have been used as drugs are recorded. The use of drugs from the human body that is not contrary to morality is recorded in detail. Those drugs that are cruel or foul [惨忍邪穢] are not recorded in detail. But all of them are listed in this category. (tr. Luo 2003: 4133)

Li does not give prescriptions for 12 of the 35 human drugs, which he considered "cruel or foul".

Li Shizhen sharply criticized medicinal usage of bone and flesh.

In ancient times, people thought it a benevolent deed to bury discarded human bones. Such people thought that they would be rewarded with good. But some alchemists [方伎] collect human bones and use them as a drug with the hope of making a profit from them. Should this be done to those who save people from diseases? Even dogs do not eat the bones of dogs. Why should a human eat the bones of other humans? (52.27, tr. Luo 2003: 4178-9)

Under the 52.34 human flesh entry, Li denounces two earlier pharmacopeias. Chen Cangqi's (early 8th century) *Bencao Shiyi* prescribes flesh as a good drug for *láozhài* 癆瘵 "consumptive and infectious diseases", and Li Shizhen (tr. Luo 2003: 4188) says, "Our bodies, skin, and hair are inherited from our parents and should be well protected. Even when parents are seriously ill, how can they bear to eat the flesh of their offspring? This is a practice followed only by stupid, foolish folk." Li Shizhen (tr. Luo 2003: 4189) quotes Tao Jiucheng's (8th century) *Chuogeng Lu*, "In ancient and present-day warfare, soldiers have eaten human flesh, calling it Xiangrou (meaning "imagine it as meat") or Liangjiaoyang (meaning meat of sheep with two legs")", and comments, "This is done by bandits and thieves without human hearts. Such damned villains!"

For such a renowned physician and herbalist, Li Shizhen was sometimes credulous. The "penis" entry (52.32) gives the common term *yīnjīng* 陰莖 "Yin stalk" and says,

Li Shizhen: A man's penis is not a drug. The book *Chuogeng Lu* by Tao Jiucheng: Mr. Shen in Hangzhou was once caught in the act of raping a woman. He cut off part of his penis as a self-punishment. But the wound bled incessantly and did not heal for a month thereafter. Someone told him to find the amputated part of his penis. He found it, pounded it into powder, and took the powder by mouth with wine. After a few days, the wound healed. This might be a useful reference to those whose genitals are physically damaged. So it is recorded here for reference. (tr. Luo 2003: 4187)

Luo's "those whose genitals are physically damaged" euphemistically translates the original metaphor *cánshì* 蠶室 "silkworm nursery; (traditional) prison where the punishment of castration was inflicted". Compare Cooper & Sivin's (1973: 263) version, "Contemplating this story, it would seem that those 'who go down to the silkworm room' [who are administratively sentenced to castration] should not be ignorant of this method, so I append it here."

In some *Bencao gangmu* contexts concerning human drugs, Li Shizhen would accept the traditional theory but deny the contemporary practice. Under the human breath or *qi* section (52.23, tr. Luo 2003: 4176), Li says a "very effective" method for treating an elderly person who is suffering from cold and deficiency in the lower body is to have a boy or girl blow air through a cloth into the navel. However, he notes that contemporary "Taoist alchemists [術家] have advocated the following way of using this energy. Let a maiden breathe air into the nostrils, umbilicus, and penis of an old man. This will provide a connection between the three Dantians (the elixir fields at the upper, middle and lower regions of the body)." Li Shizhen moralistically warns, "This is a small skill practiced by alchemists. If this is not done exactly as stipulated, such practice can only bring harm to the person."

Scientific Analysis

Lu Gwei-djen and Joseph Needham, historians of science and technology in China, analyzed urinary steroid hormones in the first serious scientific study (1964) of Chinese human drugs. They researched early references to the concentrated sex hormone preparations (52.11) *nibaiyin* 溺白垽 "white urinary sediment" and (52.12) *qiushi* 秋石 "processed urinary sediment", which Li Shizhen says were respectively first recorded in the (659) *Xinxiu bencao* and in the (1567) *Bencao mengchuan* materia medica (Lu & Needham1964: 108-109). The Chinese use of urine as a medicine, especially for impotence and other sexual disorders, has a long history. The *Book of the Later Han* described three Daoist *fangshi* "adepts; magicians" who lived in the late 2nd century; Gan Shi 甘始, Dongguo Yannian 東郭延年, and Feng Junda 封君達 (tr. Lu & Needham 1964: 106) "were all expert at following the techniques of [Rong Cheng 容成, a semi-legendary figure associated with sexual physiology] in commerce with women. They could also drink urine and sometimes used to hang upside down. They were careful and sparing of their seminal essence and (inherited) [*qi*], and they did not boast with great words of their powers." Based upon the *Bencao gangmu* list of six methods processing urine to produce *qiushi*, Lu & Needham (1964: 116) conclude that from the 11th century onwards, Chinese alchemists, physicians, and iatro-chemists were successfully making quasi-empirical preparations of active substances with androgens and estrogens, a technique that modern biochemists did not develop until the early 20th century.

The physician William C. Cooper and the sinologist Nathan Sivin (1973) chose what the Chinese call *rényào* 人藥 "human drugs" as a pilot experiment sample for pharmacologically analyzing the efficacy of drugs used in TCM. In contrast to many traditional Chinese plant, animal, and mineral pharmaceuticals with uncertain active constituents, the chemical composition of the human body and parts is well known, and "their therapeutic effectiveness, or lack of it, can be objectively, if approximately, estimated without reference to their Chinese context." (Cooper & Sivin 1973: 203). They selected 8 widely used human drugs from the 37 listed in *Bencao gangmu* chapter 52: human hair, nails, teeth, milk, blood, semen, saliva, and bone. For each substance, Cooper and Sivin first analyzed the *Bencao gangmu* information about drug preparation and use, and then commented on the known chemical composition of the human drug and other ingredients in the prescriptions.

Cooper & Sivin (1973: 259-60, Table 8.1) applied the criteria of clinical pharmacology to analyze the possible medicinal value of the *Bencao gangmu* pharmacopeia's human drug prescriptions for 66 diseases, 58 (88%) of which prescribe one or more ancillary ingredients. Fifty (76%) diseases treated would not have been relieved strictly by known properties of the prescription constituents or their combinations, and the other sixteen (24%) diseases might possibly be benefited from the human drug, another in-gredient, or their synergistic combination.

These 24% conceivably beneficial human drug prescriptions can be divided into pos-itive and possible types. First, positive specific benefits for the ailments could come from effects of three (5%) human drug prescriptions alone (all for human blood, e.g., 52.17.3 drink blood mixed with water for internal hemorrhage from wounds, Cooper & Sivin 1973: 241), two (3%) ancillary ingredients alone (52.15.11 [not breast milk but] desiccant tung oil is "miraculously effective" for calf sores, 1973: 233). Second, uncer-tain or nonspecific therapeutic benefits include five human drugs (e.g., 52.6.14 pow-dered left-hand fingernails and rush pith form a sticky mass applied to the canthus for removing foreign bodies in the eye, Cooper & Sivin 1973: 224), three (5%) ancillary in-gredients (52.6.11 pack and roast a silkworm cocoon with a man's fingernail trimmings and a boy's hair for ulcerated hemorrhoids, 1973: 222), and three combinations of them (52.15.7 human milk and copper coins cooked in a copper vessel for trachoma could form copper sulfate, which has a mild antibacterial effect for eye infections, 1973:232).

The authors conclude (1973: 259) that less than 8% of all these disorders could have been "positively cured by known pharmacological effects of the remedies cited", and raise the question of psychosomatic or social effects of human drugs in folk medicine.

Ritual Aspects

Having demonstrated that the effectiveness of most *Bencao gangmu* human drug pre-scriptions was not attributable to pharmacognosy, Cooper & Sivin examined whether the symbolic aspects of magic and ritual in Chinese folk medicine could explain why pharmacopoeias continue to list human drugs. Within their sample of 8 human drugs, prescriptions mention two dozen symbolic ritual procedures (1973: 265). Sympathetic magic, for example, could explain using blood to treat blood loss (52.17.3 above) and attempting to treat bone damage with bone (52.27.1). Li Shizhen quotes the (9th centu-ry) *Miscellaneous Morsels from Youyang*.

The book *Youyang Zaju*: Once a military man in Jingzhou had an injured tibia. Doctor Zhang Qizheng treated him with a kind of medicinal wine, which was taken orally. A small segment of broken bone in the wounded tibia was taken out and a kind of medic-inal ointment was applied externally. The injury was cured. The patient kept the small piece of bone from his tibia under his bed. But two years later there was a recurrence. Doctor Zhang said that the bone from the tibia was cold now. He searched for the bone and found it under the man's bed. He washed the bone with hot water, wrapped it in silk fabric, and kept in a good place. After that the pain was gone. This shows the in-terrelationship between the bone left under the bed and the pain. How can we say a withered bone has no sense? People should be aware of this. (tr. Luo 2003: 4179)

Prescription 52.27.4 (tr. Luo 2003: 4171) specifies using a dead child's bone: "To treat bone fractures: Bone of infant, calcined, and muskmelon seed, stir-fried. Grind the above ingredients into powder, and take the powder by mouth with good wine. It stops the pain right away."

Demonic possession and demonic medicine are ancient Chinese beliefs (Unschuld 1986: 29-46). For example, the *Bencao gangmu* (52.28) says "bregma; skull bone" is good for treating several tuberculosis-like diseases that are supposedly caused by evil spirits. The (sometimes synonymous) names of these sicknesses are difficult to translate, as shown by the following renderings by Cooper & Sivin (1973), Luo (2003), and Zhang & Unschuld (2014):

- *chuánshī* 傳尸 "cadaver vector disease", "consumptive and infectious disease", "corpse [evil] transmission"

- *shīzhù* 尸疰 "cadaver fixation disease", "consumptive and infectious disease", "corpse attachment-illness"

- *gǔzhēng* 骨蒸 "bone-steaming disease", "consumptive disease with general debility", "bone steaming"

- *guǐ[qì]zhù* 鬼[氣]疰 [no 1973 translation], "consumptive disease of unknown cause", "demon [qi] attachment-illness"

Li Shizhen quotes Chen Cangqi's explanation (tr. Luo 2003: 4180) that when a piece of skull is cleaned, simmered in a young boy's urine, and then buried in a pit, "This will infuse the drug with a soul". Li also quotes Yang Shiying that the *shizhu* disease "is caused by a ghost that hides within a person's body and does not come out. So the disease is a prolonged one. When treated with human skull top, the ghost's soul will be dispelled from the person's body and the syndrome may subside." Cooper & Sivin (1973: 251) note that the *guzheng* "bone-steaming disease" or *chuanshi* "cadaver vector disease", "passes from one member of a family to another, sapping their strength and killing them in turn. The name comes from the patient's feeling of feverishness ("steaming") in the marrow of his bones. The syndrome as described in classic medical works corresponds on the whole to that of pulmonary tuberculosis." However, they also (1973: 257) say that whether this demon disease really meant pulmonary tuberculosis or some other debilitating infectious disease is really not pertinent "because bone would be ineffective in the treatment of any infectious process."

Prescription 52.28.1 (tr. Luo 2003: 4180-4181) *Tianlingaisan* "Powder of human Skull Top", which is said to be "good for killing worms in a consumptive disease", mentions seeing a *chuanshi*. First, take "one piece of human skull top two fingers wide, simmer the drug with Tanxiang/sandalwood, then stir-fry with Su/butter. Then chant incantations." Fifteen herbal ingredients are added with the skull bone into a decoction, which will cause the patient to defecate "worms of strange shapes". Cooper & Sivin (tr. 1973: 250) translate the chant that Luo omits, "This incantation is recited seven times in one breath: "Divine Father Thunder, Sage Mother Lightning, if you meet a cadaver vector you must control it. Quickly, quickly, as ordered by the law." This same prescription (tr. Luo 2003: 4181) also mentions Daoistic ritual purification, "Before the drug is processed, one who prepares the drug should abstain from meat and wine and should stay in a clean, quiet room far away from the patient, so that he cannot smell it. When the drug is prepared, keep away chickens, dogs, cats and other animals, as well as sons in mourning and women. The room should be kept clear of all ugly and dirty things."

Prescription 52.28.2 (tr. Luo 2003: 4181) is for treating *guzheng* "bone-steaming disease": "To treat consumptive disease with general debility and hectic fever due to Yin deficiency: Stir-fry a piece of human skull the size of a comb until it turns yellow. Then simmer it in five sheng of water until two sheng are left. Drink the decoction in three drafts. This is a drug that will cure the patient very effectively."

Two other cases of human-drug treatments for demonic medicine are *sānshī* 三尸 "Three Corpses; demonic spirits believed to live in the human body and hasten death" and *gǔdú* 蠱毒 *gu poisoning*; a poison produced by venomous insects; cast a black magic spirit possession over someone".

The first *Bencao gangmu* prescription for human nails is not from Chinese medical texts but from Daoist rituals for expelling what (Cooper & Sivin (1973: 220) describe as the "Three Corpse-Worms 三尸, the chief of the "inner gods" who are to the individual microcosm what the celestial bureaucracy is to the cosmos." Prescription 52.6.1, the 斬 三尸法 "Method of Beheading the Three Corpses", involves supernaturally cutting the nails in accordance with the traditional 60-day sexagenary cycle in the Chinese calendar and Chinese astrology.

To kill Sanshi. The book *Taishang Xuanke*: Cut fingernails on Gengchen [17th] days and cut toenails on Jiawu [31st] days. Burn the nails into ash on the 16th day of the seventh month of the year. Take the ash by mouth with water. In this way all the Sanshi and the nine worms will turn into ash. It is also said that on the days of Jiayin [51st], Sanshi will invade the hands. Trim the fingernails on those days. Sanshi will invade the feet on the days of Jiawu [31st] so trim the toenails on those days. (tr. Luo 3003: 4146)

Luo footnotes that Daoists believe *sanshi* to be "a kind of spirit haunting a patient. It may also be manifested as subcutaneous nodes appearing on three portions of the body cavity."

Gudu-poisoning diseases are supposedly treatable with four human drugs: dandruff, teeth, feces, and placenta. For instance (52.29.6, tr. Luo 2003: 4186), "To treat Gudu (disease caused by noxious agents produced by various parasites), no matter whether caused by a herb, a snake, or a dung beetle: It seems as if such things enter into the throat, causing terrible pain and making the patient feel as if he is dying. Wash a Ziheche/placenta hominis/dried human placenta and cut it into slices. Dry the slices in the sun and grind them into powder. Wash down one qianbi [an ancient coin] of the powder each time with boiled water."

Modern Medicine

Present day Chinese doctors and herbalists continue to prescribe human drugs, despite their lack of proven efficacy. Cooper & Sivin note that a modern TCM pharmacognosy handbook (Nanking 1960: 1270-1273) lists 634 medicinal substances, including 5 from humans: placenta, fingernails, ashed hair, urine, and urine sediment.

Four centuries after Li Shizhen considered the bioethical and biomedical dilemmas of using human drugs, 20th-century technological and medical advances have raised new related questions of organ transplants, transplantation medicine, organ trade, tissue banks, human cloning, and the commodification of human body parts (Awaya 1999, Nie 2002, Scheper-Hughes and Wacquant 2002).

References

- Nigel Wiseman; Ye Feng (2002-08-01). Introduction to English Terminology of Chinese Medicine. ISBN 9780912111643. Retrieved 10 June 2011.

- Scheper-Hughes, Nancy; Wacquant, Loïc J. D., eds. (2002). Commodifying Bodies. Thousand Oaks: Sage. ISBN 978-0-7619-4034-0.

- Robson, Barry & Baek, O.K. (2009). The Engines of Hippocrates: From the Dawn of Medicine to Medical and Pharmaceutical Informatics. John Wiley & Sons. p. 50. ISBN 9780470289532.

- Unschuld, Pual (2003). Huang Di Nei Jing: Nature, Knowledge, Imagery in an Ancient Chinese Medical Text. University of California Press. p. 286. ISBN 978-0-520-92849-7.

- Saad, Bashar & Said, Omar (2011). Greco-Arab and Islamic Herbal Medicine: Traditional System, Ethics, Safety, Efficacy, and Regulatory Issues. John Wiley & Sons. p. 80. ISBN 9780470474211.

- Green, James (2000). The Herbal Medicine Maker's Handbook: A Home Manual. Chelsea Green Publishing. p. 168. ISBN 9780895949905.

- Engel, Cindy (2002). Wild Health: How Animals Keep Themselves Well and What We Can Learn From Them. Houghton Mifflin. ISBN 0-618-07178-4.

- State Pharmacopoeia Commission of the PRC (2005). "Pharmacopoeia of The People's Republic of China (Volume I)". Chemical Industry Press. ISBN 7117069821

- Taylor, Mark (1998). Chinese Patent Medicines: A Beginner's Guide. Global Eyes International Press. ISBN 0-9662973-0-X.

- Nie, Jing-Bao (2002). "Confucian Bioethics". Philosophy and Medicine. 61: 167–206. doi:10.1007/0-306-46867-0_7. ISBN 0-7923-5723-X.

3

Plants used in Traditional Chinese Medicine

Herbs are an important component of Chinese medicine and certain herbs such as Camellia sinensis and liquorice are used in an everyday sense in cooking, for instance. These herbs contain medicinal properties that can benefit the human body. The major categories of Chinese medicinal plants are dealt with great details in the chapter.

Camellia Sinensis

Camellia sinensis is a species of evergreen shrub or small tree whose leaves and leaf buds are used to produce tea. It is of the genus *Camellia* (Chinese: 茶花; pinyin: *Cháhuā, literally: "tea flower"*) of flowering plants in the family Theaceae. Common names include "tea plant", "tea shrub", and "tea tree" (not to be confused with *Melaleuca alternifolia*, the source of tea tree oil, or *Leptospermum scoparium*, the New Zealand teatree).

Two major varieties are grown: *Camellia sinensis* var. *sinensis* for Chinese teas, and *Camellia sinensis* var. *assamica* for Indian Assam teas. White tea, yellow tea, green tea, oolong, pu-erh tea and black tea are all harvested from one or the other, but are processed differently to attain varying levels of oxidation. Kukicha (twig tea) is also harvested from *Camellia sinensis*, but uses twigs and stems rather than leaves.

Nomenclature and Taxonomy

The name *Camellia* is taken from the Latinized name of Rev. Georg Kamel, SJ (1661–1706), a Moravian-born Jesuit lay brother, pharmacist, and missionary to the Philippines.

Carl Linnaeus chose his name in 1753 for the genus to honor Kamel's contributions to botany (although Kamel did not discover or name this plant, or any *Camellia*, and Linnaeus did not consider this plant a *Camellia* but a *Thea*).

Robert Sweet shifted all formerly *Thea* species to the *Camellia* genus in 1818. The name *sinensis* means *from China* in Latin.

Four varieties of *Camellia sinensis* are recognized. Of these, *C. sinensis* var. *sinensis* and *C. sinensis* var. *assamica* (JW Masters) Kitamura are most commonly used for tea, and *C. sinensis* var. *pubilimba* Hung T. Chang and *C. sinensis* var. *dehungensis* (Hung T. Chang & BH Chen) TL Ming are sometimes used locally.

Cultivars

Cultivars of *C. sinensis* include:

- Benifuuki
- Fushun
- Kanayamidori
- Meiryoku
- Saemidori
- Okumidori
- Yabukita

Description

Camellia sinensis is native to East Asia, the Indian Subcontinent and Southeast Asia, but it is today cultivated across the world in tropical and subtropical regions.

Camellia sinensis is an evergreen shrub or small tree that is usually trimmed to below 2 m (6.6 ft) when cultivated for its leaves. It has a strong taproot. The flowers are yellow-white, 2.5–4 cm (0.98–1.57 in) in diameter, with 7 to 8 petals.

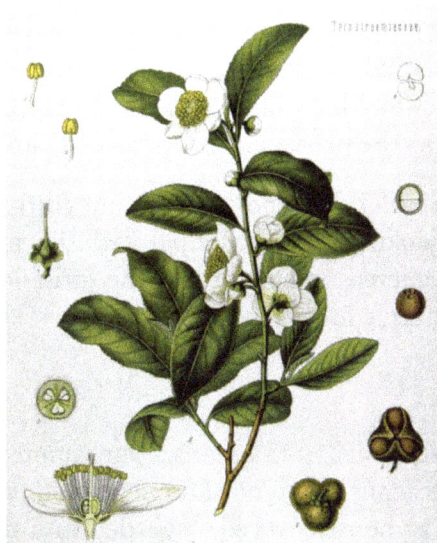

Camellia sinensis plant, with cross-section of the flower (lower left) and seeds (lower right)

The seeds of *Camellia sinensis* and *Camellia oleifera* can be pressed to yield tea oil, a sweetish seasoning and cooking oil that should not be confused with tea tree oil, an essential oil that is used for medical and cosmetic purposes, and originates from the leaves of a different plant.

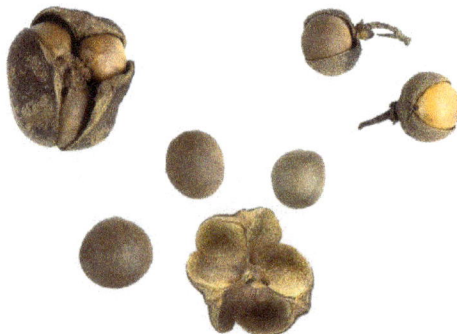

Camellia sinensis - MHNT

The leaves are 4–15 cm (1.6–5.9 in) long and 2–5 cm (0.79–1.97 in) broad. Fresh leaves contain about 4% caffeine, as well as related compounds including theobromine. The young, light green leaves are preferably harvested for tea production; they have short white hairs on the underside. Older leaves are deeper green. Different leaf ages produce differing tea qualities, since their chemical compositions are different. Usually, the tip (bud) and the first two to three leaves are harvested for processing. This hand picking is repeated every one to two weeks.

Cultivation

Camellia sinensis is mainly cultivated in tropical and subtropical climates, in areas with at least 127 cm. (50 inches) of rainfall a year. Tea plants prefer a rich and moist growing location in full to part sun, and can be grown in hardiness zones 7 – 9. However, the clonal one is commercially cultivated from the equator to as far north as Cornwall on the UK mainland. Many high quality teas are grown at high elevations, up to 1,500 meters (4,900 feet), as the plants grow more slowly and acquire more flavour.

Tea plants will grow into a tree if left undisturbed, but cultivated plants are pruned to waist height for ease of plucking. Two principal varieties are used, the small-leaved Chinese variety plant (*C. sinensis sinensis*) and the large-leaved Assamese plant (*C. sinensis assamica*), used mainly for black tea.

Chinese Teas

The Chinese plant (sometimes called *C. sinensis* var. *sinensis*) is a small-leafed bush with multiple stems that reaches a height of some 3 meters. It is native to southeast China. The first tea plant to be discovered, recorded and used to produce tea three thousand years ago, it yields some of the most popular teas.

C. sinensis var. *waldenae* was considered a different species, *Camellia waldenae* by SY Hu, but it was later identified as a variety of *C. sinensis*. This variety is commonly called Waldenae Camellia. It is seen on Sunset Peak and Tai Mo Shan in Hong Kong. It is also distributed in Guangxi province, China.

Indian Teas

Three main kinds of tea are produced in India:

- Assam comes from the northeastern section of the country. This heavily forested region is home to much wildlife, including the rhinoceros. Tea from here is rich and full-bodied. It was in Assam that the first tea estate was established, in 1837.

- Darjeeling, from the cool and wet Darjeeling region, tucked in the foothills of the Himalayas. Tea plantations reach 2,200 metres. The tea is delicately flavoured, and considered to be one of the finest teas in the world. The Darjeeling plantations have 3 distinct harvests, termed 'flushes', and the tea produced from each flush has a unique flavour. First (spring) flush teas are light and aromatic, while the second (summer) flush produces tea with a bit more bite. The third, or autumn flush gives a tea that is lesser in quality.

- Nilgiri, from a southern region of India almost as high as Darjeeling. Grown at elevations between 1,000 and 2,500 metres, Nilgiri teas are subtle and rather gentle, and are frequently blended with other, more robust teas.

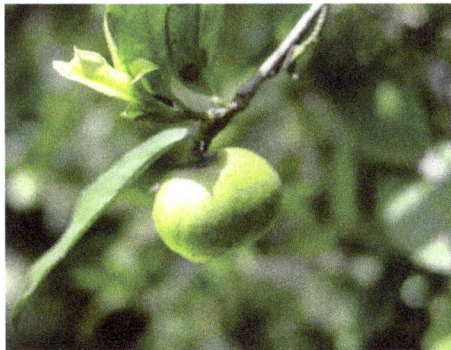

Seed-bearing fruit of *Camellia sinensis*

Pests and Diseases

Tea leaves are eaten by some herbivores, like the caterpillars of the willow beauty (*Peribatodes rhomboidaria*), a geometer moth.

Health Effects

The leaves have been used in traditional Chinese medicine and other medical systems to treat asthma (functioning as a bronchodilator), angina pectoris, peripheral vascular disease, and coronary artery disease.

Among other interesting bioactivities, (-)-catechin from *C. sinensis* was shown to act as agonist of PPARgamma, nuclear receptor that is a current pharmacological target for the treatment of diabetes type 2.

Tea may have some negative impacts on health, such as over-consumption of caffeine, and the presence of oxalates in tea.

Datura Stramonium

Datura stramonium, known by the common names Jimson weed or Devil's snare, is a plant in the nightshade family. It is believed to have originated in Mexico, but has now become naturalized in many other regions. Other common names for *D. stramonium* include thornapple and moon flower, and it has the Spanish name *toloache*. Other names for the plant include hell's bells, devil's trumpet, devil's weed, *tolguacha*, Jamestown weed, stinkweed, locoweed, pricklyburr, and devil's cucumber.

Datura has been used in traditional medicine to relieve asthma symptoms and as an analgesic during surgery or bonesetting. It is also a powerful hallucinogen and deliriant, which is used spiritually for the intense visions it produces. However, the tropane alkaloids responsible for both the medicinal and hallucinogenic properties are fatally toxic in only slightly higher amounts than the medicinal dosage, and careless use often results in hospitalizations and deaths.

Description

Datura stramonium is a foul-smelling, erect, annual, freely branching herb that forms a bush up to 60 to 150 cm (2 to 5 ft) tall.

The root is long, thick, fibrous and white. The stem is stout, erect, leafy, smooth, and pale yellow-green. The stem forks off repeatedly into branches, and each fork forms a leaf and a single, erect flower.

The leaves are about 8 to 20 cm (3–8 in) long, smooth, toothed, soft, and irregularly undulated. The upper surface of the leaves is a darker green, and the bottom is a light green. The leaves have a bitter and nauseating taste, which is imparted to extracts of the herb, and remains even after the leaves have been dried.

Datura stramonium generally flowers throughout the summer. The fragrant flowers are trumpet-shaped, white to creamy or violet, and 6 to 9 cm (2 ½–3 ½ in) long, and grow on short stems from either the axils of the leaves or the places where the branches fork. The calyx is long and tubular, swollen at the bottom, and sharply angled, surmounted by five sharp teeth. The corolla, which is folded and only partially open, is white, funnel-shaped, and has prominent ribs. The flowers open at night, emitting a pleasant fragrance, and are fed upon by nocturnal moths.

The egg-shaped seed capsule is 3 to 8 cm (1–3 in) in diameter and either covered with spines or bald. At maturity, it splits into four chambers, each with dozens of small, black seeds.

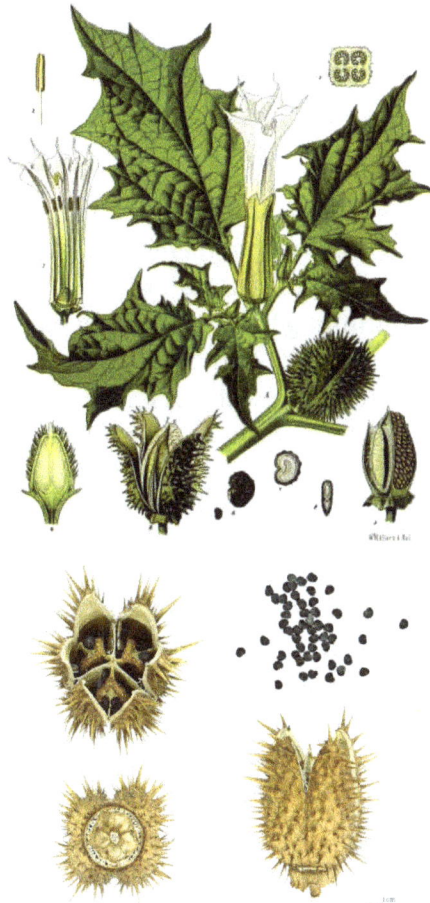

Fruits and seeds – MHNT

Range and Habitat

Datura stramonium is native to North America, but was spread to the Old World early. It was scientifically described and named by Swedish botanist Carl Linnaeus in 1753, although it had been described a century earlier by herbalists, such as Nicholas Culpeper. Today, it grows wild in all the world's warm and moderate regions, where it is found along roadsides and at dung-rich livestock enclosures. In Europe, it is found as a weed on wastelands and in garbage dumps.

The seed is thought to be carried by birds and spread in their droppings. Its seeds can lie dormant underground for years and germinate when the soil is disturbed. People who discover it growing in their gardens, and are worried about its toxicity, have been advised to dig it up or have it otherwise removed.

Toxicity

All parts of *Datura* plants contain dangerous levels of the tropane alkaloids atropine, hyoscyamine, and scopolamine, which are classified as deliriants, or anticholinergics. The risk of fatal overdose is high among uninformed users, and many hospitalizations occur amongst recreational users who ingest the plant for its psychoactive effects.

The amount of toxins varies widely from plant to plant. As much as a 5:1 variation can be found between plants, and a given plant's toxicity depends on its age, where it is growing, and the local weather conditions. Additionally, within a given datura plant, toxin concentration varies by part and even from leaf to leaf. When the plant is younger, the ratio of scopolamine to atropine is about 3:1; after flowering, this ratio is reversed, with the amount of scopolamine continuing to decrease as the plant gets older. In traditional cultures, a great deal of experience with and detailed knowledge of *Datura* was critical to minimize harm. An individual datura seed contains about 0.1 mg of atropine, and the approximate fatal dose for adult humans is >10 mg atropine or >2–4 mg scopolamine.

Datura intoxication typically produces delirium (as contrasted to hallucination), hyperthermia, tachycardia, bizarre behavior, and severe mydriasis with resultant painful photophobia that can last several days. Pronounced amnesia is another commonly reported effect. The onset of symptoms generally occurs around 30 to 60 minutes after ingesting the herb. These symptoms generally last from 24 to 48 hours, but have been reported in some cases to last as long as two weeks.

As with other cases of anticholinergic poisoning, intravenous physostigmine can be administered in severe cases as an antidote.

Use in Traditional Medicine

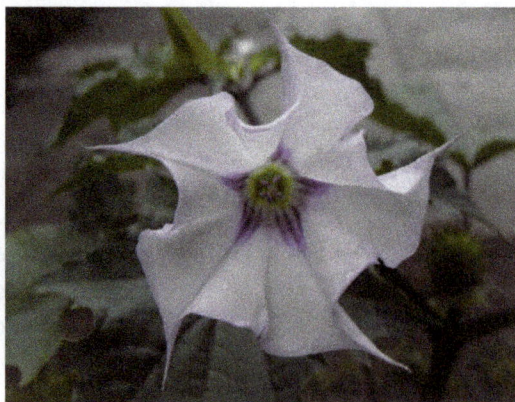

D. stramonium var. *tatula*, flower (front)

In traditional Ayurvedic medicine in India, datura has long been used for asthma symptoms. The active agent is atropine. The leaves are generally smoked either in a cigarette or a pipe. During the late 18th century, James Anderson, the English Physician General of the East India Company, learned of the practice and popularized it in Europe.

John Gerard's *Herball* (1597) states that "the juice of Thornapple, boiled with hog's grease, cureth all inflammations whatsoever, all manner of burnings and scaldings, as well of fire, water, boiling lead, gunpowder, as that which comes by lightning and that in very short time, as myself have found in daily practice, to my great credit and profit."

The Zuni once used datura as an analgesic, to render patients unconscious while broken bones were set. The Chinese also used it in this manner, as a form of anaesthesia during surgery.

Spiritual Uses

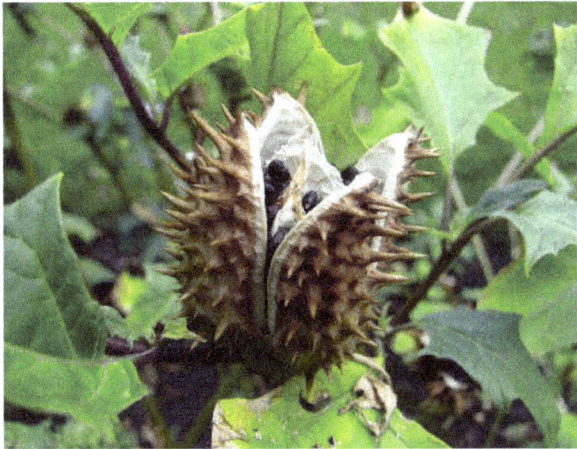

Datura seedpod, opening up to release seeds inside

The ancient inhabitants of what is today central and southern California used to ingest the small black seeds of datura to "commune with deities through visions". Across the Americas, other indigenous peoples such as the Algonquin, Navajo, Cherokee, Marie Galente, and Luiseño also used this plant in sacred ceremonies for its hallucinogenic properties. In Ethiopia, some students and *debtrawoch* (lay priests), use *D. stramonium* to "open the mind" to be more receptive to learning, and creative and imaginative thinking.

In his book, *The Serpent and the Rainbow*, Canadian ethnobotanist Wade Davis identified *D. stramonium*, called "zombi cucumber" in Haiti, as a central ingredient of the concoction vodou priests use to create zombies.

The common name "datura" has its roots in ancient India, where the plant is considered particularly sacred—believed to be a favorite of the Hindu god Shiva Nataraja.

Cultivation

Datura prefers rich, calcareous soil. Adding nitrogen fertilizer to the soil will increase the concentration of alkaloids present in the plant. Datura can be grown from seed, which is sown with several feet between plants. Datura is sensitive to frost, so should be sheltered during cold weather. The plant is harvested when the fruits are ripe, but still green. To harvest, the entire plant is cut down, the leaves are stripped from the plant, and everything is left to dry. When the fruits begin to burst open, the seeds are harvested. For intensive plantations, leaf yields of 1,100 to 1,700 kilograms per hectare (1,000 to 1,500 lb/acre) and seed yields of 780 kg/ha (700 lb/acre) are possible.

Etymology

The genus name is derived from the plant's Hindi name धतूरा *dhatūra*. *Stramonium* is originally from Greek, *strychnos* «nightshade» and *maniakos* «mad».

In the United States, the plant is called jimson weed, or more rarely Jamestown weed; it got this name from the town of Jamestown, Virginia, where British soldiers consumed it while attempting to suppress Bacon's Rebellion. They spent 11 days in altered mental states:

The James-Town Weed (which resembles the Thorny Apple of Peru, and I take to be the plant so call'd) is supposed to be one of the greatest coolers in the world. This being an early plant, was gather'd very young for a boil'd salad, by some of the soldiers sent thither to quell the rebellion of Bacon (1676); and some of them ate plentifully of it, the effect of which was a very pleasant comedy, for they turned natural fools upon it for several days: one would blow up a feather in the air; another would dart straws at it with much fury; and another, stark naked, was sitting up in a corner like a monkey, grinning and making mows [grimaces] at them; a fourth would fondly kiss and paw his companions, and sneer in their faces with a countenance more antic than any in a Dutch droll. In this frantic condition they were confined, lest they should, in their folly, destroy themselves—though it was observed that all their actions were full of innocence and good nature. Indeed, they were not very cleanly; for they would have wallowed in their own excrements, if they had not been prevented. A thousand such simple tricks they played, and after eleven days returned themselves again, not remembering anything that had passed.

– *The History and Present State of Virginia*, 1705

Liquorice

Liquorice, or licorice, is the root of *Glycyrrhiza glabra* from which a sweet flavour can be extracted. The liquorice plant is a herbaceous perennial legume native to southern Europe and parts of Asia, such as India. It is not botanically related to anise, star anise, or fennel, which are sources of similar flavouring compounds.

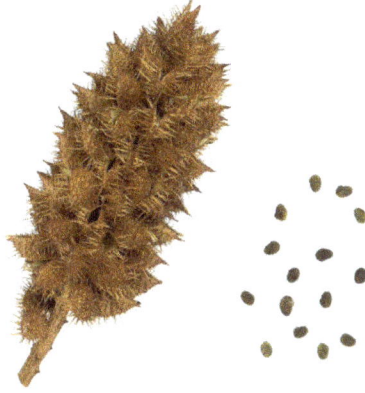

Glycyrrhiza glabra - MHNT

Most liquorice is used as a flavouring agent for tobacco, particularly US blend cigarettes, to which liquorice lends a natural sweetness and a distinctive flavour and makes it easier to inhale the smoke by creating bronchodilators, which open up the lungs. Liquorice flavours are also used as candies or sweeteners, particularly in some European and Middle Eastern countries. Liquorice extracts have a number of medical uses, and they are also used in herbal and folk medications. Excessive consumption of liquorice (more than 2 mg/kg/day of pure glycyrrhizinic acid, a liquorice component) may result in adverse effects, and overconsumption should be suspected clinically in patients presenting with otherwise unexplained hypokalemia and muscle weakness.

Etymology

The word *liquorice* is derived (via the Old French *licoresse*) from the Greek (*glukurrhiza*), meaning "sweet root", from (*glukus*), "sweet" + (*rhiza*), "root", the name provided by Dioscorides. It is usually spelled *liquorice* in British usage, but *licorice* in the United States and Canada.

Description

It is a herbaceous perennial, growing to 1 m in height, with pinnate leaves about 7–15 cm (2.8–5.9 in) long, with 9–17 leaflets. The flowers are 0.8–1.2 cm ($\frac{1}{3}$–$\frac{1}{2}$ in) long, purple to pale whitish blue, produced in a loose inflorescence. The fruit is an oblong pod, 2–3 cm ($\frac{3}{4}$–1$\frac{1}{6}$ in) long, containing several seeds. The roots are stoloniferous.

Chemistry

The scent of liquorice root comes from a complex and variable combination of compounds, of which anethole is up to 3% of total volatiles. Much of the sweetness in liquorice comes from glycyrrhizin, which has a sweet taste, 30–50 times the sweetness of sugar. The sweetness is very different from sugar, being less instant, tart, and lasting longer.

The isoflavene glabrene and the isoflavane glabridin, found in the roots of liquorice, are phytoestrogens.

Cultivation and Uses

Liquorice, which grows best in well-drained soils in deep valleys with full sun, is harvested in the autumn two to three years after planting. Countries producing liquorice include India, Iran, Afghanistan, the People's Republic of China, Pakistan, Iraq, Azerbaijan, Uzbekistan, Turkmenistan,Turkey, and England.

The world's leading manufacturer of liquorice products is M&F Worldwide, which manufactures more than 70% of the worldwide liquorice flavours sold to end users.

Tobacco

Most liquorice is used as a flavouring agent for tobacco. For example, M&F Worldwide reported in 2011 that about 63% of its liquorice product sales are to the worldwide tobacco industry for use as tobacco flavour enhancing and moistening agents in the manufacture of American blend cigarettes, moist snuff, chewing tobacco, and pipe tobacco. American blend cigarettes made up a larger portion of worldwide tobacco consumption in earlier years, and the percentage of liquorice products used by the tobacco industry was higher in the past. M&F Worldwide sold approximately 73% of its liquorice products to the tobacco industry in 2005. A consultant to M&F Worldwide's predecessor company stated in 1975 that it was believed that well over 90% of the total production of liquorice extract and its derivatives found its way into tobacco products.

Liquorice provides tobacco products with a natural sweetness and a distinctive flavour that blends readily with the natural and imitation flavouring components employed in the tobacco industry. It represses harshness and is not detectable as liquorice by the consumer. Tobacco flavourings such as liquorice also make it easier to inhale the smoke by creating bronchodilators, which open up the lungs. Chewing tobacco requires substantially higher levels of liquorice extract as emphasis on the sweet flavour appears highly desirable.

Food and Candy

Liquorice flavour is found in a wide variety of candies or sweets. In most of these candies, the taste is reinforced by aniseed oil so the actual content of liquorice is very low. Liquorice confections are primarily purchased by consumers in the European Union.

In the Netherlands, liquorice candy (*drop*) is one of the most popular forms of sweets. It is sold in many forms. Mixing it with mint, menthol, aniseed, or laurel is quite popular. Mixing it with ammonium chloride (*salmiak*) is also popular. The most popular liquorice, known in the Netherlands as *zoute drop* (salty liquorice), actually contains very little salt, i.e., sodium chloride. The salty taste is probably due to ammonium chloride and the blood pressure-raising effect is due to glycyrrhizin. Strong, salty sweets are also popular in Nordic countries.

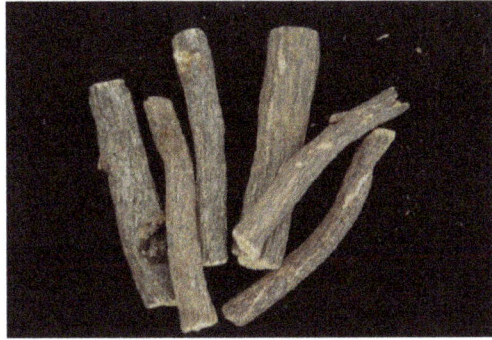
Dried sticks of liquorice root

Pontefract in Yorkshire was the first place where liquorice mixed with sugar began to be used as a sweet in the same way it is in the modern day. Pontefract cakes were originally made there. In County Durham, Yorkshire, and Lancashire, it is colloquially known as 'Spanish', supposedly because Spanish monks grew liquorice root at Rievaulx Abbey near Thirsk.

In Italy (particularly in the south), Spain, and France, liquorice is popular in its natural form. The root of the plant is simply dug up, washed, dried, and chewed as a mouth freshener. Throughout Italy, unsweetened liquorice is consumed in the form of small black pieces made only from 100% pure liquorice extract; the taste is bitter. In Calabria a popular liqueur is made from pure liquorice extract.

Liquorice is also very popular in Syria and Egypt, where it is sold as a drink, in shops as well as street vendors. It is used for its expectorant qualities in folk medicine in Egypt.

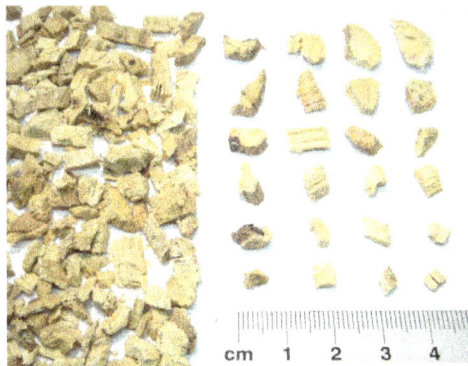
Liquorice root chips

Dried liquorice root can be chewed as a sweet. Black liquorice contains about 100 calories per ounce (15 kJ/g).

Liquorice is used by brewers to flavour and colour porter classes of beers, and the enzymes in the root also stabilize the foam heads produced by beers brewed with it.

Medicine

Glycyrrhizin has also demonstrated antiviral, antimicrobial, anti-inflammatory, hepatoprotective, and blood pressure-increasing effects *in vitro* and *in vivo*, as is supported by the finding that intravenous glycyrrhizin (as if it is given orally very little of the original drug makes it into circulation) slows the progression of viral and autoimmune hepatitis. In one clinical trial liquorice demonstrated promising activity, when applied topically, against atopic dermatitis. Additionally, liquorice may be effective in treating hyperlipidaemia (a high amount of fats in the blood). Liquorice has also demonstrated efficacy in treating inflammation-induced skin hyperpigmentation. Liquorice may also be useful in preventing neurodegenerative disorders and dental caries.

The antiulcer, laxative, antidiabetic, anti-inflammatory, immunomodulatory, antitumour and expectorant properties of liquorice have been investigated.

The compound glycyrrhizin (or glycyrrhizic acid), found in liquorice, has been proposed as being useful for liver protection in tuberculosis therapy, but evidence does not support this use, which may in fact be harmful.

Folk Medicine

In traditional Chinese medicine, liquorice (甘草) is believed to "harmonize" the ingredients in a formula and to carry the formula to the 12 "regular meridians". Liquorice has been traditionally known and used as medicine in Ayurveda for rejuvenation. Liquorice extract is used as a home remedy for skin lightening.

Toxicity

Its major dose-limiting toxicities are corticosteroid in nature, because of the inhibitory effect its chief active constituents, glycyrrhizin and enoxolone, have on cortisol degradation and include oedema, hypokalaemia, weight gain or loss, and hypertension.

The United States Food and Drug Administration believes that foods containing liquorice and its derivatives (including glycyrrhizin) are safe if not consumed excessively. Other jurisdictions have suggested no more than 100 mg to 200 mg of glycyrrhizin per day, the equivalent of about 70 to 150 g (2.5 to 5.3 oz) of liquorice.

Catharanthus Roseus

Catharanthus roseus, commonly known as the Madagascar periwinkle, rosy periwinkle or teresita as it is usually named in the southern part of México, specifically in Champotón, Campeche and Mérida, is a species of flowering plant in the dogbane family Apocynaceae. It is native and endemic to Madagascar, but grown elsewhere as an ornamental and medicinal plant, a source of the drugs vincristine and vinblastine, used to treat cancer. Other English names include Vinca, Cape periwinkle, rose periwinkle, rosy periwinkle, and "old-maid". It was formerly included in the genus *Vinca* as *Vinca rosea*.

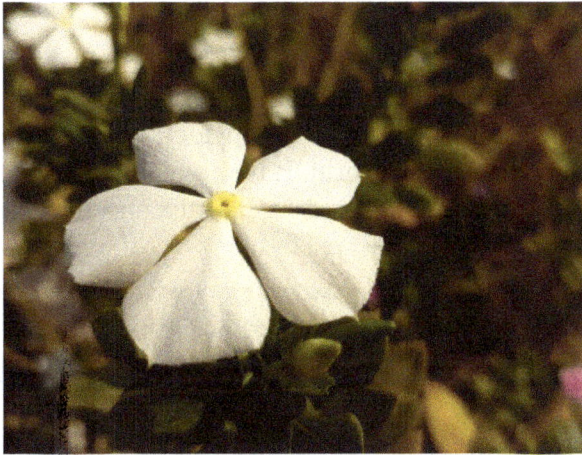

A Catharanthus Roseus flower in Hyderabad, Pakistan

Synonyms

Two varieties are recognized

- *Catharanthus roseus* var. *roseus*

  Synonymy for this variety

  Catharanthus roseus var. *angustus* Steenis ex Bakhuizen f.

  Catharanthus roseus var. *albus* G.Don

  Catharanthus roseus var. *occellatus* G.Don

  Catharanthus roseus var. *nanus*Markgr.

  Lochnera rosea f. alba (G.Don) Woodson

  Lochnera rosea var. *ocellata* (G.Don) Woodson

- *Catharanthus roseus var. angustus* (Steenis) Bakh. f.

Synonymy for this variety

Catharanthus roseus var. *nanus* Markgr.

Lochnera rosea var. *angusta* Steenis

Description

It is an evergreen subshrub or herbaceous plant growing 1 m tall. The leaves are oval to oblong, 2.5–9 cm long and 1–3.5 cm broad, glossy green, hairless, with a pale mid-rib and a short petiole 1–1.8 cm long; they are arranged in opposite pairs. The flowers are white to dark pink with a darker red centre, with a basal tube 2.5–3 cm long and a corolla 2–5 cm diameter with five petal-like lobes. The fruit is a pair of follicles 2–4 cm long and 3 mm broad.

In the wild, it is an endangered plant; the main cause of decline is habitat destruction by slash and burn agriculture. It is also however widely cultivated and is naturalised in subtropical and tropical areas of the world. It is so well adapted to growth in Australia, that it is listed as a noxious weed in Western Australia and the Australian Capital Territory, and also in parts of eastern Queensland.

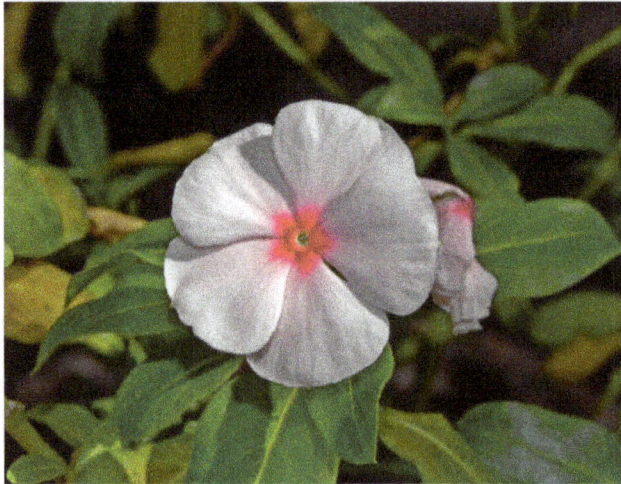

Pale Pink with Red Centre Cultivar

Cultivation and Uses

The species has long been cultivated for herbal medicine and as an ornamental plant. In Ayurveda (Indian traditional medicine) the extracts of its roots and shoots, though poisonous, is used against several diseases. In traditional Chinese medicine, extracts from it have been used against numerous diseases, including diabetes, malaria, and Hodgkin's lymphoma. Many of the vinca alkaloids were first isolated from *Catharanthus roseus*. The substances vinblastine and vincristine extracted from the plant are used in the treatment of leukemia and Hodgkin's lymphoma.

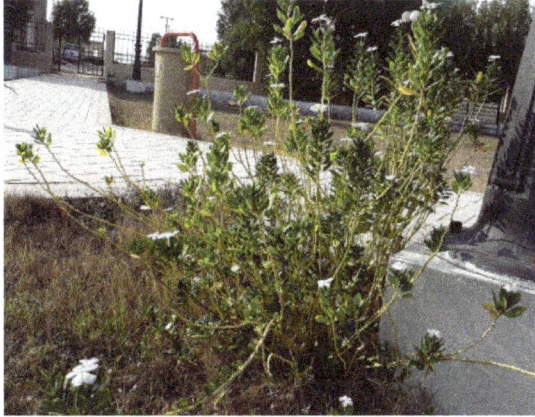

A Periwinkle shrub in Hyderabad, Pakistan

This conflict between historical indigenous use, and recent patents on *C.roseus*-derived drugs by western pharmaceutical companies, without compensation, has led to accusations of biopiracy.

C. roseus can be extremely toxic if consumed orally by humans, and is cited (under its synonym *Vinca rosea*) in Louisiana State Act 159.

As an ornamental plant, it is appreciated for its hardiness in dry and nutritionally deficient conditions, popular in subtropical gardens where temperatures never fall below 5 °C to 7 °C, and as a warm-season bedding plant in temperate gardens. It is noted for its long flowering period, throughout the year in tropical conditions, and from spring to late autumn, in warm temperate climates. Full sun and well-drained soil are preferred. Numerous cultivars have been selected, for variation in flower colour (white, mauve, peach, scarlet and reddish-orange), and also for tolerance of cooler growing conditions in temperate regions. Notable cultivars include 'Albus' (white flowers), 'Grape Cooler' (rose-pink; cool-tolerant), the Ocellatus Group (various colours), and 'Peppermint Cooler' (white with a red centre; cool-tolerant).

C. roseus is used in plant pathology as an experimental host for phytoplasmas. This is because it is easy to infect with a large majority of phytoplasmas, and also often has very distinctive symptoms such as phyllody and significantly reduced leaf size.

Chemical Constituents

Rosinidin is an anthocyanidin pigment found in the flowers of *C. roseus*.

Vincristine and vinblastine, chemotherapy medications used to treat a number of types of cancers, are also found in the plant.

Other Names

C. roseus is known as "Noyon Tora" (Assamese:নয়নতৰা) in Assamese, "noyontara"

(Bengali: নয়নতারা) in Bengali, *sadaphuli* (Marathi: सदाफुली) in Marathi, "Tapak Dara" in Indonesian, *boa-noite* ("good night") and *maria-sem-vergonha* ("shameless maria", name shared with *Impatiens* and *Thunbergia alata*) in Portuguese (American), *vinca-de-madagáscar*, *vinca-de-gato* ("cats' vinca"), vinca-branca (white vinca), vinca or *boa-noite* in Portuguese (European), *vinca del Cabo*, *vinca rosa* ("pink vinca") or *vinca rosada* ("roseous vinca") in Spanish, *putica* ("little whore") in Venezuela, *nithyakalyani* in Tamil (Tamil: **நித்யகல்யாணி பூ**), "barmasi" in Gujarati, "İzmir Güzeli" in Turkish (meaning Symrna beauty) indicating the city that has the best climate conditions to flourish in Turkey, and "Dhafnaki" in Greece and Cyprus (meaning little Daphne), in Cambodia ផ្កាកង្ហារ (phkar kanghar).

References

- Murray, edited by Joseph E. Pizzorno, Jr., Michael T. (2012). Textbook of natural medicine (4th ed.). Edinburgh: Churchill Livingstone. p. 628. ISBN 978-1-4377-2333-5.

- Culpeper, Nicholas (n.d.; 20th century edition of 1653 publication), Culpeper's Complete Herbal, Slough: W Foulsham & Co Ltd, pp. 368–369, ISBN 0-572-00203-3.

- Preissel, Ulrike & Hans-Georg Preissel (2002). Brugmansia and Datura: Angel's Trumpets and Thorn Apples. Firefly Books. pp. 124–125. ISBN 1-55209-598-3.

- AJ Giannini,Drugs of Abuse--Second Edition. Los Angeles, Practice Management Information Corporation, pp.48-51. ISBN 1-57066-053-0.

- Nellis, David W. (1997). Poisonous Plants and Animals of Florida and the Caribbean. Pineapple Press. p. 237. ISBN 9781561641116.

- Freye, Enno (21 September 2009). Pharmacology and Abuse of Cocaine, Amphetamines, Ecstasy and Related Designer Drugs. Springer Netherlands. pp. 217–218. ISBN 978-90-481-2447-3.

- Pennachio, Marcello et al. (2010). Uses and Abuses of Plant-Derived Smoke: Its Ethnobotany As Hallucinogen, Perfume, Incense, and Medicine. Oxford University Press. p. 7. ISBN 9780195370010.

- Goldfrank, Lewis R.; Flommenbaum, Neil (2006). Goldfrank's Toxicologic Emergencies. McGraw-Hill Professional. p. 677. ISBN 9780071479141.

- Turner, Matt W. (2009). Remarkable Plants of Texas: Uncommon Accounts of Our Common Natives. University of Texas Press. p. 209. ISBN 9780292718517.

- Nellis, David W. (1997). Poisonous Plants and Animals of Florida and the Caribbean. Pineapple Press. p. 238. ISBN 9781561641116.

- Davis, Wade (1997). The Serpent and the Rainbow: a Harvard scientist's astonishing journey into the secret societies of Haitian voodoo, zombis and magic. Simon & Schuster. p. . ISBN 9780684839295.

- Molvaer, Reidulf Knut (1995). Socialization and Social Control in Ethiopia. Otto Harrassowitz Verlag. p. 259. ISBN 9783447036627.

- Balakrishna, Acharya (2006). Ayurveda: Its Principles & Philosophies. New Delhi, India: Divya prakashan. p. 206. ISBN 8189235567.

Acupuncture: An Overview

In order to completely understand Chinese traditional medicine, it is necessary to understand acupuncture. The insertion of needles in the skin or muscles of a person is known as acupuncture, in traditional Chinese medicine it aims at affecting the flow of Qi. According to the tradition it eases pain and treats various diseases.

Acupuncture

Acupuncture is a form of pseudoscience and alternative medicine involving thin needles being inserted into the body. It is a key component of traditional Chinese medicine (TCM). TCM theory and practice are not based upon scientific knowledge, and acupuncture is commonly described as without scientific basis. There is a diverse range of acupuncture theories, involving different philosophies. Techniques vary depending on the country. The method used in TCM is likely the most widespread in the US. It is most often used for pain relief, though it is also used for a wide range of other conditions. It is generally only used in combination with other forms of treatment.

The conclusions of many trials and numerous systematic reviews of acupuncture are largely inconsistent. An overview of Cochrane reviews found that acupuncture is not effective for a wide range of conditions, and they suggest it may be effective for only chemotherapy-induced nausea/vomiting, postoperative nausea/vomiting, and idiopathic headache. An overview of high-quality Cochrane reviews suggests that acupuncture may alleviate certain kinds of pain. A systematic review of systematic reviews found little evidence of acupuncture's effectiveness in treating pain. The evidence suggests that short-term treatment with acupuncture does not produce long-term benefits. Some research results suggest acupuncture can alleviate pain, though the majority of research suggests that acupuncture's effects are mainly due to placebo. A systematic review concluded that the analgesic effect of acupuncture seemed to lack clinical relevance and could not be clearly distinguished from bias.

Acupuncture is generally safe when done by an appropriately trained practitioner using clean needle technique and single-use needles. When properly delivered, it has a low rate of mostly minor adverse effects. Accidents and infections are associated with infractions of sterile technique or neglect of the practitioner. A review stated that the reports of infection transmission increased significantly in the prior decade. The most frequently reported adverse events were pneumothorax and infections. Since serious adverse events continue to be reported, it is recommended that acupuncturists be trained sufficiently to reduce the risk. A meta-analysis found that acupuncture for chronic low back pain was cost-effective as an adjunct to standard care, while a systematic review found insufficient evidence for the cost-effectiveness of acupuncture in the treatment of chronic low back pain.

Scientific investigation has not found any histological or physiological evidence for traditional Chinese concepts such as *qi*, meridians, and acupuncture points,[n 1] and many modern practitioners no longer support the existence of life force energy (*qi*) flowing through meridians, which was a major part of early belief systems. Acupuncture is believed to have originated around 100 BC in China, around the time *The Yellow Emperor's Classic of Internal Medicine* (Huangdi Neijing) was published, though some experts suggest it could have been practiced earlier. Over time, conflicting claims and belief systems emerged about the effect of lunar, celestial and earthly cycles, yin and yang energies, and a body's "rhythm" on the effectiveness of treatment. Acupuncture grew and diminished in popularity in China repeatedly, depending on the country's political leadership and the favor of rationalism or Western medicine. Acupuncture spread first to Korea in the 6th century AD, then to Japan through medical missionaries, and then to Europe, starting with France. In the 20th century, as it spread to the United States and Western countries, the spiritual elements of acupuncture that conflict with Western beliefs were abandoned in favor of tapping needles into nerves.

Clinical Practice

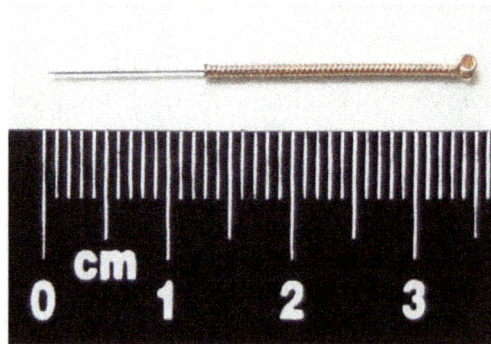

One type of acupuncture needle

Acupuncture is a form of alternative medicine. It is commonly used for pain relief, though it is also used to treat a wide range of conditions. The majority of people who seek out acupuncture do so for musculoskeletal problems, including low back pain, shoulder stiffness, and knee pain. Acupuncture is generally only used in combination with other forms of treatment. For example, American Society of Anesthesiologists states it may be considered in the treatment for nonspecific, noninflammatory low back pain only in conjunction with conventional therapy.

Acupuncture is the insertion in the skin of thin needles. According to the Mayo Foundation for Medical Education and Research (Mayo Clinic), a typical session entails lying still while approximately five to twenty needles are inserted; for the majority of cases, the needles will be left in place for ten to twenty minutes. It can be associated with the application of heat, pressure, or laser light. Classically, acupuncture is individualized and based on philosophy and intuition, and not on scientific research. There is also a non-invasive therapy developed in early 20th century Japan using an elaborate set of "needles" for the treatment of children (*shōnishin* or *shōnihari*).

Clinical practice varies depending on the country. A comparison of the average number of patients treated per hour found significant differences between China (10) and the United States (1.2). Chinese herbs are often used. There is a diverse range of acupuncture approaches, involving different philosophies. Although various different techniques of acupuncture practice have emerged, the method used in traditional Chinese medicine (TCM) seems to be the most widely adopted in the US. Traditional acupuncture involves needle insertion, moxibustion, and cupping therapy, and may be accompanied by other procedures such as feeling the pulse and other parts of the body and examining the tongue. Traditional acupuncture involves the belief that a "life force" (*qi*) circulates within the body in lines called meridians. The main methods practiced in the UK are TCM and Western medical acupuncture. The term Western medical acupuncture is used to indicate an adaptation of TCM-based acupuncture which focuses less on TCM. The Western medical acupuncture approach involves using acupuncture after a medical diagnosis. Limited research has compared the contrasting acupuncture systems used in various countries for determining different acupuncture points and thus there is no defined standard for acupuncture points.

In traditional acupuncture, the acupuncturist decides which points to treat by observing and questioning the patient to make a diagnosis according to the tradition used. In TCM, the four diagnostic methods are: inspection, auscultation and olfaction, inquiring, and palpation. Inspection focuses on the face and particularly on the tongue, including analysis of the tongue size, shape, tension, color and coating, and the absence or presence of teeth marks around the edge. Auscultation and olfaction involves listening for particular sounds such as wheezing, and observing body odor. Inquiring involves focusing on the "seven inquiries": chills and fever; perspiration; appetite, thirst and taste; defecation and urination; pain; sleep; and menses and leukorrhea. Palpation is focusing on feeling the body for tender *"A-shi"* points and feeling the pulse.

Needles

The most common mechanism of stimulation of acupuncture points employs penetration of the skin by thin metal needles, which are manipulated manually or the needle may be further stimulated by electrical stimulation (electroacupuncture). Acupuncture needles are typically made of stainless steel, making them flexible and preventing them from rusting or breaking. Needles are usually disposed of after each use to prevent contamination. Reusable needles when used should be sterilized between applications.

Needles vary in length between 13 to 130 millimetres (0.51 to 5.12 in), with shorter needles used near the face and eyes, and longer needles in areas with thicker tissues; needle diameters vary from 0.16 mm (0.006 in) to 0.46 mm (0.018 in), with thicker needles used on more robust patients. Thinner needles may be flexible and require tubes for insertion. The tip of the needle should not be made too sharp to prevent breakage, although blunt needles cause more pain.

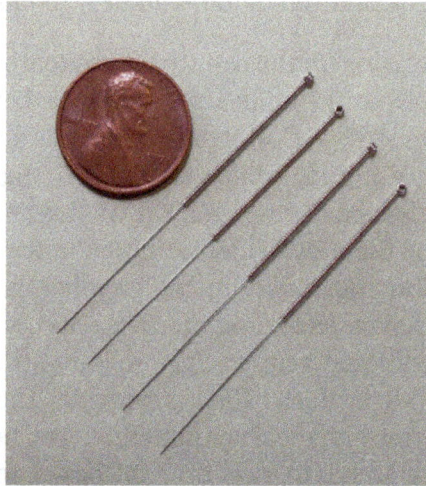

Acupuncture needles

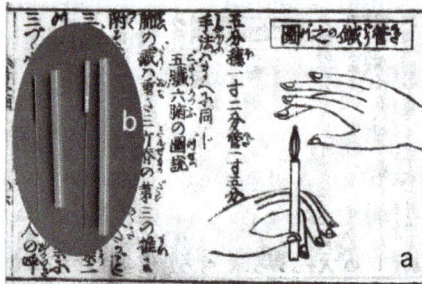

Traditional and modern Japanese guiding tube needles

Apart from the usual filiform needle, other needle types include three-edged needles and the Nine Ancient Needles. Japanese acupuncturists use extremely thin needles that are used superficially, sometimes without penetrating the skin, and surrounded by a guide tube (a 17th-century invention adopted in China and the West). Korean acupuncture uses copper needles and has a greater focus on the hand.

Needling Technique

Insertion

The skin is sterilized and needles are inserted, frequently with a plastic guide tube. Needles may be manipulated in various ways, including spinning, flicking, or moving up and down relative to the skin. Since most pain is felt in the superficial layers of the skin, a quick insertion of the needle is recommended. Often the needles are stimulated by hand in order to cause a dull, localized, aching sensation that is called *de qi*, as well as "needle grasp," a tugging feeling felt by the acupuncturist and generated by a mechanical interaction between the needle and skin. Acupuncture can be painful. The skill level of the acupuncturist may influence how painful the needle insertion is, and a sufficiently skilled practitioner may be able to insert the needles without causing any pain.

De-qi Sensation

De-qi (Chinese: 得气; pinyin: *dé qì*; "arrival of qi") refers to a sensation of numbness, distension, or electrical tingling at the needling site which might radiate along the corresponding meridian. If *de-qi* can not be generated, then inaccurate location of the acupoint, improper depth of needle insertion, inadequate manual manipulation, or a very weak constitution of the patient can be considered, all of which are thought to decrease the likelihood of successful treatment. If the *de-qi* sensation does not immediately occur upon needle insertion, various manual manipulation techniques can be applied to promote it (such as "plucking", "shaking" or "trembling").

Once *de-qi* is achieved, further techniques might be utilized which aim to "influence" the *de-qi*; for example, by certain manipulation the *de-qi* sensation allegedly can be conducted from the needling site towards more distant sites of the body. Other techniques aim at "tonifying" (Chinese: 补; pinyin: *bǔ*) or "sedating" (Chinese: 泄; pinyin: *xiè*) qi. The former techniques are used in deficiency patterns, the latter in excess patterns. *De qi* is more important in Chinese acupuncture, while Western and Japanese patients may not consider it a necessary part of the treatment.

Related Practices

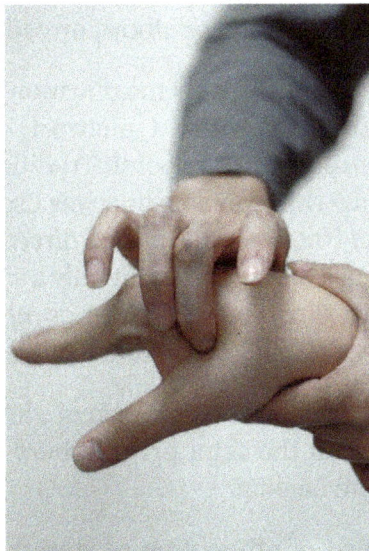

Acupressure being applied to a hand.

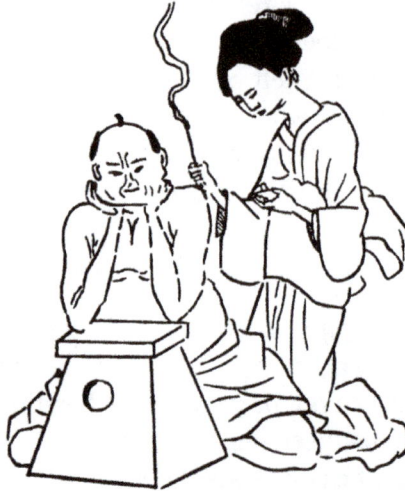

Japanese moxibustion

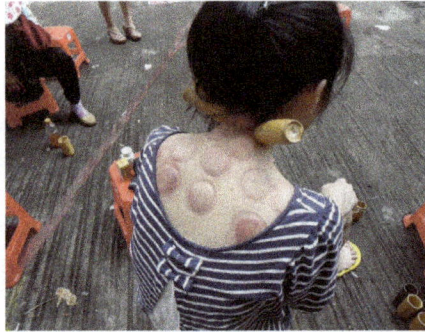

A woman receiving fire cupping in China.

- Acupressure, a non-invasive form of bodywork, uses physical pressure applied to acupressure points by the hand or elbow, or with various devices.

- Acupuncture is often accompanied by moxibustion, the burning of cone-shaped preparations of moxa (made from dried mugwort) on or near the skin, often but not always near or on an acupuncture point. Traditionally, acupuncture was used to treat acute conditions while moxibustion was used for chronic diseases. Moxibustion could be direct (the cone was placed directly on the skin and allowed to burn the skin, producing a blister and eventually a scar), or indirect (either a cone of moxa was placed on a slice of garlic, ginger or other vegetable, or a cylinder of moxa was held above the skin, close enough to either warm or burn it).

- Cupping therapy is an ancient Chinese form of alternative medicine in which a local suction is created on the skin; practitioners believe this mobilizes blood flow in order to promote healing.

- Tui na is a TCM method of attempting to stimulate the flow of *qi* by various bare-handed techniques that do not involve needles.

- Electroacupuncture is a form of acupuncture in which acupuncture needles are attached to a device that generates continuous electric pulses (this has been described as "essentially transdermal electrical nerve stimulation [TENS] masquerading as acupuncture").

- Fire needle acupuncture also known as fire needling is a technique which involves quickly inserting a flame-heated needle into areas on the body.

- Sonopuncture is a stimulation of the body similar to acupuncture using sound instead of needles. This may be done using purpose-built transducers to direct a narrow ultrasound beam to a depth of 6–8 centimetres at acupuncture meridian points on the body. Alternatively, tuning forks or other sound emitting devices are used.

- Acupuncture point injection is the injection of various substances (such as drugs, vitamins or herbal extracts) into acupoints.

- Auriculotherapy, commonly known as ear acupuncture, auricular acupuncture, or auriculoacupuncture, is considered to date back to ancient China. It involves inserting needles to stimulate points on the outer ear. The modern approach was developed in France during the early 1950s. There is no scientific evidence that it can cure disease; the evidence of effectiveness is negligible.

- Scalp acupuncture, developed in Japan, is based on reflexological considerations regarding the scalp. Hand acupuncture, developed in Korea, centers around assumed reflex zones of the hand. Medical acupuncture attempts to integrate reflexological concepts, the trigger point model, and anatomical insights (such as dermatome distribution) into acupuncture practice, and emphasizes a more formulaic approach to acupuncture point location.

- Cosmetic acupuncture is the use of acupuncture in an attempt to reduce wrinkles on the face.

- Bee venom acupuncture is a treatment approach of injecting purified, diluted bee venom into acupoints.

- A 2006 review of veterinary acupuncture found that there is insufficient evidence to "recommend or reject acupuncture for any condition in domestic animals". Rigorous evidence for complementary and alternative techniques is lacking in veterinary medicine but evidence has been growing.

Effectiveness

Sham Acupuncture and Research

It is difficult but not impossible to design rigorous research trials for acupuncture. Due to acupuncture's invasive nature, one of the major challenges in efficacy research is in the design of an appropriate placebo control group. For efficacy studies to determine whether acupuncture has specific effects, "sham" forms of acupuncture where the patient, practitioner, and analyst are blinded seem the most acceptable approach. Sham acupuncture uses non-penetrating needles or needling at non-acupuncture points, e.g. inserting needles on meridians not related to the specific condition being studied, or in places not associated with meridians. The under-performance of acupuncture in such trials may indicate that therapeutic effects are due entirely to non-specific effects, or that the sham treatments are not inert, or that systematic protocols yield less than optimal treatment.

A 2014 *Nature Reviews Cancer* review article found that "contrary to the claimed mechanism of redirecting the flow of *qi* through meridians, researchers usually find that it generally does not matter where the needles are inserted, how often (that is, no dose-response effect is observed), or even if needles are actually inserted. In other words, 'sham' or 'placebo' acupuncture generally produces the same effects as 'real' acupuncture and, in some cases, does better." A 2013 meta-analysis found little evidence that the effectiveness of acupuncture on pain (compared to sham) was modified by the location of the needles, the number of needles used, the experience or technique of the practitioner, or by the circumstances of the sessions. The same analysis also suggested that the number of needles and sessions is important, as greater numbers improved the outcomes of acupuncture compared to non-acupuncture controls. There has been little systematic investigation of which components of an acupuncture session may be important for any therapeutic effect, including needle placement and depth, type and intensity of stimulation, and number of needles used. The research seems to suggest that needles do not need to stimulate the traditionally specified acupuncture points or penetrate the skin to attain an anticipated effect (e.g. psychosocial factors).

A response to "sham" acupuncture in osteoarthritis may be used in the elderly, but placebos have usually been regarded as deception and thus unethical. However, some physicians and ethicists have suggested circumstances for applicable uses for placebos such as it might present a theoretical advantage of an inexpensive treatment without adverse reactions or interactions with drugs or other medications. As the evidence for most types of alternative medicine such as acupuncture is far from strong, the use of alternative medicine in regular healthcare can present an ethical question.

Using the principles of evidence-based medicine to research acupuncture is controversial, and has produced different results. Some research suggests acupuncture can alleviate pain but the majority of research suggests that acupuncture's effects are mainly due to placebo. Evidence suggests that any benefits of acupuncture are short-lasting. There is insufficient evidence to support use of acupuncture compared to mainstream medical treatments. Acupuncture is not better than mainstream treatment in the long term.

Publication Bias

Publication bias is cited as a concern in the reviews of randomized controlled trials (RCTs) of acupuncture. A 1998 review of studies on acupuncture found that trials originating in China, Japan, Hong Kong, and Taiwan were uniformly favourable to acupuncture, as were ten out of eleven studies conducted in Russia. A 2011 assessment of the quality of RCTs on TCM, including acupuncture, concluded that the methodological quality of most such trials (including randomization, experimental control, and blinding) was generally poor, particularly for trials published in Chinese journals (though the quality of acupuncture trials was better than the trials testing TCM remedies). The study also found that trials published in non-Chinese journals tended to be of higher quality. Chinese authors use more Chinese studies, which have been demonstrated to be uniformly positive. A 2012 review of 88 systematic reviews of acupuncture published in Chinese journals found that less than half of these reviews reported testing for publication bias, and that the majority of these reviews were published in journals with impact factors of zero.

Specific Conditions

Pain

The conclusions of many trials and numerous systematic reviews of acupuncture are largely inconsistent with each other. A 2011 overview of high-quality Cochrane reviews suggests that acupuncture is effective for certain types of pain. A 2011 systematic review of systematic reviews found that for reducing pain, real acupuncture was no better than sham acupuncture, and concluded that numerous reviews have shown little convincing evidence that acupuncture is an effective treatment for reducing pain. The same review found that neck pain was one of only four types of pain for which a positive effect was suggested, but cautioned that the primary studies used carried a considerable risk of bias. A 2009 overview of Cochrane reviews found acupuncture is not effective for a wide range of conditions, and suggested that it may be effective for only chemotherapy-induced nausea/vomiting, postoperative nausea/vomiting, and idiopathic headache.

A 2014 systematic review suggests that the nocebo effect of acupuncture is clinically relevant and that the rate of adverse events may be a gauge of the nocebo effect. According to the 2014 *Miller's Anesthesia* book, "when compared with placebo, acupuncture treatment has proven efficacy for relieving pain". A 2012 meta-analysis conducted by the Acupuncture Trialists' Collaboration found "relatively modest" efficiency of acupuncture (in comparison to sham) for the treatment of four different types of chronic pain (back and neck pain, knee osteoarthritis, chronic headache, and shoulder pain) and on that basis concluded that it "is more than a placebo" and a reasonable referral option. Commenting on this meta-analysis, both Edzard Ernst and David Colquhoun said the results were of negligible clinical significance. Edzard Ernst later stated that "I fear that, once we manage to eliminate this bias [that operators are not blind] ... we might find that the effects of acupuncture exclusively are a placebo response." Andrew Vickers, lead author of the original 2012 paper and chair of the *Acupuncture Trialists' Collaboration*, rejects that analysis, stating that the differences between acupuncture and sham acupuncture are statistically significant.

A 2010 systematic review suggested that acupuncture is more than a placebo for commonly occurring chronic pain conditions, but the authors acknowledged that it is still unknown if the overall benefit is clinically meaningful or cost-effective. A 2010 review found real acupuncture and sham acupuncture produce similar improvements, which can only be accepted as evidence against the efficacy of acupuncture. The same review found limited evidence that real acupuncture and sham acupuncture appear to produce biological differences despite similar effects. A 2009 systematic review and meta-analysis found that acupuncture had a small analgesic effect, which appeared to lack any clinical importance and could not be discerned from bias. The same review found that it remains unclear whether acupuncture reduces pain independent of a psychological impact of the needling ritual. A 2016 Cochrane review found moderate quality evidence that real acupuncture was more effective than sham acupuncture or inactive for short-term relief of neck pain measured either upon completion of treatment or at short-term follow-up.

Low Back

A 2013 meta-analysis found that acupuncture was better than no treatment for reducing lower back pain, but not better than sham acupuncture, and concluded that the effect of acupuncture "is likely to be produced by the nonspecific effects of manipulation". A 2013 systematic review found supportive evidence that real acupuncture may be more effective than sham acupuncture with respect to relieving lower back pain, but there were methodological limitations with the studies. A 2013 systematic review found that acupuncture may be effective for nonspecific lower back pain, but the authors noted there were limitations in the studies examined, such as heterogeneity in study characteristics and low methodological quality in many studies. A 2012 systematic review found some supporting evidence that acupuncture was more effective than no treatment for chronic non-specific low back pain; the evidence was conflicting comparing the effectiveness over other treatment approaches. A 2011 overview of Cochrane reviews found inconclusive evidence regarding acupuncture efficacy in treating low back pain. A 2011 systematic review of systematic reviews found that "for chronic low back pain, individualized acupuncture is not better in reducing symptoms than formula acupuncture or sham acupuncture with a toothpick that does not penetrate the skin." A 2010 review found that sham acupuncture was as effective as real acupuncture for chronic low back pain. The specific therapeutic effects of acupuncture were small, whereas its clinically relevant benefits were mostly due to contextual and psychosocial circumstances. Brain imaging studies have shown that traditional acupuncture and sham acupuncture differ in their effect on limbic structures, while at the same time showed equivalent analgesic effects. A 2005 Cochrane review found insufficient evidence to recommend for or against either acupuncture or dry needling for acute low back pain. The same review found low quality evidence for pain relief and improvement compared to no treatment or sham therapy for chronic low back pain only in the short term immediately after treatment. The same review also found that acupuncture is not more effective than conventional therapy and other alternative medicine treatments.

Headaches and Migraines

Two separate 2016 Cochrane reviews found that acupuncture could be useful in the prophylaxis of tension-type headaches and episodic migraines. The 2016 Cochrane review evaluating acupuncture for episodic migraine prevention concluded that true acupuncture had a small effect beyond sham acupuncture and found moderate-quality evidence to suggest that acupuncture is at least similarly effective to prophylactic medications for this purpose. A 2012 review found that acupuncture has demonstrated benefit for the treatment of headaches, but that safety needed to be more fully documented in order to make any strong recommendations in support of its use. A 2009 Cochrane review of the use of acupuncture for migraine prophylaxis treatment concluded that "true" acupuncture was no more efficient than sham acupuncture, but "true" acupuncture appeared to be as effective as, or possibly more effective than routine care in the treatment of migraines, with fewer adverse effects than prophylactic drug treatment. The same review stated that the specific points chosen to needle may be of limited importance. A 2009 Cochrane review found insufficient evidence to support acupuncture for tension-type headaches. The same review found evidence that suggested that acupuncture might be considered a helpful non-pharmacological approach for frequent episodic or chronic tension-type headache.

Osteoarthritis

A 2014 review concluded that "current evidence supports the use of acupuncture as an alternative to traditional analgesics in osteoarthritis patients." As of 2014, a meta-analysis showed that acupuncture may help osteoarthritis pain but it was noted that the effects were insignificant in comparison to sham needles. A 2013 systematic review and network meta-analysis found that the evidence suggests that acupuncture may be considered one of the more effective physical treatments for alleviating pain due to knee osteoarthritis in the short-term compared to other relevant physical treatments, though much of the evidence in the topic is of poor quality and there is uncertainty about the efficacy of many of the treatments. A 2012 review found "the potential beneficial action of acupuncture on osteoarthritis pain does not appear to be clinically relevant." A 2010 Cochrane review found that acupuncture shows statistically significant benefit over sham acupuncture in the treatment of peripheral joint osteoarthritis; however, these benefits were found to be so small that their clinical significance was doubtful, and "probably due at least partially to placebo effects from incomplete blinding".

Extremity Conditions

A 2014 systematic review found moderate quality evidence that acupuncture was more effective than sham acupuncture in the treatment of lateral elbow pain. A 2014 systematic review found that although manual acupuncture was effective at relieving short-term pain when used to treat tennis elbow, its long-term effect in relieving pain was "unremarkable". A 2007 review found that acupuncture was significantly better than sham acupuncture at treating chronic knee pain; the evidence was not conclusive due to the lack of large, high-quality trials.

A 2011 overview of Cochrane reviews found inconclusive evidence regarding acupuncture efficacy in treating shoulder pain and lateral elbow pain.

Nausea and Vomiting and Post-operative Pain

A 2014 overview of systematic reviews found insufficient evidence to suggest that acupuncture is an effective treatment for postoperative nausea and vomiting (PONV) in a clinical setting. A 2013 systematic review concluded that acupuncture might be beneficial in prevention and treatment of PONV. A 2009 Cochrane review found that stimulation of the P6 acupoint on the wrist was as effective (or ineffective) as antiemetic drugs and was associated with minimal side effects. The same review found "no reliable evidence for differences in risks of postoperative nausea or vomiting after P6 acupoint stimulation compared to antiemetic drugs."

A 2014 overview of systematic reviews found insufficient evidence to suggest that acupuncture is effective for surgical or post-operative pain. For the use of acupuncture for post-operative pain, there was contradictory evidence. A 2014 systematic review found supportive but limited evidence for use of acupuncture for acute post-operative pain after back surgery. A 2014 systematic review found that while the evidence suggested acupuncture could be an effective treatment for postoperative gastroparesis, a firm conclusion could not be reached because the trials examined were of low quality.

Allergies

Acupuncture is an unproven treatment for allergic-immunologic conditions. A 2015 meta-analysis suggests that acupuncture might be a good option for people with allergic rhinitis (AR), and a number of randomized clinical trials (RCTs) support the use of acupuncture for AR and itch. There is some evidence that acupuncture might have specific effects on perennial allergic rhinitis (PAR), though all of the efficacy studies were small and conclusions should be made with caution. There is mixed evidence for the symptomatic treatment or prevention of AR. For seasonal allergic rhinitis (SAR), the evidence failed to demonstrate specific effects for acupuncture. Using acupuncture to treat other allergic conditions such as contact eczema, drug rashes, or anaphylaxis is not recommended.

Cancer-related Conditions

A 2015 Cochrane review found that there is insufficient evidence to determine whether acupuncture is an effective treatment for cancer pain in adults. A 2014 systematic review found that acupuncture may be effective as an adjunctive treatment to palliative care for cancer patients. A 2013 overview of reviews found evidence that acupuncture could be beneficial for people with cancer-related symptoms, but also identified few rigorous trials and high heterogeneity between trials. A 2012 systematic review of randomised clinical trials (RCTs) using acupuncture in the treatment of cancer pain found that the number and quality of RCTs was too low to draw definite conclusions.

A 2014 systematic review reached inconclusive results with regard to the effectiveness of acupuncture for treating cancer-related fatigue. A 2013 systematic review found that acupuncture is an acceptable adjunctive treatment for chemotherapy-induced nausea and vomiting, but that further research with a low risk of bias is needed. A 2013 systematic review found that the quantity and quality of available RCTs for analysis were too low to draw valid conclusions for the effectiveness of acupuncture for cancer-related fatigue. A 2012 systematic review and meta-analysis found very limited evidence regarding acupuncture compared with conventional intramuscular injections for the treatment of hiccups in cancer patients. The methodological quality and amount of RCTs in the review was low.

Dyspepsia

A 2015 systematic review and meta-analysis found some evidence that acupuncture was effective for FD, but also called for further well-designed, long-term studies to be conducted to evaluate its efficacy for this condition. A 2014 Cochrane review found that "it remains unknown whether manual acupuncture or electroacupuncture is more effective or safer than other treatments" for functional dyspepsia (FD).

Fertility and Childbirth

A 2014 systematic review and meta-analysis found poor quality evidence for use of acupuncture in infertile men to improve sperm motility, sperm concentration, and the pregnancy rate; the evidence was rated as insufficient to draw any conclusion regarding efficacy. A 2013 Cochrane review found no evidence of acupuncture for improving the success of *in vitro* fertilization (IVF). A 2013 systematic review found no benefit of adjuvant acupuncture for IVF on pregnancy success rates. A 2012 systematic review found that acupuncture may be a useful adjunct to IVF, but its conclusions were rebutted after reevaluation using more rigorous, high quality meta-analysis standards. A 2012 systematic review and meta-analysis found that acupuncture did not significantly improve the outcomes of in vitro fertilization. A 2011 overview of systematic reviews found that the evidence that acupuncture was effective was not compelling for most gynecologic conditions. The exceptions to this conclusion included the use of acupuncture during embryo transfer as an adjunct to in vitro fertilization.

Rheumatological Conditions

A 2013 Cochrane review found low to moderate evidence that acupuncture improves pain and stiffness in treating people with fibromyalgia compared with no treatment and standard care. A 2012 review found "there is insufficient evidence to recommend acupuncture for the treatment of fibromyalgia." A 2010 systematic review found a small pain relief effect that was not apparently discernible from bias; acupuncture is not a recommendable treatment for the management of fibromyalgia on the basis of this review.

A 2012 review found that the effectiveness of acupuncture to treat rheumatoid arthritis is "sparse and inconclusive." A 2005 Cochrane review concluded that acupuncture use to treat rheumatoid arthritis "has no effect on ESR, CRP, pain, patient's global assessment, number of swollen joints, number of tender joints, general health, disease activity and reduction of analgesics." A 2010 overview of systematic reviews found insufficient evidence to recommend acupuncture in the treatment of most rheumatic conditions, with the exceptions of osteoarthritis, low back pain, and lateral elbow pain.

Stroke

A 2014 overview of systematic reviews and meta-analyses found that the evidence does not demonstrate acupuncture helps reduce the rates of death or disability after a stroke or improve other aspects of stroke recovery, such as poststroke motor dysfunction, but the evidence suggests it may help with poststroke neurological impairment and dysfunction such as dysphagia, which would need to be confirmed with future rigorous studies. A 2012 review found evidence of benefit for acupuncture combined with exercise in treating shoulder pain after stroke. A 2010 systematic review found that acupuncture was not effective as a treatment for functional recovery after a stroke. A 2012 overview of systematic reviews found inconclusive evidence supporting the effectiveness of acupuncture for stroke.

A 2015 systematic review found limited evidence that the method of *Xingnao Kaiqiao* needling had a better effect than *Xingnao Kaiqiao* alone or combined with other treatments in reducing disability rate for ischemic stroke, and that the long-term effect was better than traditional acupuncture or combination treatment. A 2014 meta-analysis found tentative evidence for acupuncture in cerebral infarction, a type of ischemic stroke, but the authors noted the trials reviewed were often of poor quality. A 2008 Cochrane review found that evidence was insufficient to draw any conclusion about the effect of acupuncture on dysphagia after acute stroke. A 2006 Cochrane review found no clear evidence for acupuncture on subacute or chronic stroke. A 2005 Cochrane review found no clear evidence of benefit for acupuncture on acute stroke.

Sleep

A 2016 systematic review and meta-analysis found that acupuncture was "associated with a significant reduction in sleep disturbances in women experiencing menopause-related sleep disturbances."

Other Conditions

For the following conditions, the Cochrane Collaboration or other reviews have concluded there is no strong evidence of benefit: alcohol dependence, angina pectoris, ankle sprain, Alzheimer's disease, attention deficit hyperactivity disorder, autism, asthma, bell's palsy, traumatic brain injury, carpal tunnel syndrome, chronic obstructive pulmonary disease, cardiac arrhythmias, cerebral hemorrhage, cocaine dependence, constipation, depression, diabetic peripheral neuropathy, drug detoxification, dry eye, primary dysmenorrhoea, enuresis, endometriosis, epilepsy, erectile dysfunction, essential hypertension, glaucoma, gynaecological conditions (except possibly fertility and nausea/vomiting), hot flashes, hypoxic ischemic encephalopathy in neonates, insomnia, induction of childbirth, irritable bowel syndrome, labor pain, lumbar spinal stenosis, major depressive disorders in pregnant women, musculoskeletal disorders of the extremities, myopia, obesity, obstetrical conditions, Parkinson's disease, polycystic ovary syndrome, premenstrual syndrome, preoperative anxiety, psychological symptoms associated with opioid addiction, restless legs syndrome, schizophrenia, sensorineural hearing loss, smoking cessation, stress urinary incontinence, acute stroke, stroke rehabilitation, temporomandibular joint dysfunction, tennis elbow, labor induction, tinnitus, uremic itching, uterine fibroids, vascular dementia, and whiplash.

Moxibustion and Cupping

A 2010 overview of systematic reviews found that moxibustion was effective for several conditions but the primary studies were of poor quality, so there persists ample uncertainty, which limits the conclusiveness of their findings. A 2012 systematic review suggested that cupping therapy seems to be effective for herpes zoster and various other conditions but due to the high risk of publication bias, larger studies are needed to draw definitive conclusions.

Safety

Adverse Events

Acupuncture is generally safe when administered by an experienced, appropriately trained practitioner using clean-needle technique and sterile single-use needles. When improperly delivered it can cause adverse effects. Accidents and infections are associated with infractions of sterile technique or neglect on the part of the practitioner. To reduce the risk of serious adverse events after acupuncture, acupuncturists should be trained sufficiently. People with serious spinal disease, such as cancer or infection, are not good candidates for acupuncture. Contraindications to acupuncture (conditions that should not be treated with acupuncture) include coagulopathy disorders (e.g. hemophilia and advanced liver disease), warfarin use, severe psychiatric disorders (e.g. psychosis), and skin infections or skin trauma (e.g. burns). Further, electroacupuncture should be avoided at the spot of implanted electrical devices (such as pacemakers).

A 2011 systematic review of systematic reviews (internationally and without language restrictions) found that serious complications following acupuncture continue to be reported. Between 2000 and 2009, ninety-five cases of serious adverse events, including five deaths, were reported. Many such events are not inherent to acupuncture but are due to malpractice of acupuncturists. This might be why such complications have not been reported in surveys of adequately-trained acupuncturists. Most such reports originate from Asia, which may reflect the large number of treatments performed there or a relatively higher number of poorly trained Asian acupuncturists. Many serious adverse events were reported from developed countries. These included Australia, Austria, Canada, Croatia, France, Germany, Ireland, the Netherlands, New Zealand, Spain, Sweden, Switzerland, the UK, and the US. The number of adverse effects reported from the UK appears particularly unusual, which may indicate less under-reporting in the UK than other countries. Reports included 38 cases of infections and 42 cases of organ trauma. The most frequent adverse events included pneumothorax, and bacterial and viral infections.

A 2013 review found (without restrictions regarding publication date, study type or language) 295 cases of infections; mycobacterium was the pathogen in at least 96%. Likely sources of infection include towels, hot packs or boiling tank water, and reusing reprocessed needles. Possible sources of infection include contaminated needles, reusing personal needles, a person's skin containing mycobacterium, and reusing needles at various sites in the same person. Although acupuncture is generally considered a safe procedure, a 2013 review stated that the reports of infection transmission increased significantly in the prior decade, including those of mycobacterium. Although it is recommended that practitioners of acupuncture use disposable needles, the reuse of sterilized needles is still permitted. It is also recommended that thorough control practices for preventing infection be implemented and adapted.

The *Xingnao Kaiqiao* approach appears to be a safe form of treatment. Fainting was the most frequent adverse event. Fainting while being treated, hematoma, and pain while being treated are associated with individual physical differences and with needle manipulation.

English-language

A 2013 systematic review of the English-language case reports found that serious adverse events associated with acupuncture are rare, but that acupuncture is not without risk. Between 2000 and 2011 the English-language literature from 25 countries and regions reported 294 adverse events. The majority of the reported adverse events were relatively minor, and the incidences were low. For example, a prospective survey of 34,000 acupuncture treatments found no serious adverse events and 43 minor ones, a rate of 1.3 per 1000 interventions. Another survey found there were 7.1% minor adverse events, of which 5 were serious, amid 97,733 acupuncture patients. The most common adverse effect observed was infection (e.g. mycobacterium), and the majority of infections were bacterial in nature, caused by skin contact at the needling site. Infection has also resulted from skin contact with unsterilized equipment or with dirty towels in an unhygienic clinical setting. Other adverse complications included five reported cases of spinal-cord injuries (e.g. migrating broken needles or needling too deeply), four brain injuries, four peripheral nerve injuries, five heart injuries, seven other organ and tissue injuries, bilateral hand edema, epithelioid granuloma, pseudolymphoma, argyria, pustules, pancytopenia, and scarring due to hot-needle technique. Adverse reactions from acupuncture, which are unusual and uncommon in typical acupuncture practice, included syncope, galactorrhoea, bilateral nystagmus, pyoderma gangrenosum, hepatotoxicity, eruptive lichen planus, and spontaneous needle migration.

A 2013 systematic review found 31 cases of vascular injuries caused by acupuncture, three resulting in death. Two died from pericardial tamponade and one was from an aortoduodenal fistula. The same review found vascular injuries were rare, bleeding and pseudoaneurysm were most prevalent. A 2011 systematic review (without restriction in time or language), aiming to summarize all reported case of cardiac tamponade after acupuncture, found 26 cases resulting in 14 deaths, with little doubt about causality in most fatal instances. The same review concluded cardiac tamponade was a serious, usually fatal, though theoretically avoidable complication following acupuncture, and urged training to minimize risk.

A 2012 review found a number of adverse events were reported after acupuncture in the UK's National Health Service (NHS) but most (95%) were not severe, though miscategorization and under-reporting may alter the total figures. From January 2009 to December 2011, 468 safety incidents were recognized within the NHS organizations. The adverse events recorded included retained needles (31%), dizziness (30%), loss of consciousness/unresponsive (19%), falls (4%), bruising or soreness at needle site (2%), pneumothorax (1%) and other adverse side effects (12%). Acupuncture practitioners should know, and be prepared to be responsible for, any substantial harm from treatments. Some acupuncture proponents argue that the long history of acupuncture suggests it is safe. However, there is an increasing literature on adverse events (e.g. spinal-cord injury).

Acupuncture seems to be safe in people getting anticoagulants, assuming needles are used at the correct location and depth. Studies are required to verify these findings. The evidence suggests that acupuncture might be a safe option for people with allergic rhinitis.

Chinese, South Korean, and Japanese-language

A 2010 systematic review of the Chinese-language literature found numerous acupuncture-related adverse events, including pneumothorax, fainting, subarachnoid hemorrhage, and infection as the most frequent, and cardiovascular injuries, subarachnoid hemorrhage, pneumothorax, and recurrent cerebral hemorrhage as the most serious, most of which were due to improper technique. Between 1980 and 2009, the Chinese-language literature reported 479 adverse events. Prospective surveys show that mild, transient acupuncture-associated adverse events ranged from 6.71% to 15%. In a study with 190,924 patients, the prevalence of serious adverse events was roughly 0.024%. Another study showed a rate of adverse events requiring specific treatment of 2.2%, 4,963 incidences among 229,230 patients. Infections, mainly hepatitis, after acupuncture are reported often in English-language research, though are rarely reported in Chinese-language research, making it plausible that acupuncture-associated infections have been underreported in China. Infections were mostly caused by poor sterilization of acupuncture needles. Other adverse events included spinal epidural hematoma (in the cervical, thoracic and lumbar spine), chylothorax, injuries of abdominal organs and tissues, injuries in the neck region, injuries to the eyes, including orbital hemorrhage, traumatic cataract, injury of the oculomotor nerve and retinal puncture, hemorrhage to the cheeks and the hypoglottis, peripheral motor-nerve injuries and subsequent motor dysfunction, local allergic reactions to metal needles, stroke, and cerebral hemorrhage after acupuncture.

A causal link between acupuncture and the adverse events cardiac arrest, pyknolepsy, shock, fever, cough, thirst, aphonia, leg numbness, and sexual dysfunction remains uncertain. The same review concluded that acupuncture can be considered inherently safe when practiced by properly trained practitioners, but the review also stated there is a need to find effective strategies to minimize the health risks. Between 1999 and 2010, the Republic of Korean-literature contained reports of 1104 adverse events. Between the 1980s and 2002, the Japanese-language literature contained reports of 150 adverse events.

Children and Pregnancy

Although acupuncture has been practiced for thousands of years in China, its use in pediatrics in the United States did not become common until the early 2000s. In 2007, the National Health Interview Survey (NHIS) conducted by the National Center For Health Statistics (NCHS) estimated that approximately 150,000 children had received acupuncture treatment for a variety of conditions.

Acupuncture can potentially improve a number of common pediatric issues, including gastrointestinal issues, reflux, colic, asthma, allergies, ADHD, and headaches, however, its safety has been debated. In 2008 a study determined that the use of acupuncture-needle treatment on children was "questionable" due to the possibility of adverse side-effects and the pain manifestation differences in children versus adults. The study also includes warnings against practicing acupuncture on infants, as well as on children who are over-fatigued, very weak, or have over-eaten.

When used on children, acupuncture is considered safe when administered by well-trained, licensed practitioners using sterile needles; however, a 2011 review found there was limited research to draw definite conclusions about the overall safety of pediatric acupuncture. The same review found 279 adverse events, 25 of them serious. The adverse events were mostly mild in nature (e.g. bruising or bleeding). The prevalence of mild adverse events ranged from 10.1% to 13.5%, an estimated 168 incidences among 1,422 patients. On rare occasions adverse events were serious (e.g. cardiac rupture or hemoptysis); many might have been a result of substandard practice. The incidence of serious adverse events was 5 per one million, which included children and adults.

When used during pregnancy, the majority of adverse events caused by acupuncture were mild and transient, with few serious adverse events. The most frequent mild adverse event was needling or unspecified pain, followed by bleeding. Although two deaths (one stillbirth and one neonatal death) were reported, there was a lack of acupuncture-associated maternal mortality. Limiting the evidence as certain, probable or possible in the causality evaluation, the estimated incidence of adverse events following acupuncture in pregnant women was 131 per 10,000. Although acupuncture is not contraindicated in pregnant women, some specific acupuncture points are particularly sensitive to needle insertion; these spots, as well as the abdominal region, should be avoided during pregnancy.

Moxibustion and Cupping

Four adverse events associated with moxibustion were bruising, burns and cellulitis, spinal epidural abscess, and large superficial basal cell carcinoma. Ten adverse events were associated with cupping. The minor ones were keloid scarring, burns, and bullae; the serious ones were acquired hemophilia A, stroke following cupping on the back and neck, factitious panniculitis, reversible cardiac hypertrophy, and iron deficiency anemia.

Cost-effectiveness

A 2013 meta-analysis found that acupuncture for chronic low back pain was cost-effective as a complement to standard care, but not as a substitute for standard care except in cases where comorbid depression presented. The same meta-analysis found there was no difference between sham and non-sham acupuncture. A 2011 systematic review found insufficient evidence for the cost-effectiveness of acupuncture in the treatment of chronic low back pain. A 2010 systematic review found that the cost-effectiveness of acupuncture could not be concluded. A 2012 review found that acupuncture seems to be cost-effective for some pain conditions.

Risk of Forgoing Conventional Medical Care

As with other alternative medicines, unethical or naïve practitioners may induce patients to exhaust financial resources by pursuing ineffective treatment. Profession ethical codes set by accrediting organizations such as the National Certification Commission for Acupuncture and Oriental Medicine require practitioners to make "timely referrals to other health care professionals as may be appropriate." Stephen Barrett states that there is a "risk that an acupuncturist whose approach to diagnosis is not based on scientific concepts will fail to diagnose a dangerous condition".

Conceptual Basis

Traditional

Acupuncture is a substantial part of traditional Chinese medicine (TCM). Early acupuncture beliefs relied on concepts that are common in TCM, such as a life force energy called *qi*. *Qi* was believed to flow from the body's primary organs (zang-fu organs) to the "superficial" body tissues of the skin, muscles, tendons, bones, and joints, through channels called meridians. Acupuncture points where needles are inserted are mainly (but not always) found at locations along the meridians. Acupuncture points not found along a meridian are called extraordinary points and those with no designated site are called "A-shi" points.

In TCM, disease is generally perceived as a disharmony or imbalance in energies such as yin, yang, *qi*, xuě, zàng-fŭ, meridians, and of the interaction between the body and the environment. Therapy is based on which "pattern of disharmony" can be identified. For example, some diseases are believed to be caused by meridians being invaded with an excess of wind, cold, and damp. In order to determine which pattern is at hand, practitioners examine things like the color and shape of the tongue, the relative strength of pulse-points, the smell of the breath, the quality of breathing, or the sound of the voice. TCM and its concept of disease does not strongly differentiate between the cause and effect of symptoms.

Purported Scientific Basis

Scientific research has not supported the existence of *qi*, meridians, or yin and yang.[n 1] A *Nature* editorial described TCM as "fraught with pseudoscience", with the majority of its treatments having no logical mechanism of action. Quackwatch states that "TCM theory and practice are not based upon the body of knowledge related to health, disease, and health care that has been widely accepted by the scientific community. TCM practitioners disagree among themselves about how to diagnose patients and which treatments should go with which diagnoses. Even if they could agree, the TCM theories are so nebulous that no amount of scientific study will enable TCM to offer rational care."

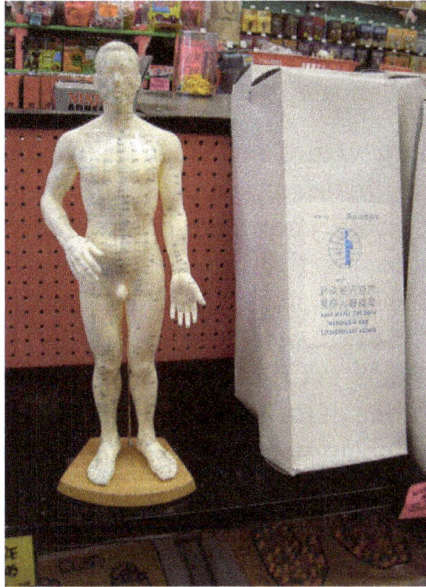

Modern acupuncture model

Some modern practitioners support the use of acupuncture to treat pain, but have abandoned the use of *qi*, meridians, *yin*, *yang* and other energies based in mysticism, as explanatory frameworks. The use of *qi* as an explanatory framework has been decreasing in China, even as it becomes more prominent during discussions of acupuncture in the US. Academic discussions of acupuncture still make reference to pseudoscientific concepts such as *qi* and meridians despite the lack of scientific evidence. Many within the scientific community consider attempts to rationalize acupuncture in science to be quackery, pseudoscience and "theatrical placebo". Academics Massimo Pigliucci and Maarten Boudry describe it as a "borderlands science" lying between science and pseudoscience.

Many acupuncturists attribute pain relief to the release of endorphins when needles penetrate, but no longer support the idea that acupuncture can affect a disease. It is a generally held belief within the acupuncture community that acupuncture points and meridians structures are special conduits for electrical signals but no research has established any consistent anatomical structure or function for either acupuncture points or meridians.[n 1] Human tests to determine whether electrical continuity was significantly different near meridians than other places in the body have been inconclusive.

Some studies suggest acupuncture causes a series of events within the central nervous system, and that it is possible to inhibit acupuncture's analgesic effects with the opioid antagonist naloxone. Mechanical deformation of the skin by acupuncture needles appears to result in the release of adenosine. The anti-nociceptive effect of acupuncture may be mediated by the adenosine A1 receptor. A 2014 *Nature Reviews Cancer* review article found that since the key mouse studies that suggested acupuncture relieves pain via the local release of adenosine, which then triggered close-by A1 receptors "caused more tissue damage and inflammation relative to the size of the animal in mice than in humans, such studies unnecessarily muddled a finding that local inflammation can result in the local release of adenosine with analgesic effect."

It has been proposed that acupuncture's effects in gastrointestinal disorders may relate to its effects on the parasympathetic and sympathetic nervous system, which have been said to be the "Western medicine" equivalent of "yin and yang". Another mechanism whereby acupuncture may be effective for gastrointestinal dysfunction involves the promotion of gastric peristalsis in subjects with low initial gastric motility, and suppressing peristalsis in subjects with active initial motility. Acupuncture has also been found to exert anti-inflammatory effects, which may be mediated by the activation of the vagus nerve and deactivation of inflammatory macrophages. Neuroimaging studies suggest that acupuncture stimulation results in deactivation of the limbic brain areas and the default mode network.

History

Origins

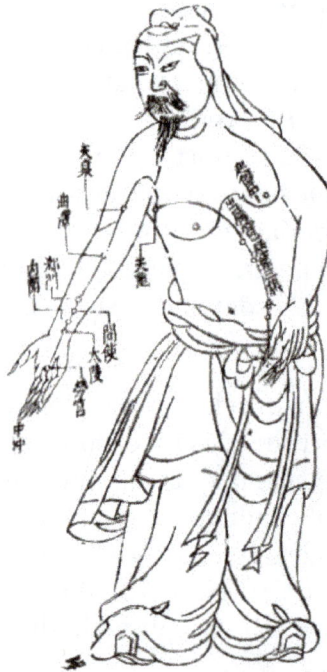

Acupuncture chart from the Ming dynasty (c. 1368–1644)

Acupuncture, along with moxibustion, is one of the oldest practices of Traditional Chinese Medicine. Most historians believe the practice began in China, though there are some conflicting narratives on when it originated. Academics David Ramey and Paul Buell said the exact date acupuncture was founded depends on the extent dating of ancient texts can be trusted and the interpretation of what constitutes acupuncture.

According to an article in *Rheumatology*, the first documentation of an "organized system of diagnosis and treatment" for acupuncture was in *The Yellow Emperor's Classic of Internal Medicine* (Huangdi Neijing) from about 100 BC. Gold and silver needles found in the tomb of Liu Sheng from around 100 BC are believed to be the earliest archeological evidence of acupuncture, though it is unclear if that was their purpose. According to Dr. Plinio Prioreschi, the earliest known historical record of acupuncture is the Shih-Chi ("Record of History"), written by a historian around 100 BC. It is believed that this text was documenting what was established practice at that time.

Alternate Theories

The 5,000-year-old mummified body of Ötzi the Iceman was found with 15 groups of tattoos, many of which were located at points on the body where acupuncture needles are used for abdominal or lower back problems. Evidence from the body suggests Otzi suffered from these conditions. This has been cited as evidence that practices similar to acupuncture may have been practiced elsewhere in Eurasia during the early Bronze Age; however, *The Oxford Handbook of the History of Medicine* calls this theory "speculative". It is considered unlikely that acupuncture was practiced before 2000 BC. The Ötzi the Iceman's tattoo marks suggest to some experts that an acupuncture-like treatment was previously used in Europe 5 millennia ago.

Acupuncture may have been practiced during the Neolithic era, near the end of the stone age, using sharpened stones called Bian shi.[70] Many Chinese texts from later eras refer to sharp stones called "plen", which means "stone probe", that may have been used for acupuncture purposes.[70] The ancient Chinese medical text, Huangdi Neijing, indicates that sharp stones were believed at-the-time to cure illnesses at or near the body's surface, perhaps because of the short depth a stone could penetrate.[71] However, it is more likely that stones were used for other medical purposes, such as puncturing a growth to drain its pus. The *Mawangdui* texts, which are believed to be from the 2nd century BC, mention the use of pointed stones to open abscesses, and moxibustion, but not for acupuncture. It is also speculated that these stones may have been used for bloodletting, due to the ancient Chinese belief that illnesses were caused by demons within the body that could be killed or released. It is likely bloodletting was an antecedent to acupuncture.

According to historians Lu Gwei-djen and Joseph Needham, there is substantial evidence that acupuncture may have begun around 600 BC. Some hieroglyphs and pictographs from that era suggests acupuncture and moxibustion were practiced. However, historians Gwei-djen and Needham said it was unlikely a needle could be made out of the materials available in China during this time period.[71-72] It is possible Bronze was used for early acupuncture needles. Tin, copper, gold and silver are also possibilities, though they are considered less likely, or to have been used in fewer cases.[69] If acupuncture was practiced during the Shang dynasty (1766 to 1122 BC), organic materials like thorns, sharpened bones, or bamboo may have been used.[70] Once methods for producing steel were discovered, it would replace all other materials, since it could be used to create a very fine, but sturdy needles.[74] Gwei-djen and Needham noted that all the ancient materials that could have been used for acupuncture and which often produce archeological evidence, such as sharpened bones, bamboo or stones, were also used for other purposes. An article in *Rheumatology* said that the absence of any mention of acupuncture in documents found in the tomb of Ma-Wang-Dui from 198 BC suggest that acupuncture was not practiced by that time.

Belief Systems

Several different and sometimes conflicting belief systems emerged regarding acupuncture. This may have been the result of competing schools of thought. Some ancient texts referred to using acupuncture to cause bleeding, while others mixed the ideas of blood-letting and spiritual ch'i energy. Over time, the focus shifted from blood to the concept of puncturing specific points on the body, and eventually to balancing Yin and Yang energies as well. According to Dr. David Ramey, no single "method or theory" was ever predominantly adopted as the standard. At the time, scientific knowledge of medicine was not yet developed, especially because in China dissection of the deceased was forbidden, preventing the development of basic anatomical knowledge.

It is not certain when specific acupuncture points were introduced, but the autobiography of Pien Chhio from around 400–500 BC references inserting needles at designated areas. Bian Que believed there was a single acupuncture point at the top of one's skull that he called the point "of the hundred meetings." Texts dated to be from 156–186 BC document early beliefs in channels of life force energy called meridians that would later be an element in early acupuncture beliefs.

Ramey and Buell said the "practice and theoretical underpinnings" of modern acupuncture were introduced in the *The Yellow Emperor's Classic* (Huangdi Neijing) around 100 BC. It introduced the concept of using acupuncture to manipulate the flow of life energy (*qi*) in a network of meridian (channels) in the body. The network concept was made up of acu-tracts, such as a line down the arms, where it said acupoints were located. Some of the sites acupuncturists use needles at today still have the same names as those given to them by the *Yellow Emporer's Classic*. Numerous additional documents were published over the centuries introducing new acupoints. By the 4th century AD, most of the acupuncture sites in use today had been named and identified.

Early Development in China

Establishment and Growth

In the first half of the 1st century AD, acupuncturists began promoting the belief that acupuncture's effectiveness was influenced by the time of day or night, the lunar cycle, and the season. The Science of the Yin-Yang Cycles (*Yün Chhi Hsüeh*) was a set of beliefs that curing diseases relied on the alignment of both heavenly (thien) and earthly (ti) forces that were attuned to cycles like that of the sun and moon. There were several different belief systems that relied on a number of celestial and earthly bodies or elements that rotated and only became aligned at certain times. According to Needham and Gwei-djen, these "arbitrary predictions" were depicted by acupuncturists in complex charts and through a set of special terminology.

Acupuncture needles during this period were much thicker than most modern ones and often resulted in infection. Infection is caused by a lack of sterilization, but at that time it was believed to be caused by use of the wrong needle, or needling in the wrong place, or at the wrong time. Later, many needles were heated in boiling water, or in a flame. Sometimes needles were used while they were still hot, creating a cauterizing effect at the injection site. Nine needles were recommended in the *Chen Chiu Ta Chheng* from 1601, which may have been because of an ancient Chinese belief that nine was a magic number.

Other belief systems were based on the idea that the human body operated on a rhythm and acupuncture had to be applied at the right point in the rhythm to be effective. In some cases a lack of balance between Yin and Yang were believed to be the cause of disease.

In the 1st century AD, many of the first books about acupuncture were published and recognized acupuncturist experts began to emerge. The *Zhen Jiu Jia Yi Jing*, which was published in the mid-3rd century, became the oldest acupuncture book that is still in existence in the modern era. Other books like the *Yu Kuei Chen Ching*, written by the Director of Medical Services for China, were also influential during this period, but were not preserved. In the mid 7th century, Sun Simiao published acupuncture-related diagrams and charts that established standardized methods for finding acupuncture sites on people of different sizes and categorized acupuncture sites in a set of modules.

Acupuncture became more established in China as improvements in paper led to the publication of more acupuncture books. The Imperial Medical Service and the Imperial Medical College, which both supported acupuncture, became more established and created medical colleges in every province. The public was also exposed to stories about royal figures being cured of their diseases by prominent acupuncturists. By time *The Great Compendium of Acupuncture and Moxibustion* was published during the Ming dynasty (1368–1644 AD), most of the acupuncture practices used in the modern era had been established.

Decline

By the end of the Song dynasty (1279 AD), acupuncture had lost much of its status in China. It became rarer in the following centuries, and was associated with less prestigious professions like alchemy, shamanism, midwifery and moxibustion. Additionally, by the 18th century, scientific rationality was becoming more popular than tradition-al superstitious beliefs. By 1757 a book documenting the history of Chinese medicine called acupuncture a "lost art". Its decline was attributed in part to the popularity of prescriptions and medications, as well as its association with the lower classes.

In 1822, the Chinese Emperor signed a decree excluding the practice of acupunc-ture from the Imperial Medical Institute. He said it was unfit for practice by gentle-men-scholars. In China acupuncture was increasingly associated with lower-class, il-literate practitioners. It was restored for a time, but banned again in 1929 in favor of science-based Western medicine. Although acupuncture declined in China during this time period, it was also growing in popularity in other countries.

International Expansion

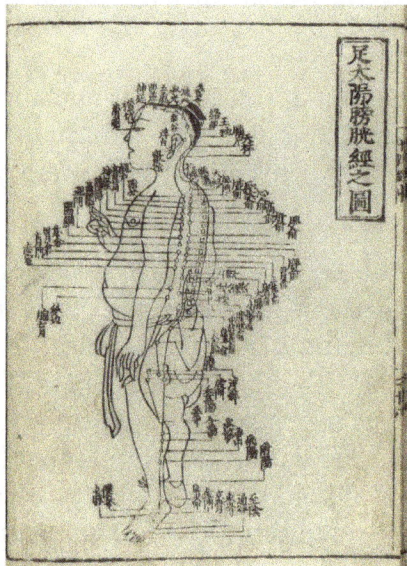

Acupuncture chart from *Shisi jing fahui* (Expression of the Fourteen Meridians) written by Hua Shou (fl. 1340s, Ming dynasty). Japanese reprint by Suharaya Heisuke (Edo, 1. year Kyōhō = 1716).

Korea is believed to be the first country in Asia that acupuncture spread to outside of China. Within Korea there is a legend that acupuncture was developed by emperor Da-ngun, though it is more likely to have been brought into Korea from a Chinese colonial prefecture in 514 AD. Acupuncture use was commonplace in Korea by the 6th century. It spread to Vietnam in the 8th and 9th centuries. As Vietnam began trading with Ja-pan and China around the 9th century, it was influenced by their acupuncture practices as well. China and Korea sent "medical missionaries" that spread traditional Chinese medicine to Japan, starting around 219 AD. In 553, several Korean and Chinese citizens were appointed to re-organize medical education in Japan and they incorporated acu-puncture as part of that system.[264] Japan later sent students back to China and estab-lished acupuncture as one of five divisions of the Chinese State Medical Administration System.

Acupuncture began to spread to Europe in the second half of the 17th century. Around this time the surgeon-general of the Dutch East India Company met Japanese and Chinese acupuncture practitioners and later encouraged Europeans to further investigate it. He published the first in-depth description of acupuncture for the European audience and created the term "acupuncture" in his 1683 work *De Acupunctura*. France was an early adopter among the West due to the influence of Jesuit missionaries, who brought the practice to French clinics in the 16th century. The French doctor Louis Berlioz (the father of the composer Hector Berlioz) is usually credited with being the first to experiment with the procedure in Europe in 1810, before publishing his findings in 1816.

By the 19th century, acupuncture had become commonplace in many areas of the world. Americans and Britains began showing interest in acupuncture in the early 20th century. Western practitioners abandoned acupuncture's traditional beliefs in spiritual energy, pulse diagnosis, and the cycles of the moon, sun or the body's rhythm. Diagrams of the flow of spiritual energy, for example, conflicted with the West's own anatomical diagrams. It adopted a new set of ideas for acupuncture based on tapping needles into nerves. In Europe it was speculated that acupuncture may allow or prevent the flow of electricity in the body, as electrical pulses were found to make a frog's leg twitch after death.

The West eventually created a belief system based on Travell trigger points that were believed to inhibit pain. They were in the same locations as China's spiritually identified acupuncture points, but under a different nomenclature. The first elaborate Western treatise on acupuncture was published in 1683 by Willem ten Rhijne.

Modern Era

In China, the popularity of acupuncture rebounded in 1949 when Mao Zedong took power and sought to unite China behind traditional cultural values. It was also during this time that many Eastern medical practices were consolidated under the name Traditional Chinese Medicine (TCM).

New practices were adopted in the 20th century, such as using a cluster of needles, electrified needles, or leaving needles inserted for up to a week. A lot of emphasis developed on using acupuncture on the ear. Acupuncture research organizations were founded in the 1950s and acupuncture services became available in modern hospitals. China, where acupuncture was believed to have originated, was increasingly influenced by Western medicine. Meanwhile, acupuncture grew in popularity in the US. The US Congress created the Office of Alternative Medicine in 1992 and the National Institutes of Health (NIH) declared support for acupuncture for some conditions in November 1997. In 1999, the National Center for Complementary and Alternative Medicine was created within the NIH. Acupuncture became the most popular alternative medicine in the US.

Politicians from the Chinese Communist Party said acupuncture was superstitious and conflicted with the party's commitment to science. Communist Party Chairman Mao Zedong later reversed this position, arguing that the practice was based on scientific principles.

In 1971, a *New York Times* reporter published an article on his acupuncture experiences in China, which led to more investigation of and support for acupuncture. The US President Richard Nixon visited China in 1972. During one part of the visit, the delegation was shown a patient undergoing major surgery while fully awake, ostensibly receiving acupuncture rather than anesthesia. Later it was found that the patients selected for the surgery had both a high pain tolerance and received heavy indoctrination before the operation; these demonstration cases were also frequently receiving morphine surreptitiously through an intravenous drip that observers were told contained only fluids and nutrients. One patient receiving open heart surgery while awake was ultimately found to have received a combination of three powerful sedatives as well as large injections of a local anesthetic into the wound. After the National Institute of Health expressed support for acupuncture for a limited number of conditions, adoption in the US grew further. In 1972 the first legal acupuncture center in the US was established in Washington DC and in 1973 the American Internal Revenue Service allowed acupuncture to be deducted as a medical expense.

In 2006, a BBC documentary *Alternative Medicine* filmed a patient undergoing open heart surgery allegedly under acupuncture-induced anesthesia. It was later revealed that the patient had been given a cocktail of anesthetics.

Adoption

Acupuncture is popular in China, the US, Australia, and Europe including all five Nordic countries, though less so in Finland. It is most heavily practiced in China and is one of the most common alternative medicine practices in Europe.[45] In Switzerland, acupuncture has become the most frequently used alternative medicine since 2004. In the United Kingdom, a total of 4 million acupuncture treatments were administered in 2009. Acupuncture is used in most pain clinics and hospices in the UK. An estimated 1 in 10 adults in Australia used acupuncture in 2004. In Japan, it is estimated that 25 percent of the population will try acupuncture at some point, though in most cases it is not covered by public health insurance. Users of acupuncture in Japan are more likely to be elderly and to have a limited education. Approximately half of users surveyed indicated a likelihood to seek such remedies in the future, while 37% did not. Less than one percent of the US population reported having used acupuncture in the early 1990s. By the early 2010s, more than 14 million Americans reported having used acupuncture as part of their health care.

In the US, acupuncture is increasingly (as of 2014) used at academic medical centers, and is usually offered through CAM centers or anesthesia and pain management services. Examples include those at Harvard University, Stanford University, Johns Hopkins University, and UCLA. This usage has been criticized owing to there being little scientific evidence for explicit effects, or the mechanisms for its supposed effectiveness, for any condition that is discernible from placebo. Acupuncture has been called 'theatrical placebo', and David Gorski argues that when acupuncture proponents advocate 'harnessing of placebo effects' or work on developing 'meaningful placebos', they essentially concede it is little more than that.

The use of acupuncture in Germany increased by 20% in 2007, after the German acupuncture trials supported its efficacy for certain uses. In 2011, there were more than one million users, and insurance companies have estimated that two-thirds of German users are women. As a result of the trials, German public health insurers began to cover acupuncture for chronic low back pain and osteoarthritis of the knee, but not tension headache or migraine. This decision was based in part on socio-political reasons. Some insurers in Germany chose to stop reimbursement of acupuncture because of the trials. For other conditions, insurers in Germany were not convinced that acupuncture had adequate benefits over usual care or sham treatments. Highlighting the results of the placebo group, researchers refused to accept a placebo therapy as efficient.

Regulation

There are various government and trade association regulatory bodies for acupuncture in the United Kingdom, the United States, Saudi Arabia, Australia, Japan, Canada, and in European countries and elsewhere. The World Health Organization recommends that before being licensed or certified, an acupuncturist receive 200 hours of specialized training if they are a physician and 2,500 hours for non-physicians; many governments have adopted similar standards.

In China, the practice of acupuncture is regulated by the Chinese Medicine Council that was formed in 1999 by the Legislative Council. It includes a licensing exam and registration, as well as degree courses approved by the board. Canada has acupuncture licensing programs in the provinces of British Columbia, Ontario, Alberta and Quebec; standards set by the Chinese Medicine and Acupuncture Association of Canada are used in provinces without government regulation. Regulation in the US began in the 1970s in California, which was eventually followed by every state but Wyoming and Idaho. Licensing requirements vary greatly from state to state. The needles used in acupuncture are regulated in the US by the Food and Drug Administration. In some states acupuncture is regulated by a board of medical examiners, while in others by the board of licensing, health or education.

In Japan, acupuncturists are licensed by the Minister of Health, Labour and Welfare after passing an examination and graduating from a technical school or university. Australia regulates Chinese medical traditions through the Chinese Medicine Board of Australia and the Public Health (Skin Penetration) Regulation of 2000. It restricts the use of words like "Acupuncture" and "Registered Acupuncturist". At least 28 countries in Europe have professional associations for acupuncturists. In France, the Académie Nationale de Médecine (National Academy of Medicine) has regulated acupuncture since 1955.

Acupuncture Point

Acupuncture points (Chinese: 腧穴 or Chinese: 穴位, also called acupoints) are locations on the body that are the focus of acupuncture, acupressure, sonopuncture and laser acupuncture treatment. In Traditional Chinese Medicine, several hundred acupuncture points are claimed to be located along what practitioners call meridians. There are also numerous "extra points" not associated with a particular meridian.

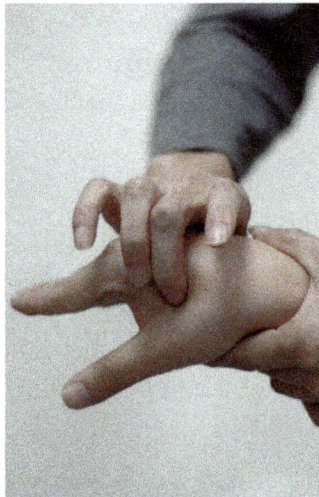

Point LI-4 known in Chinese as 合谷 (hégǔ)

Scientific evidence for the efficacy of either meridians or acupuncture points is mixed; overall reviews indicate evidence is not yet sufficiently compelling while others support the efficacy of some points for managing specific symptoms, such as labour pain or nausea.

Theory

Acupoints in treatment may or may not be in the same area of the body as the targeted symptom. The Traditional Chinese Medicine (TCM) theory for the selection of such points and their effectiveness is that they work by stimulating the meridian system to bring about relief by rebalancing yin, yang and qi (also spelled "chi" or "ki"). This theory is based on the paradigm of TCM and has no analogue in western medicine.

Body acupoints are generally located using a measurement unit, called the cun, that is calibrated according to their proportional distances from various landmark points on the body. Acupoint location usually depends on specific anatomical landmarks that can be palpated. Many of these basic points are rarely used. Some points are considered therapeutically more valuable than others, and are used very frequently for a wide array of health conditions.

Points tend to be located where nerves enter a muscle, the midpoint of the muscle, or at the enthesis where the muscle joins with the bone. Location by palpation for tenderness is also a common way of locating acupoints. Points may also be lo-cated by feeling for subtle differences in temperature on the skin surface or over the skin surface, as well as changes in the tension or "stickiness" of the skin and tissue. There is no scientific proof that this method works and some practitioners disagree with the method.

Body acupoints are referred to either by their traditional name, or by the name of the meridian on which they are located, followed by a number to indicate what order the point is in on the meridian. A common point on the hand, for example, is named *Hegu*, and referred to as LI 4 which means that it is the fourth point on the Large Intestine meridian.

Acupuncture points often have allusive, poetic names that developed over the course of centuries, often involving synonyms to ensure similar points are located on the appro-priate limb. A total of 360 points are generally recognized, but the number of points has changed over the centuries. Roughly 2/3 of the points are considered "yang", while the remaining 1/3 are considered "yin".

Scientific Research

Overall there is only preliminary evidence to suggest acupuncture points exist.

A 1997 NIH consensus statement has observed that "Despite considerable efforts to understand the anatomy and physiology of the 'acupuncture points', the definition and characterization of these points remains controversial. Even more elusive is the basis of some of the key traditional Eastern medical concepts such as the circulation of Qi, the meridian system, and the five phases theory, which are difficult to reconcile with contemporary biomedical information but continue to play an important role in the evaluation of patients and the formulation of treatment in acupuncture."

There are several theories for how acupuncture works or what acupuncture points are, but none of these theories have been proven. Acupuncture points may exhibit low elec-trical resistance and impedance but this evidence is mixed, and limited by poor-quality studies with small sample sizes and multiple confounding factors.

Efficacy of P6 Point Against Nausea with Vomiting

A meta-analysis of 40 trials suggested that stimulation of the P6 acupuncture point (located on the wrist) was effective for prophylactic treatment of postoperative nausea and vomiting, with minimal side-effects. The study also said: "The risks of postoperative nausea and vomiting were similar after P6 acupoint stimulation and antiemetic drugs."

Standardization

The World Health Organization (WHO) convened a Working Group on the Standardization of Acupuncture Nomenclature in 1982, with meetings of experts in 1984, 1985 and 1987, resulting in a standardized nomenclature for 361 classical acupuncture points organized according to the fourteen meridians, eight extra meridians, 48 extra points, and scalp acupuncture points. A proposed standard was published by WHO in 1991, and a *Standard Acupuncture Nomenclature* was published in 1993.

Acupressure

Acupressure is an alternative medicine technique similar in principle to acupuncture. It is based on the concept of life energy which flows through "meridians" in the body. In treatment, physical pressure is applied to acupuncture points with the aim of clearing blockages in these meridians. Pressure may be applied by hand, by elbow, or with various devices.

Some medical studies have suggested that acupressure may be effective at helping manage nausea and vomiting, for helping lower back pain, tension headaches, stomach ache, among other things, although such studies have been found to have a high likelihood of bias. Like many alternative medicines, it may benefit from a placebo effect.

According to Quackwatch acupressure is a dubious practice, and its practitioners use irrational methods.

Background

Acupoints used in treatment may or may not be in the same area of the body as the targeted symptom. The traditional Chinese medicine (TCM) theory for the selection of such points and their effectiveness is that they work by stimulating the meridian system to bring about relief by rebalancing yin, yang and qi (also spelled "chi").

Many East Asian martial arts also make extensive study and use of acupressure for self-defense and health purposes, (chin na, tui na). The points or combinations of points are said to be used to manipulate or incapacitate an opponent. Also, martial artists regularly massage their own acupressure points in routines to remove supposed blockages from their own meridians, claiming to thereby enhance their circulation and flexibility and keeping the points "soft" or less vulnerable to an attack.

Efficacy

A 2011 systematic review of acupressure's effectiveness at treating symptoms found that 35 out of 43 randomized controlled trials had concluded that acupressure was effective at treating certain symptoms; however, the nature of these 43 studies "indicated a significant likelihood of bias." The authors of this systematic review concluded that this "review of clinical trials from the past decade did not provide rigorous support for the efficacy of acupressure for symptom management. Well-designed, randomized controlled studies are needed to determine the utility and efficacy of acupressure to manage a variety of symptoms in a number of patient populations."

A 2011 Cochrane review of four trials using acupuncture and nine studies using acupressure to control pain in childbirth concluded that "acupuncture or acupressure may help relieve pain during labour, but more research is needed". Another Cochrane Collaboration review found that massage provided some long-term benefit for low back pain, and stated: *It seems that acupressure or pressure point massage techniques provide more relief than classic (Swedish) massage, although more research is needed to confirm this.*

P6 Acupuncture Point

An acupressure wristband that is claimed to relieve the symptoms of motion sickness and other forms of nausea provides pressure to the P6 acupuncture point, a point that has been extensively investigated. The Cochrane Collaboration reviewed the use of P6 for nausea and vomiting, and found it to be effective for reducing post-operative nausea, but not vomiting. The Cochrane review included various means of stimulating P6, including acupuncture, electro-acupuncture, transcutaneous nerve stimulation, laser stimulation, acustimulation device and acupressure; it did not comment on whether one or more forms of stimulation were more effective. EBM reviewer Bandolier said that P6 in two studies showed 52% of patients with control having a success, compared with 75% with P6.

Quackwatch includes acupressure in a list of methods which have no "rational place" as massage therapy and states that practitioners "may also use irrational diagnostic methods to reach diagnoses that do not correspond to scientific concepts of health and disease."

Theory

A variant system known as two point acupressure attempts to bypass a blockage of vital flow by using one acupoint to create a link with one of the collateral meridians, and then using one additional acupoint to stimulate or reduce the flow around the obstruction.

Criticism

Clinical use of acupressure frequently relies on the conceptual framework of Traditional Chinese Medicine (TCM). There is no physically verifiable anatomical or histological basis for the existence of acupuncture points or meridians. Proponents reply that TCM is a prescientific system that continues to have practical relevance. Acupuncturists tend to perceive TCM concepts in functional rather than structural terms (e.g., as being useful in guiding evaluation and care of patients).

Instruments

There are several different instruments for applying nonspecific pressure by rubbing, rolling, or applying pressure on the reflex zones of the body. The acuball is a small ball made of rubber with protuberances that is heatable. It is used to apply pressure and relieve muscle and joint pain. The energy roller is a small cylinder with protuberances. It is held between the hands and rolled back and forth to apply acupressure. The foot roller (also "krupa chakra") is a round, cylindrical roller with protuberances. It is placed on the floor and the foot is rolled back and forth over it. The power mat (also pyramid mat) is a mat with small pyramid-shaped bumps that you walk on. The spine roller is a bumpy roller containing magnets that is rolled up and down the spine. The Teishein is one of the original nine classical acupuncture needles described in the original texts of acupuncture. Even though it is described as an acupuncture needle it did not pierce the skin. It is used to apply rapid percussion pressure to the points being treated.

Pressure Point

A pressure point (Chinese: 穴位; Japanese: *kyūsho* 急所 "vital point, tender spot"; Sinhala: නිල/මර්ම ස්ථාන *Nila/Marma Sthana* (in Angampora); Telugu: మర్మ స్థానం *Marma Sthanam*; Malayalam: മർമ്മം *marmam*; Tamil: **வர்மம்** *varmam*) derives from the meridian points in Traditional Chinese Medicine and Indian Ayurveda and Siddha medicine, and the field of martial arts, and refers to an area on the human body that may produce significant pain or other effects when manipulated in a specific manner.

 The concept of pressure points spread through the South Indian martial art called Varma kalai, which is a martial art that concentrates on the body's pressure points. The concept of pressure points is also present in the old school Japanese martial arts; in a 1942 article in the *Shin Budo magazine*, Takuma Hisa asserted the existence of a tradition attributing the first development of pressure-point attacks to Shinra Saburō Minamoto no Yoshimitsu (1045–1127).

Hancock and Higashi (1905) published a book which pointed out a number of vital points in Japanese martial arts.

Accounts of pressure-point fighting appeared in Chinese Wuxia fiction novels and became known by the name of Dim Mak, or "Death Touch", in western popular culture in the 1960s.

While it is undisputed that there are sensitive points on the human body where even comparatively weak pressure may induce significant pain or serious injury, the association of *kyūsho* with notions of Death is controversial.

Types

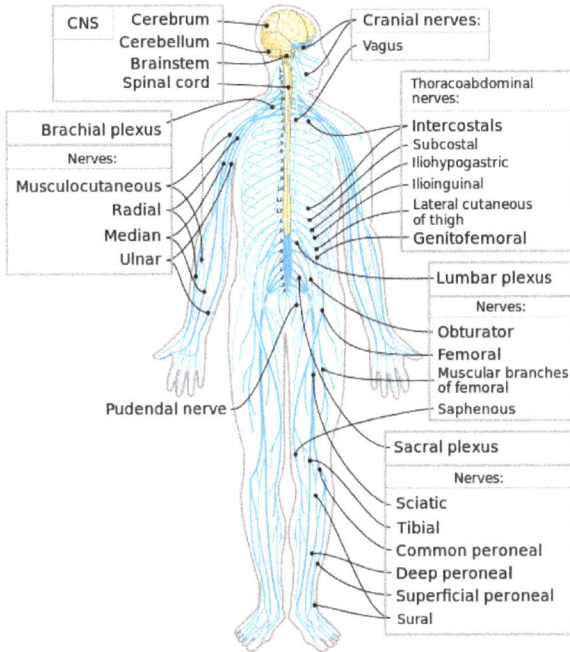

The nervous system.

There are several types of pressure points — each is applied differently and each creates a different effect. "Pain points", for example, use tendons, ligaments, and muscles; the goal is to temporarily immobilize the target, or, at the very least, to distract them. "Reflex points" produce involuntary movements, for example, causing the hand to release its grip, the knees to buckle, the target to gag, or even for the person to be knocked unconscious. Most pressure points are located on pathways on the nervous system.These points are called Meridians.

Pain

Some pressure points produce pain when struck, pressed, or rubbed, depending on the point itself. These points are also referred to as nerve centers. While the distraction of pain might offer sufficient advantage in a fight or flight, the body has a pain withdrawal reflex, whereby it reacts to pain by moving away from the source. Martial artists can use this reflex with minimal effort.

Blood Pressure

The baroreceptors in the carotid artery are pressure-sensitive, supplying the brain with information to control systemic blood pressure. Pressure against this region will send signals that indicate that blood pressure is too high, leading to a lowering of blood pressure.

Break

There are certain areas that are likely to lead to a break if struck effectively, such as:

- the floating ribs.
- the philtrum.
- the side of the knee.
- the jaw.
- the joints.

Reflex

There are points that, when struck, result in specific reflexes, such as:

- the base of throat strike results in gag reflex.
- Tendon reflex like Golgi organ strike, a relatively gentle strike to the Golgi tendon at the back of the elbow, which triggers a reflex that immediately relaxes the tendon, allowing the elbow to bend more easily in the wrong direction. If this is directly followed by a solid strike to the elbow joint, the elbow can be broken with significantly less effort than it could through brute force.

Concussion

The brain is a sensitive organ which floats in *cerebrospinal fluid*. The fluid is a safety mechanism that allows the head to take substantial impact without resulting in concussion, although such an impact could still cause permanent brain damage. However, it is possible to deliver a blow using artful techniques so that even these protections can be effectively eliminated, causing disorientation or instantaneous knockout. The most commonly taught technique involves a strike just below the occipital ridge, at the correct angle, in the correct direction. Another well-known point with this effect is the chin or lower jaw, giving rise to the boxing expression a "glass jaw".

List of Acupuncture Points

This article provides a comprehensive list of acupuncture points, locations on the body used in acupuncture, acupressure, and other treatment systems based on Traditional Chinese Medicine (TCM).

Human body meridians

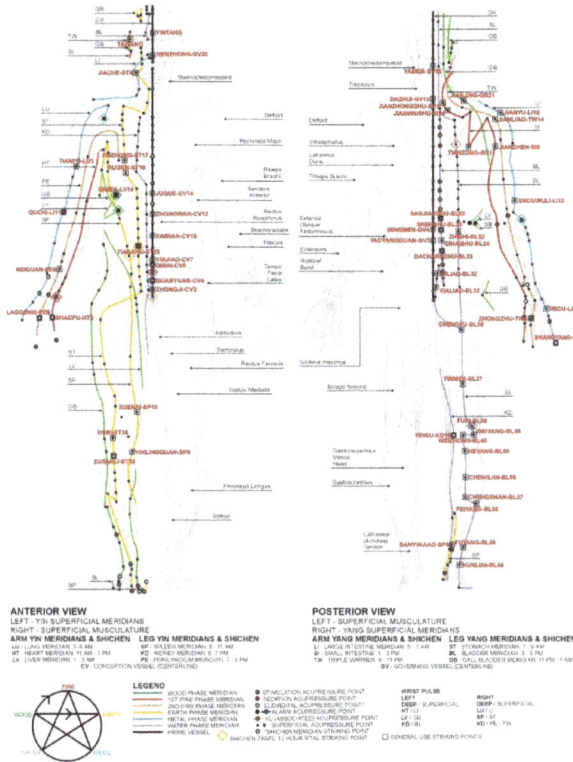

System of main meridians with acupuncture point locations

Locations and Basis

More than four hundred acupuncture points have been described, with the majority located on one of the main meridians, pathways which run throughout the body and according to Traditional Chinese Medicine (TCM) transport life energy (qi, 氣). TCM recognizes twenty meridians, cutaneous and subcutaneous in nature, which have branching sub-meridians believed to affect surrounding tissues. Twelve of these major meridians, commonly referred to as "the primary meridians", are bilateral and are associated with internal organs. The remaining eight meridians are designated as "extraordinary", and are also bilateral except for three, one that encircles the body near the waist, and two that run along the midline of the body. Only those two extraordinary meridians that run along the midline contain their own points, the remaining six comprise points from the aforementioned twelve primary meridians. There are also points that are not located on the fourteen major meridians but do lie in the complete nexus referred to as *jing luo* (經絡). Such outliers are often referred to as "extra points".

Although many hypotheses have been proposed, the anatomical and physiological basis for acupuncture points and meridians remains elusive. Hypotheses include neural signaling, with possible involvement of opioid peptides, glutamate, and adenosine, and correspondence to responsive parts in the central nervous system; or mechanical signaling, with involvement of connective tissue (fascia), and mechanical wave activation of the calcium ion channel to beta-endorphin secretion. In practice, acupuncture points are located by a combination of anatomical landmarks, palpation, and feedback from the patient.

Twelve Primary Meridians:

Code	Name	English	Pinyin	Han Geul 한글	Romaji	Vietnamese	Alternative names
LU		Lung				Thủ thái âm phế	
LI		Large Intestine				Thủ dương minh đại trường	
ST		Stomach				Túc dương minh vị	
SP		Spleen				Túc thái âm tỳ	
HT		Heart				Thủ thiếu âm tâm	
SI		Small Intestine				Thủ thái dương tiểu trường	
BL		Bladder				Túc thái dương bàng quang	
KI		Kidney				Túc thiếu âm thận	
PC		Pericardium				Thủ quyết âm tâm bào	
TE		Triple Energizer				Thủ thiếu dương tam tiêu	
GB		Gallbladder				Túc thiếu dương đởm	
LV		Liver				Túc quyết âm can	

Eight Extraordinary Meridians 奇經八脈 (奇经八脉), qí jīng bā mài (qí jīng bā mò):

Code		Name	English	Pinyin	Han Geul 한글	Romaji	Vietnamese	Alternative names
GV	督脈 (督脉)	Dumai	Governing Vessel	dū mài			Đốc mạch	
CV	任脈 (任脉)	Renmai	Conception Vessel	rén mài			Nhâm mạch	
TV	衝脈 (冲脉)	Chongmai	Thrusting Vessel	chòng mài			Xung mạch	

BV	帶 脈 (帶脉)	Daimai	Belt Vessel	dài mài			Đới mạch	
YinHV	陰 蹻 脈 (陰 跷 脉)	Yinqiao-mai	Yin Heel Vessel	yīn qiāo mài			Âm kiều	
YangHV	陽 蹻 脈 (陽 跷 脉)	Yangqiao-mai	Yang Heel Vessel	yáng qiāo mài			Dương kiều	
YinLV	陰 維 脈 (陰 维 脉)	Yinwei-mai	Yin Link Vessel	yīn wéi mài			Âm duy	
YangLV	陽 維 脈 (陽 维 脉)	Yangwei-mai	Yang Link Vessel	yáng wéi mài			Dương duy	

Nomenclature

In east Asian countries practitioners commonly refer to acupuncture points by their traditional names. Some points have several names. When acupuncture was adopted in the western world, a standard nomenclature was developed to unambiguously identify the acupuncture points on meridians. This model achieved wide acceptance and today virtually every book on acupuncture refers to acupuncture points using it. The World Health Organization (WHO) published *A Proposed Standard International Acupuncture Nomenclature Report* in 1991, listing 361 classical acupuncture points organized according to the fourteen meridians, eight extra meridians, 48 extra points, and scalp acupuncture points, and published *Standard Acupuncture Nomenclature* in 1993, focused on the 361 classical acupuncture points. Each acupuncture point is identified by the meridian on which it is located and its number in the point sequence on that channel. For example, *Lu-9* identifies the 9th acupuncture point on the lung meridian, *tài yuān* (太淵) or *gui xin* (鬼心), two names used for this same point. The only glitch with this unique systemized method can be found on the urinary bladder meridian, where the outer line of 14 points found on the back near the spine are inserted in one of two ways; following the last point of the inner line along the spine (會陽) and resuming with the point found in the crease of the buttocks (承扶), or following the point in the center of the crease of the knee (委中) and resuming with the point just below that (合陽), found in the bifurcation of the gastrocnemius muscle. Although classification of the extra points often tries to utilize a similar shortcut method, where a numbered sequence along an assigned body part is used, there is no commonly agreed-upon system and therefore universal identification of these points relies on the original naming system of traditional Chinese characters.

The above figure and the tables below follow the standard numbering scheme to identify the acupuncture points of the main channels. For extra points the tables follow the numbering scheme found in *A Manual of Acupuncture*.

Lung Meridian

Abbreviated as LU, described in Chinese as 手太阴肺经穴 or 手太陰肺經 "The Lung channel of Hand Taiyin".

Point		Name	English	Pinyin	Han Geul 한글	Romaji	Viet-namese	Alternative names
LU-1	中府	Zhongfu	Middle Palace	zhōng fǔ	jung bu 중부	chū fu	Trung phủ	
LU-2	雲門	Yunmen	Cloud Gate	yún mén	un mun 운문	un mon?	Vân môn	
LU-3	天府 (?)	Tianfu	Palace of Heaven	tiān fǔ(?)	cheon bu 천부	tem pu(?)	Thiên phủ	
LU-4	俠白 (?)	Xiabai	Clasping the White	xiá bái(?)	hyeop baek 협백	kyō haku?	Hiệp bạch	
LU-5	尺澤	Chize	Cubit Marsh	chǐ zé	cheok taek 척택	shaku taku	Xích trạch	
LU-6	孔最 (?)	Kongzui	Maximum Opening	kǒng zuì	gong choe 공최	kō sai	Khổng tối	
LU-7	列缺	Lieque	Broken Sequence	liè quē	yeol gyeol 열결	rek ketsu	Liệt khuyết	
LU-8	經渠	Jingqu	Channel Gutter	jīng qú	gyeong geo 경거	kei kyo	Kinh cừ	
LU-9	太淵	Taiyuan	Supreme Abyss	tài yuān	tae yeon 태연	tai en	Thái uyên	
LU-10	魚際	Yuji	Fish Border	yú jì	eo jae 어재	gyo sai	Ngư tế	
LU-11	少商	Shaoshang	Lesser Shang	shào shāng	so sang 소상	shō shō	Thiếu thương	

Large Intestine Meridian

Abbreviated as LI or CO (colon), described in Chinese as 手阳明大肠经穴 or 手陽明大腸經 "The Large Intestine channel of Hand Yangming".

Point		Name	English	Pinyin	Han Geul 한글	Romaji	Vietnam-ese	Alterna-tive names
LI-1	商陽	Shangyang	Shang Yang	shāng yáng	sang yang 상양	shō yō	Thương dương	
LI-2	二間 (?)	Erjian	Second Space	èr jiān	i gan 이간	ji kan	Nhị gian	
LI-3	三間 (?)	Sanjian	Third Space	sān jiān(?)	sam gan 삼간	san kan(?)	Tam gian	
LI-4	合谷	He Gu	Joining Valley	hé gǔ	hap gok 합곡	gō koku	Hiệp cốc	
LI-5	陽谿	Yangxi	Yang Stream	yáng xī	yang gye 양계	yō kei	Dương khê	
LI-6	偏歷	Pianli	Veering Passage	piān lì	pyeon ryeok 편력	hen reki	Thiên lịch	
LI-7	溫溜	Wenliu	Warm Flow	wēn liū	ol lyu 온류	on rū	Ôn lưu	

LI-8	下廉 (?)	Xialian	Lower Angle	xià lián(?)	ha ryeom 하렴	ge ren(?)	Hạ liêm	
LI-9	上廉 (?)	Shanglian	Upper Angle	shàng lián(?)	sang nyeom 상렴	jō ren?	Thượng liêm	
LI-10	手三里	Shousanli	Arm Three Miles	shǒu sān lǐ	[su] sam ni [수] 삼리	te san ri	Thủ tam lý	
LI-11	曲池	Quchi	Pool at the Crook	qū chí	gok ji 곡지	kyoku chi	Khúc trì	
LI-12	肘髎 (?)	Zhouliao	Elbow Crevice	zhǒu liáo(?)	ju ryo 주료	chū ryō?	Trửu liêu	
LI-13	手五里(?)	Shouwuli	Arm Five Miles	shǒu wǔ lǐ(?)	[su] o ri [수] 오리	te no go ri?	(Thủ) ngũ lý	
LI-14	臂臑	Binao	Upper Arm	bì nào	bi noe 비뇌	hi ju	Tí nhu	
LI-15	肩髃	Jianyu	Shoulder Bone	jiān yú	gyeon u 견우	ken gū	Kiên ngung	
LI-16	巨骨	Jugu	Great Bone	jù gǔ	geo gol 거골	ko kotsu	Ngự cốt	
LI-17	天鼎 (?)	Tianding	Heaven's Tripod	tiān dǐng	cheon jeong 천정	ten tei	Thiên đỉnh	
LI-18	扶突 (?)	Futu	Support the Prominence	fú tū(?)	bu dol 부돌	fu tot-su(?)	Phù đột	
LI-19	口禾髎	Kouheliao	Mouth Grain Crevice	kǒu hé liáo	hwa ryo 화료	ka ryō(?)	Hòa liêu	
LI-20	迎香	Yingxiang	Welcome Fragrance	yíng xiāng	yeong hyang 영향	gei ko	Nghênh hương	'gei gō'

Stomach Meridian

Abbreviated as ST, described in Chinese as 足阳明胃经穴 or 足陽明胃經 "The Stomach channel of Foot Yangming".

Point		Name	English	Pinyin	Han Geul 한글	Roma-ji	Vietnamese	Alternative names
St-1	承泣	Chengqi	Container of Tears	chéng qì	seung eup 승읍	shō kyū	Thừa khấp	
St-2	四白 (?)	Sibai	Four Whites	sì bái	sa baek 사백	shi haku	Tứ bạch	
St-3	巨髎	Juliao	Great Crevice	jù liáo	geo ryo 거료	ko ryō	Cự liêu	
St-4	地倉	Dicang	Earth Granary	dì cāng	ji chang 지창	chi so	Địa thương	
St-5	大迎	Daying	Great Welcome	dà yíng	dae yeo-ng 대영	da gei	Đại nghênh	

St-6	頰車	Jiache	Jaw Bone	jiá chē	hyeop geo 협거	kyō sha	Giáp xa	
St-7	下關	Xiaguan	Below the Joint	xià guān	ha gwan 하관	ge kan	Hạ quan	
St-8	頭維	Touwei	Head's Binding	tóu wéi	du yu 두유	zu i	Đầu duy	
St-9	人迎	Renying	Man's Welcome	rén yíng	in yeong 인영	jin gei	Nhân nghênh	Tianwuhui (Heaven's Five Meetings)
St-10	水突(?)	Shuitu	Water Prominence	shⲅi tū(?)	su dol 수돌	sui tot-su(?)	Thủy đột	
St-11	氣舍	Qishe	Abode of Qi	qì shè	gi sa 기사	ki sha(?)	Khí xá	
St-12	缺盆	Quepen	Empty Basin	quē pén	gyeol bun 결분	ketsu bon	Khuyết bồn	
St-13	氣戶	Qihu	Qi Door	qì hù	gi ho 기호	ki ko(?)	Khí hộ	
St-14	庫房(?)	Kufang	Storehouse	kù fáng(?)	go bang 고방	ko bō?	Khố phòng	
St-15	屋翳(?)	Wuyi	Room Screen	wū yì(?)	ok ye 옥예	o kuei?	Ốc ế	
St-16	膺窗(?)	Yingchuang	Breast Window	yìng chuāng?	eung chang 응창	yō sō?	Ưng song	
St-17	乳中(?)	Ruzhong	Middle of the Breast	rⲅzhōng(?)	yu jung 유중	nyū chū?	Nhũ trung	
St-18	乳根	Rugen	Root of the Breast	rⲅgēn	yu geun 유근	nyū kon?	Nhũ căn	
St-19	不容(?)	Burong	Not Contained	bù róng	bul yong 불용	fu yō	Bất dung	"Uncontainable" refers to vomiting
St-20	承滿(?)	Chengman	Supporting Fullness	chéng mⲅn	seng man 승만	shō man	Thừa mãn	
St-21	梁門(?)	Liangmen	Beam Gate	liáng mén	yang mun 양문	ryō mon	Lương môn	
St-22	關門	Guanmen	Pass Gate	guān mén	gwan mun 관문	kan mon?	Quan môn	
St-23	太乙(?)	Taiyi	Supreme Unity	tài yⲅ(?)	tae eul 태을	tai itsu(?)	Thái ất	
St-24	滑肉門(?)	Huaroumen	Slippery Flesh Gate	huá ròu mén	hwal yung mun 활육문	katsu niku mon	Hoạt nhục môn	

St-25	天樞	Tianshu	Heaven's Pivot	tiān shū	cheon chu 천추	ten sū	Thiên xu	
St-26	外陵 (?)	Wailing	Outer Mound	wài líng(?)	woe neung 외릉	gai ryō?	Ngoại lăng	
St-27	大巨 (?)	Daju	The Great	dà jù	dae geo 대거	dai ko	Đại cự	
St-28	水道 (?)	Shuidao	Water Passage	shuǐ dào?	su do 수도	sui do(?)	Thủy đạo	Left ST 28 = Baomen "Gate of Uterus"; Right ST 28 = Zihu "Child's Door - Sun Si Miao
St-29	歸來 (归来)	Guilai	Return	guī lái?	gui rae 귀래	ki rai(?)	Qui lai	
St-30	氣沖	Qichong	Rushing Qi	qì chōng	gi chung 기충	ki shō	Khí xung	
St-31	髀關	Biguan	Thigh Gate	bì guān	bi gwan 비관	hi kan(?)	Bễ quan	
St-32	伏兔 (?)	Futu	Crouching Rabbit	fú tù	bok to 복토	fuku to	Phục thỏ	
St-33	阴市 (?)	Yinshi	Yin Market	yīn shì(?)	eum si 음시	in shi(?)	Âm thị	
St-34	梁丘 (?)	Liangq-iu	Ridge Mound	liáng qiu	yang gu 양구	ryō kyū	Lương khâu	
St-35	犊鼻 (?)	Dubi	Calf's Nose	dú bí	dok bi 독비	toku bi	Độc tị	
St-36	足三里	Zusanli	Leg Three Miles	zú sān lǐ	[jok] sam ni [족]삼리	ashi san ri	Túc tam lý	
St-37	上巨虛	Shangjuxu	Upper Great Void	shàng jù xū	sang geo heo 상거허	jō ko kyu	Thượng cự hư	
St-38	條口 (?)	Tiaokou	Lines Opening	tiáo kǒu(?)	jo gu 조구	jō kō?	Điều khẩu	
St-39	下巨虛	Xiajuxu	Lower Great Void	xià jù xū	ha geo heo 하거허	ge ko kyu?	Hạ cự hư	
St-40	豐隆	Fen-glong	Abundant Bulge	fēng lóng	pung nyung 풍륭	hō ryū	Phong long	
St-41	解谿	Jiexi	Stream Divide	jiě xī	hae gye 해계	kai kei	Giải khê	
St-42	沖陽	Chong-yang	Rushing Yang	chōng yáng	chung yang 충양	shō yō	Xung dương	

St-43	陷谷 (?)	Xiangu	Sunken Valley	xiàn gǔ(?)	ham gok 함곡	kan koku(?)	Hãm cốc	
St-44	内庭	Neiting	Inner Courtyard	nèi tíng	nae jeong 내정	nai tei(?)	Nội đình	
St-45	厲兌	Lidui	Strict Ex-change	lì duì	ye tae 예 태	rei da	Lệ đoài	

Spleen Meridian

Abbreviated as SP, described in Chinese as 足太阴脾经穴 or 足太陰脾經 "The Spleen channel of Foot Taiyin".

Point		Name	English	Pinyin	Han Geul 한글	Ro-maji	Vietnamese	Alterna-tive names
SP-1	隱白	Yinbai	Hidden White	yǐn bái	eun baek 은백	im paku	Ẩn bạch	'in paku'
SP-2	大都	Dadu	Great Metrop-olis	dà dū	dae do 대도	dai to	Đại đô	
SP-3	太白	Taibai	Supreme White	taì bái	tae baek 태백	tai haku	Thái bạch	
SP-4	公孫	Gongsun	Grandfather Grandson	gōng sūn	gong son 공손	kō son	Công tôn	
SP-5	商丘	Shangqiu	Shang Mound	shāng qiū	sang gu 상구	shō kyū	Thương khâu	
SP-6	三陰交	Sanyin-jiao	Three Yin Intersection	sān yīn jiāo	sam eum gyo 삼음교	san in kō	Tam âm giao	
SP-7	漏谷	Lougu	Dripping Valley	loù gǔ	nu gok 루곡	rō koku?	Lậu cốc	
SP-8	地機	Diji	Earth Pivot	dì jī	ji gi 지기	chi ki	Địa cơ	
SP-9	陰陵泉	Yinlingq-uan	Yin Mound Spring	yīn líng quán	eum neung cheon 음릉천	in ryō sen	Âm lăng tuyền	
SP-10	血海	Xuehai	Sea of Blood	xuè hǎi	hyeol hae 혈해	kek kai	Huyết hải	
SP-11	箕門	Jimen	Winnowing Gate	jī mén	gi mun 기문	ki mon	Cơ môn	
SP-12	沖門	Chong-men	Rushing Gate	chōng mén	chung mun 충문	shō mon	Xung môn	
SP-13	府舍	Fushe	Abode of the Fu	fǔ shè	bu sa 부사	fu sha	Phủ xá	
SP-14	腹結 (?)	Fujie	Abdomen Knot	fù jié(?)	bok gyeol 복결	fuk ketsu	Phúc kết	

SP-15	大横	Da heng	Great Horizontal	dà héng?	dae hoeng 대횡	dai ō	Đại hoành	
SP-16	腹哀 (?)	Fuai	Abdomen Sorrow	fù āi(?)	bok ae 복애	fuku ai	Phúc ai	
SP-17	食竇 (?)	Shidou	Food Cavity	shí dòu(?)	sik du 식두	shoku tō	Thực đậu	
SP-18	天谿	Tianxi	Heavenly Stream	tiān xī	cheon gye 천계	ten kei	Thiên khê	
SP-19	胸鄉 (?)	Xiongxiang	Chest Village	xiōng xiāng(?)	hyung hyang 흉향	kyō kyō?	Hung hương	
SP-20	周榮 (?)	Zhourong	Encircling Glory	zhōu róng(?)	ju yeong 주영	shū ei	Chu vinh	
SP-21	大包	Dabao	Great Wrapping	dà bāo	dae po 대포	tai hō	Đại bao	

Heart Meridian

Abbreviated as HE, HT or H, described in Chinese as 手少阴心经穴 or 手少陰心經 "The Heart channel of Hand Shaoyin".

Point		Name	English	Pinyin	Han Geul 한글	Ro-maji	Viet-namese	Alterna-tive names
HE-1	極泉	Jiquan	Summit Spring	jí quán	geuk cheon 극천	kyoku sen	Cực tuyền	
HE-2	青靈	Qingling	Green Spirit	qīng líng	cheong nyeo-ng 청령	sei rei(?)	Thanh linh	
HE-3	少海	Shaohai	Lesser Sea	shào hǎi	so hae 소해	shō kai	Thiếu hải	
HE-4	靈道	Lingdao	Spirit Path	líng dào(?)	ryeong do 령도	rei dō?	Linh đạo	
HE-5	通里	Tongli	Penetrating the Interior	tōng lǐ(?)	tong ni 통리	tsū ri?	Thông lý	
HE-6	陰郄	Yinxi	Yin Cleft	yīn xī	eum geuk 음극	in geki	Âm khích	
HE-7	神門	Shen-men	Spirit Gate	shén mén	sin mun 신문	shin mon	Thần môn	
HE-8	少府	Shaofu	Lesser Palace	shào fǔ(?)	so bu 소부	shō fu?	Thiếu phủ	
HE-9	少沖	Shaoc-hong	Lesser Rushing	shào chōng	so chung 소충	shō shō	Thiếu xung	

Small Intestine Meridian

Abbreviated as SI, described in Chinese as 手太阳小肠经穴 or 手太陽小腸經 "The Small Intestine channel of Hand Taiyang".

Point		Name	English	Pinyin	Han Geul 한글	Romaji	Vietnamese	Alternative names
SI-1	少澤	Shaoze	Lesser Marsh	shào zé	so taek 소택	shō taku	Thiếu trạch	
SI-2	前谷	Qiangu	Front Valley	qián gǔ	jeon gok 전곡	zen koku(?)	Tiền cốc	
SI-3	後谿	Houxi	Back Stream	hòu xī	hu gye 후계	go kei	Hậu khê	'kō kei'
SI-4	腕骨	Wangu	Wrist Bone	wàn gǔ	wan gol 완골	wan kot-su(?)	Uyển cốt	
SI-5	陽谷	Yanggu	Yang Valley	yáng gǔ(?)	yang gok 양곡	yō koku	Dương cốc	
SI-6	養老	Yanglao	Support the Aged	yǎng lǎo	yang no 양노	yō rō	Dưỡng lão	
SI-7	支正	Zhizheng	Branch of Upright	zhī zhèng(?)	ji jeong 지정	shi sei(?)	Chi chính	
SI-8	小海	Xiaohai	Small Sea	xiǎo hǎi	so hae 소해	shō kai	Tiểu hải	
SI-9	肩貞	Jianzhen	True Shoulder	jiān zhēn	gyeon jeong 견정	ken tei	Kiên trinh	
SI-10	臑俞	Naoshu	Upper arm transporter	nāo shū	noe yu 뇌유	ju yu	Nhu du	
SI-11	天宗	Tianzong	Heavenly Gathering	tiān zōng	cheon jong 천종	ten sō	Thiên tông	
SI-12	秉風	Bingfeng	Grasping the Wind	bǐng fēng	byeong pung 병풍	hei fū	Bỉnh phong	
SI-13	曲垣	Quyuan	Crooked Wall	qū yuán	gok won 곡원	kyo ku en?	Khúc viên	
SI-14	肩外俞	Jian-waishu	Outer Shoulder Transporter	jiān wài shū	gyeon oe yu 견외유	ken gai yu(?)	Kiên ngoại du	
SI-15	肩中俞	Jian-zhongshu	Middle Shoulder Transporter	jiān zhōng shū	gyeon jung yu 견중유	ken chū yu?	Kiên trung du	
SI-16	天窗	Tianch-uang	Heavenly Window	tiān chuāng	cheon chang 천창	ten sō?	Thiên song	
SI-17	天容	Tianrong	Heavenly Appearance	tiān róng(?)	cheon yong 천용	ten yō?	Thiên dung	
SI-18	顴髎	Quanliao	Cheek Bone Crevice	quán liáo	gwal lyo 관료	kan ryō	Quyền liêu	
SI-19	聽宮	Tinggong	Palace of Hearing	tīng gōng	cheong gung 청궁	chō kyū	Thính cung	

Bladder Meridian

Abbreviated as BL or UB (urinary bladder), described in Chinese as 足太阳膀胱经穴 or 足太陽膀胱經 "The Bladder channel of Foot Taiyang".

An alternative numbering scheme for the "appended part" (beginning with Bl-41 in the list below), which places the outer line along the spine after Bl-35 (會陽) instead of Bl-40 (委中), will be noted in the *Alternative names* column.

Point		Name	English	Pinyin	Han Geul 한글	Romaji	Vietnamese	Alternative names
Bl-1	睛明	Jingming	Bright Eyes	jīng míng	cheong myeong 청명	sei mei	Tình minh	
Bl-2	攢竹	Zanzhu	Gathered Bamboo	cuán zhú	chan juk 찬죽	san chiku	Toản trúc	
Bl-3	眉衝	Meichong	Eyebrows' Pouring	méi chōng	mi chung 미충	bi shō	Mi xung	
Bl-4	曲差 (?)	Quchai	Crooked Curve	qǔ chā?	gok cha 곡차	kyo kusa?	Khúc sai	
Bl-5	五處	Wuchu	Fifth Place	wǔ chǔ	o cheo 오처	go sho(?)	Ngũ xứ	
Bl-6	承光 (?)	Chengguang	Receiving Light	chéng guāng(?)	seung gwang 승광	shō kō?	Thừa quang	
Bl-7	通天 (?)	Tongtian	Heavenly Connection	tōng tiān(?)	tong cheon 통천	tsū ten	Thông thiên	
Bl-8	絡卻	Luoque	Declining Connection	luò què	nak gak 락각	rak kyaku?	Lạc khước	
Bl-9	玉枕 (?)	Yuzhen	Jade Pillow	yù zhěn(?)	ok chim 옥침	gyoku chin(?)	Ngọc chẩm	
Bl-10	天柱 (?)	Tianzhu	Celestial Pillar	tiān zhù	cheon ju 천주	ten chū	Thiên trụ	
Bl-11	大杼	Dazhu	Great Shuttle	dà zhù	dae jeo 대저	dai jo	Đại trữ	
Bl-12	風門	Fengmen	Wind Gate	fēng mén	pung mun 풍문	fū mon	Phong môn	
Bl-13	肺俞	Feishu	Lung Transporter	fèi shū	pye yu 폐유	hai yu	Phế du	
Bl-14	厥陰俞	Jueyinshu	Jueyin Transporter	jué yīn shū	gweor eum yu 궐음유	ketsu in yu	Quyết âm du	
Bl-15	心俞 (?)	Xinshu	Heart Transporter	xīn shū	sim yu 심유	shin yu	Tâm du	
Bl-16	督俞	Dushu	Governor Transporter	dū shū?	dok yu 독유	toku yu	Đốc du	

Bl-17	膈俞	Geshu	Diaphragm Transporter	gé shū	gyeok yu 격유	kaku yu	Cách du	
Bl-18	肝俞	Ganshu	Liver Transporter	gān shū	gan yu 간유	kan yu	Can du	
Bl-19	膽俞	Danshu	Gallbladder Transporter	dǎn shū	dam yu 담유	tan yu	Đởm du	
Bl-20	脾俞	Pishu	Spleen Transporter	pí shū	bi yu 비유	hi yu	Tỳ du	
Bl-21	胃俞	Weishu	Stomach Transporter	wèi shū	wi yu 위유	i yu	Vị du	
Bl-22	三焦俞	Sanjiaoshu	Sanjiao Transporter	sān jiāo shū	sam cho yu 삼초유	san shō yu	Tam tiêu du	
Bl-23	腎俞	Shenshu	Kidney Transporter	shèn shū	sim yu 신유	jin yu	Thận du	
Bl-24	氣海俞	Qihaishu	Sea of Qi Transporter	qì hǎi shū?	gi hae yu 기해유	kikai yu?	Khí hải du	
Bl-25	大腸俞	Dachangshu	Large Intestine Transporter	dà cháng shū	dae jang yu 대장유	dai chō yu	Đại trường du	
Bl-26	關元俞	Guanyuanshu	Gate of Origin Transporter	guān yuán shū	gwan won yu 관원유	kan gen yu?	Quan nguyên du	
Bl-27	小腸俞	Xiaochangshu	Small Intestine Transporter	xiǎo cháng shū	so jang yu 소장유	shō chō yu	Tiểu trường du	
Bl-28	膀胱俞 (?)	Pangguangshu	Bladder Transporter	páng guāng shū(?)	bang wang yu 방광유	bōkō yu	Bàng quang du	
Bl-29	中膂俞 (?)	Zhonglushu	Mid-Spine Transporter	zhōng lǚ shū(?)	jung nyeo nae yu 중려내유	chū ryo yu?	Trung lữ du	中膂內俞 zhōng lǚ nèi shù
Bl-30	白環俞	Baihuanshu	White Ring Transporter	bái huán shū	baek hwan yu 백환유	hak kan yu?	Bạch hoàn du	
Bl-31	上髎 (?)	Shangliao	Upper Crevice	shàng liáo(?)	sang nyo 상료	jyō ryō?	Thượng liêu	
Bl-32	次髎 (?)	Ciliao	Second Crevice	cì liáo	cha ryo 차료	ji ryō	Thứ liêu	
Bl-33	中髎 (?)	Zhongliao	Middle Crevice	zhōng liáo(?)	jung nyo 중료	chū ryō?	Trung liêu	
Bl-34	下髎 (?)	Xialiao	Lower crevice	xià liáo(?)	ha ryo 하료	ge ryō?	Hạ liêu	
Bl-35	會陽	Huiyang	Meeting of Yang	huì yáng	hoe yang 회양	e yō	Hội dương	
Bl-36	承扶 (?)	Chengfu	Hold and Support	chéng fú(?)	seung bu 승부	sho fu(?)	Thừa phù	Bl-50

Bl-37	殷門	Yinmen	Gate of Abundance	yīn mén	eun mun 은문	in mon	Ân môn	Bl-51
Bl-38	浮郄	Fuxi	Floating Cleft	fú xī	bu geuk 부극	fu geki(?)	Phù khích	Bl-52
Bl-39	委陽	Weiyang	Outside of the Crook	wěi yáng	wi yang 위양	i yō	Ủy dương	Bl-53
Bl-40	委中	Weizhong	Middle of the Crook	wěi zhōng	wi jung 위중	i chū	Ủy trung	Bl-54
Bl-41	附分	Fufen	Attached Branch	fù fēn	bu bun 부분	fu bun(?)	Phụ phân	Bl-36
Bl-42	魄戶	Pohu	Door of the Corporeal Soul	pò hù	baek ho 백호	haku ko	Phách hạ	Bl-37
Bl-43	膏肓俞	Gaohuang-shu	Vital Region Shu	gāo huāng shū	go hwang [yu] 고황 [유]	kō kō yu	Cao hoang du	Bl-38
Bl-44	神堂 (?)	Shentang	Hall of the Spirit	shén táng(?)	sin dang 신당	shin dō?	Thần đường	Bl-39
Bl-45	譩譆 (?)	Yixi	Yi Xi ?	yì xǐ?	ui hoe 의회	i ki(?)	Y hy	Bl-40
Bl-46	膈關	Geguan	Diaphragm Gate	gé guān	gyeok gwan 격관	kaku kan(?)	Cách quan	Bl-41
Bl-47	魂門	Hunmen	Gate of the Ethereal Soul	hún mén	hon mun 혼문	kon mon?	Hồn môn	Bl-42
Bl-48	陽綱	Yanggang	Yang's Key Link	yáng gāng	yang gang 양강	yō kō?	Dương cương	Bl-43
Bl-49	意舍 (?)	Yishe	Abode of Consciousness of Potentials	yì shě?	ui sa 의사	i sha(?)	Ý xá	Bl-44
Bl-50	胃倉	Weicang	Stomach Granary	wèi cāng	wi chang 위창	i sō	Vị thương	Bl-45
Bl-51	肓門	Huangmen	Vitals Gate	huāng mén	hwang mun 황문	kō mon?	Hoang môn	Bl-46
Bl-52	志室 (?)	Zhishi	Residence of the Will	zhì shì	ji sil 지실	shi shitsu	Chí thất	Bl-47
Bl-53	胞肓 (?)	Baohuang	Bladder's Vitals	bāo huāng	po hwang 포황	hō kō	Bào hoang	Bl-48
Bl-54	秩邊	Zhibian	Order's Limit	zhì biān	jil byeon 질변	chip pen	Trật biên	Bl-49
Bl-55	合陽	Heyang	Confluence of Yang	hé yáng	hap yang 합양	gō yō?	Hợp dương	
Bl-56	承筋 (?)	Chengjin	Support the Sinews	chéng jīn	seung geun 승근	shō kin	Thừa cân	
Bl-57	承山 (?)	Chengshan	Support the Mountain	chéng shān(?)	seung san 승산	shō zan	Thừa sơn	

Bl-58	飛陽	Feiyang	Soaring Up-wards	fēi yáng	bi yang 비양	hi yō	Phi dương	
Bl-59	跗陽	Fuyang	Instep Yang	fū yáng	bu yang 부양	fu yō	Phụ dương	
Bl-60	昆侖	Kunlun	Kunlun Mountains	kūn lún	gol lyun 곤륜	kon ron	Côn lôn (luân)	'崑崙' is the older writing
Bl-61	僕參	Pucan	Servant's Respect	pú cān	bok cham 복참	boku shin(?)	Bộc tham	
Bl-62	申脈	Shenmai	Extending Vessel	shēn mài	sin maek 신맥	shim myaku	Thân mạch	
Bl-63	金門	Jinmen	Golden Gate	jīn mén	geum mun 금문	kim mon	Kim môn	
Bl-64	京骨 (?)	Jinggu	Capital Bone	jīng gǔ(?)	gyeong gol 경골	kei kot-su(?)	Kinh cốt	
Bl-65	束骨 (?)	Shugu	Restraining Bone	shù gǔ(?)	sok gol 속골	sok kotsu?	Thúc cốt	
Bl-66	足通谷	Zutonggu	Foot Con-necting Valley	zú tōng gǔ	[jok] tong gok [족] 통곡	ahsi tsū koku?	Thủ thông cốc	
Bl-67	至陰	Zhiyin	Reaching Yin	zhì yīn	ji eum 지음	shi in	Chí âm	

Kidney Meridian

Abbreviated as KI or K, described in Chinese as 足少阴肾经穴 or 足少陰腎經 "The Kidney channel of Foot Shaoyin".

Point		Name	English	Pinyin	Han Geul 한글	Romaji	Viet-namese	Alternative names
Kd-1	涌泉	Yong Quan	Gushing Spring	yǒng quán	yong cheon 용천	yu sen	Dũng tuyền	
Kd-2	然谷	Rangu	Nature Valley	rán gǔ	yeon gok 연곡	nen koku	Nhiên cốc	
Kd-3	太谿	Taixi	Supreme Stream	taì xī	tae yeon 태계	tai kei	Thái khê	
Kd-4	大鐘	Dazhong	Great Bell	dà zhōng(?)	dae jong 대종	dai shō?	Đại chung	
Kd-5	水泉	Shui-quan	Water Spring	shuǐ quán	su cheon 수천	sui sen	Thủy tuyền	
Kd-6	照海	Zhaohai	Shining Sea	zhào hǎi	joh hae 조해	shō kai	Chiếu hải	
Kd-7	復溜	Fuliu	Returning Current	fù liū	bong nyu 복류	fuku ryū	Phục lưu	

Kd-8	交信	Jiaoxin	Exchange Belief	jiāo xìn(?)	gyo sin 교신	kō shin?	Giao tín	
Kd-9	築賓	Zhubin	Guest House	zhú bīn	chuk bin 축빈	chiku hin	Trúc tân	
Kd-10	陰谷	Yingu	Yin Valley	yīn gǔ	eum gok 음곡	in koku	Âm cốc	
Kd-11	橫骨	Henggu	Pubic Bone	héng gǔ	hoeng gol 횡골	ō kotsu	Hoành cốt	
Kd-12	大赫(?)	Dahe	Great Luminance	dà hè	dae hyeok 대혁	tai kaku	Đại hách	
Kd-13	氣穴	Qixue	Qi Cave	qì xué?	gi hyeol 기혈	ki ketsu	Khí huyệt	
Kd-14	四滿	Siman	Four Fullnesses	sì mǎn	sa man 사만	shi man	Tứ mãn	
Kd-15	中注(?)	Zhongzhu	Middle Flow	zhōng zhù(?)	jung ju 중주	chū chū	Trung chú	
Kd-16	肓俞	Huangshu	Vitals Transporter	huāng shū	hwang yu 황유	kō yu	Hoang du	
Kd-17	商曲(?)	Shangqu	Shang Bend	shāng qū(?)	sang gok 상곡	shō kyoku	Thương khúc	
Kd-18	石關(?)	Shiguan	Stone Pass	shí guān(?)	seok gwan 석관	seki kan	Thạch quan	
Kd-19	陰都	Yindu	Yin Metropolis	yīn dū	eum do 음도	in to	Âm đô	
Kd-20	腹通谷	Futdonggu	Abdomen Connecting Valley	fù tōng gǔ(?)	tong gok 통곡	hara no tsū koku	(Phúc) Thông cốc	
Kd-21	幽門	Youmen	Hidden Gate	yōu mén	yu mun 유문	yū mon	U môn	
Kd-22	步廊(?)	Bulang	Walking Corridor	bù láng(?)	po rang 포랑	hō ro?	Bộ lang	
Kd-23	神封	Shenfeng	Spirit Seal	shén fēng	sin bong 신봉	shim pō	Thần phong	
Kd-24	靈墟	Lingxu	Spirit Ruin	líng xū(?)	yeong heo 영허	rei kyo(?)	Linh khâu	
Kd-25	神藏	Shencang	Spirit Storehouse	shén cáng	sin jang 신장	shin zō	Thần tàng	
Kd-26	或中	Yuzhong	Comfortable Chest	yù zhōng	uk jung 옥중/hok jung 혹중	waku chū	Hoắc trung	或中 huò zhōng – obvious mistranscription
Kd-27	俞府	Shufu	Shu Mansion	shū fǔ	yu bu 유부	yu fu	Du phủ	

Pericardium Meridian

Abbreviated as PC or P, described in Chinese as 手厥阴心包经穴 or 手厥陰心包經 "The Pericardium channel of Hand Jueyin".

Point		Name	English	Pinyin	Han Geul 한글	Romaji	Vietnamese	Alternative names
Pc-1	天池	Tianchi	Heavenly Pool	tiān chí	cheon ji 천지	ten chi	Thiên trì	
Pc-2	天泉(?)	Tianquan	Heavenly Spring	tiān quán(?)	cheon cheon 천천	ten sen(?)	Thiên tuyền	
Pc-3	曲澤	Quze	Marsh at the Crook	qū zé	gok taek 곡택	kyoku taku(?)	Khúc trạch	
Pc-4	郄門	Ximen	Xi-Cleft Gate	xī mén	geung mun 극문	geki mon	Khích môn	
Pc-5	間使	Jianshi	Intermediate Messenger	jiān shǐ	gan sa 간사	kan shi(?)	Giản sử	
Pc-6	內關	Neiguan	Inner Pass	nèi guān	nae gwan 내관	nai kan	Nội quan	
Pc-7	大陵	Daling	Great Mound	dà líng	dae reung 대릉	dai ryō	Đại lăng	'tai ryō'
Pc-8	勞宮	Laogong	Palace of Toil	láo gōng	no gung 노궁	rō kyū	Lao cung	
Pc-9	中衝	Zhongchong	Middle Rushing	zhōng chōng	jung chung 중충	chū shō	Trung xung	

Triple Burner Meridian

Also known as San Jiao, triple-heater, triple-warmer or triple-energizer, abbreviated as TB or SJ and described in Chinese as 手少阳三焦经穴 or 手少陽三焦經 "The Sanjiao channel of Hand Shaoyang".

Point		Name	English	Pinyin	Han Geul 한글	Romaji	Vietnamese	Alternative names
SJ-1	關衝	Guanchong	Rushing Pass	guān chōng	gwan chung 관충	kan shō	Quan xung	
SJ-2	液門(?)	Yemen	Fluid Gate	yè mén(?)	aeng mun 액문	eki mon(?)	Dịch môn	

SJ-3	中渚 (?)	Zhongzhu	Central Islet	zhōng zhŭ	jung jeo 중저	chū sho	Trung chử	
SJ-4	陽池 (?)	Yangchi	Yang Pool	yáng chí(?)	yang ji 양지	yō chi?	Dương trì	
SJ-5	外關	Waiguan	Outer Pass	wài guān	oe gwan 외관	gai kan	Ngoại quan	
SJ-6	支溝 (?)	Zhigou	Branch Ditch	zhī gōu(?)	ji gu 지구	shi kō?	Chi câu	
SJ-7	會宗	Huizong	Ancestral Meeting	huì zōng	hui jung 회종	e sō	Hội tông	
SJ-8	三陽 絡 (?)	Sanyan-gluo	Three Yang Meeting	sān yáng luò(?)	sam yang nak 삼양락	san kyō raku?	Tam dương lạc	
SJ-9	四瀆 (?)	Sidu	Four Rivers	sì dú	sa dok 사독	shi toku	Tứ độc	
SJ-10	天井	Tianjing	Heavenly Well	tiān jĭng	cheon jeong 천정	ten sei(?)	Thiên tỉnh	TW 10
SJ-11	清冷 淵 (?)	Qin-glengyuan	Clear Cold Abyss	qīng lěng yuān(?)	cheong naeng yeon 청랭연	sei rei en?	Thanh lãng uyên	
SJ-12	消濼 (?)	Xiaoluo	Dispers-ing Luo River	xiāo luò(?)	so bak 소박	shō reki?	Tiêu lạc	
SJ-13	臑會 (?)	Naohui	Upper Arm Meeting	nào huì(?)	noe hui 뇌회	ju e	Nhu hội	
SJ-14	肩髎 (?)	Jianliao	Shoulder Crevice	jiān liáo(?)	gyeol lyo 견료	ken ryō	Kiên liêu	
SJ-15	天髎	Tianliao	Heavenly Crevice	tiān liáo	cheol lyo 천료	ten ryō	Thiên liêu	
SJ-16	天牖 (?)	Tianyou	Window of Heav-en	tiān yŏu(?)	cheon yong 천용	ten yū?	Thiên dũ	
SJ-17	翳風	Yifeng	Wind Screen	yì fēng	ye pung 예풍	ei fū	É phong	
SJ-18	契 脈?	Qimai	Spasm Vessel	qì mài?	gye maek 계맥	kei myaku(?)	Khế mạch	First charac-ter means qì/ qī (contract/ spasm)
SJ-19	顱息 (?)	Luxi	Skull's Rest	lú xī?	no sik 로식	ro soku(?)	Lư tức	
SJ-20	角孫	Jiaosun	Minute Angle	jiăo sūn	gak son 각손	kaku son	Giác tôn	
SJ-21	耳門 (?)	Ermen	Ear Gate	ěr mén(?)	i mun 이문	ji mon(?)	Nhĩ môn	

| SJ-22 | 耳和膠 | Erheliao | Ear Harmony Crevice | ěr hé liáo | hwa ryo 화료 | ji wa ryō? | (Nhĩ) Hòa liêu |
| SJ-23 | 絲竹空 | Sizhukong | Silken Bamboo Hollow | sī zhú kōng | sa juk gong 사죽공 | shi chiku kū | Ti trúc không |

Gallbladder Meridian

Abbreviated as GB, described in Chinese as 足少阳胆经穴 or 足少陽膽經 "The Gallbladder channel of Foot Shaoyang".

Point	Name		English	Pinyin	Han Geul 한글	Romaji	Vietnamese	Alternative names
Gb-1	瞳子膠	Tongziliao	Pupil Crevice	tóng zǐ liáo	dong ja ryo 동자료	dō shi ryō	Đồng tử liêu	
Gb-2	聽會	Tinghui	Meeting of Hearing	tīng huì	cheong hoe 청회	chō e	Thính hội	
Gb-3	上關	Shangguan	Above the Joint	shàng guān	sang gwan 상관/gaek ju in 객주인	kyaku shu jin	Thượng quan	客主人 kè zhǔ rén
Gb-4	頷厭	Hanyan	Jaw Serenity	hàn yàn	ha yeom 함염	gan en	Hàm yến	
Gb-5	懸顱	Xuanlu	Suspended Skull	xuán lú	hyeol lo 현로	ken ro	Huyền lư	
Gb-6	懸厘	Xuanli	Suspended Hair	xuán lí	hyeol li 현리	ken ri	Huyền ly	
Gb-7	曲鬢	Qubin	Crook of the Temple	qū bìn	gok bin 곡빈	kyoku bin(?)	Khúc tân	
Gb-8	率谷	Shuaigu	Leading Valley	shuài gǔ	sol gok 솔곡	sok koku?	Suất cốc	
Gb-9	天沖	Tianchong	Heavenly Rushing	tiān chōng	cheon chung 천충	ten shō?	Thiên xung	
Gb-10	浮白	Fubai	Floating White	fú bái	bu baek 부백	fu haku(?)	Phù bạch	
Gb-11	頭竅陰	Touqiaoyin	Yin Portals of the Head	tóu qiào yīn	[du] gyu eum [두]규음	atama kyō in	Đầu khiếu âm	
Gb-12	完骨	Wangu	Mastoid Process	wán gǔ	wan gol 완골	kan kotsu	Hoàn cốt	
Gb-13	本神	Benshen	Root of the Spirit	běn shén	bon sin 본신	hon jin	Bản thần	
Gb-14	陽白	Yangbai	Yang White	yáng bái	yang baek 양백	yō haku	Dương bạch	
Gb-15	頭臨泣	Toulinqi	Head Governor of Tears	tóu lín qì	[du] im eup [두]임읍	atama no rin kyū	Đầu lâm khấp	

Gb-16	目窗 (?)	Much-uang	Window of the Eye	mù chuāng(?)	mok chang 목창	moku sō	Mục song	
Gb-17	正營	Zhengy-ing	Upright Nutrition	zhèng yíng	jyeong yeo-ng 정영	shō ei	Chính dinh	
Gb-18	承靈	Chen-gling	Support Spirit	chéng líng	seung nyeo-ng 승령	shō rei	Thừa linh	
Gb-19	腦空	Naokong	Brain Hol-low	nǎo kōng	noe gong 뇌공	nō kū	Não không	
Gb-20	風池	Fengchi	Wind Pool	fēng chí	pung ji 풍지	fū chi	Phong trì	
Gb-21	肩井	Jianjing	Shoulder Well	jīan jǐng	gyeon jeong 견정	ken sei	Kiên tỉnh	
Gb-22	淵腋	Yuanye	Armpit Abyss	yuān yè	yeon aek 연액	en eki(?)	Uyển dịch	
Gb-23	輒筋	Zhejin	Flank Sinews	zhé jīn	cheop geun 첩근	chō kin?	Triếp cân	
Gb-24	日月	Riyue	Sun and Moon	rì yuè	il weol 일월	jitsu getsu	Nhật nguyệt	
Gb-25	京門	Jingmen	Capital Gate	jīng mén	gyeong mun 경문	kei mon	Kinh môn	
Gb-26	帶脈	Daimai	Girdling Vessel	dài mài	dae maek 대맥	tai myaku	Đới mạch	
Gb-27	五樞	Wushu	Five Pivots	wǔ shū	o chu 오추	gō sū	Ngũ khu	
Gb-28	維道	Weidao	Linking Path	wéi dào	yu do 유도	yui dō	Duy đạo	
Gb-29	居髎	Juliao	Stationary Crevice	jū liáo	geo ryo 거료	kyo ryō	Cự liêu	
Gb-30	環跳	Huantiao	Jumping Circle	huán tiào	hwan do 환도	kan chō	Hoàn khiêu	
Gb-31	風市	Fengshi	Wind Mar-ket	fēng shì	pung si 풍시	fū shi	Phong thị	
Gb-32	中瀆	Zhongdu	Middle Ditch	zhōng dú	jung dok 중독	chū toku?	Trung độc	
Gb-33	膝陽關	Xiyang-guan	Knee Yang Gate	xī yáng guān	[seul] yang gwan [슬] 양관	hiza no yō kan?	(Tất) Dương quan	
Gb-34	陽陵泉	Yan-glingq-uan	Yang Mound Spring	yáng líng quán	yang neung cheon 양 룡천	yō ryō sen	Dương lăng tuyền	
Gb-35	陽交	Yangjiao	Yang Inter-section	yáng jiāo	yang gyo 양교	yō ko	Dương giao	
Gb-36	外丘 (?)	Waiqiu	Outer Hill	wài qiū(?)	woe gu 외구	gai kyū	Ngoại khâu	
Gb-37	光明 (?)	Guang-ming	Bright Light	guāng míng(?)	gwang my-eong 광명	kō mei?	Quang minh	
Gb-38	陽輔	Yangfu	Yang Assis-tance	yáng fǔ	yang bo 양 보	yō ho	Dương phụ	

Gb-39	懸鐘	Xuan-zhong	Suspended Bell	xuán zhōng	hyeon jong 현종/jeol gol 절골	ken shō	Huyền chung	絕骨 jué gǔ
Gb-40	丘墟	Qiuxu	Mound of Ruins	qiū xū	gu heo 구허	kyū kyo	Khâu khư	
Gb-41	足臨泣	Zulinqi	Foot Governor of Tears	zú lín qì	[jok] im eup [족] 임읍	ashi no rin kyū	Túc lâm khấp	
Gb-42	地五會	Diwuhui	Earth Five Meetings	dì wǔ huì	ji o hoe 지오회	chi go e(?)	Địa ngũ hội	
Gb-43	俠谿	Xiaxi	Clamped Stream	xiá xī	hyeop gye 협계	kyō kei?	Hiệp khê	
Gb-44	足竅陰	Zuqiao-yin	Yin Portals of the Foot	zú qiào yīn	[jok] gyu eum [족] 규음	ashi no kyō in	Túc khiếu âm	

Liver Meridian

Abbreviated as LR or LV, described in Chinese as 足厥阴肝经穴 or 足厥陰肝經 "The Liver channel of Foot Jueyin".

Point		Pinyin	English	Han Geul 한글	Romaji	Vietnam-ese	Alternative names
Liv-1	大敦	dà dūn	Great and Thick	dae don 대돈	tai ton	Đại đôn	
Liv-2	行間	xíng jiān	Interval Pass	haeng gan 행간	kō kan	Hành gian	
Liv-3	太沖	tài chōng	Supreme Rush	tae chung 태충	tai shō	Thái xung	
Liv-4	中封	zhōng fēng	Middle Margin	jung bong 중봉	chū hō	Trung phong	
Liv-5	蠡溝	lǐ gōu	Gnawed Channel	yeo gu 여구	rei kō	Lãi câu	
Liv-6	中都	zhōng dū(?)	Central Capital	jung do 중도	chū to	Trung đô	
Liv-7	膝關(?)	xī guān(?)	Knee Pass	seul gwan 슬관	shitsu kan(?)	Tất quan	
Liv-8	曲泉	qū quán	Pool Spring	gok cheon 곡천	kyoku sen	Khúc tuyền	
Liv-9	陰包	yīn bāo(?)	Yin Wrapping	eum bo 음보	im pō?	Âm bao	
Liv-10	足五里(?)	zú wǔ li?	Foot Governor of Tears	[jok] o ri [족] 오리	ashi no go ri?	(Túc) Ngũ lý	
Liv-11	陰廉	yīn lián	Yin Side	eum yeom 음염	in ren(?)	Âm liêm	
Liv-12	急脈	jí mài	Swift Pulse	geum maek 금맥	kyū myaku?	Cấp mạch	
Liv-13	章門	zhāng mén	Gate of the Ordering	jang mun 장문	shō mon	Trương môn	
Liv-14	期門	qí mén	Ciclic Gate	gi mun 기문	ki mon	Kỳ môn	

Governing Vessel

Also known as Du, abbreviated as GV and described in Chinese as 督脉穴 or 督脈 "The Governing Vessel".

Point		Pinyin	English	Han Geul 한글	Romaji	Vietnamese	Alternative names
Du-1	長強	cháng qiáng	Long and Rigid	jang gang 장강	chō kyō	Trường cường	
Du-2	腰俞	yāo shū(?)	Low Back Transporter	yo yu 요유	yō yu?	Yêu du	
Du-3	腰陽關	yāo yáng guān	Low Back Yang Passage	[yo] yang gwan [요] 양관	koshi no yo kan?	(Yêu) Dương quan	
Du-4	命門	mìng mén	Life Gate	myeong mun 명문	mei mon	Mệnh môn	
Du-5	懸樞	xuán shū	Suspended Pivot	hyeon chu 현추	ken sū?	Huyền khu	
Du-6	脊中(?)	jì zhōng?	Middle of the Spine	cheok jung 척중	seki chū?	Tích trung	
Du-7	中樞	zhōng shū	Central Pivot	jung chu 중추	chū sū?	Trung khu	
Du-8	筋縮	jīn suō	Muscle Spasm	geun chuk 근축	kin shuku(?)	Cân súc	
Du-9	至陽	zhì yáng	Reaching Yang	ji yang 지양	shi yō?	Chí dương	
Du-10	靈台	líng tái	Spirit Platform	yeong dae 영대	rei dai(?)	Linh đài	
Du-11	神道(?)	shén dào(?)	Way of the Spirit	sin do 신도	shin dō	Thần đạo	
Du-12	身柱(?)	shēn zhù(?)	Body Pillar	sin ju 신주	shin chū	Thân trụ	
Du-13	陶道	táo dào	Way of the Pot	do do 도도	tō dō?	Đào đạo	
Du-14	大椎	dà zhuī	Great Vertebra	dae chu 대추	dai tsui	Đại chùy	
Du-15	啞門	yǎ mén	Mutism Gate	a mun 아문	a mon	Á môn	
Du-16	風府	fēng fǔ	Wind Palace	pung bu 풍부	fū fu	Phong phủ	
Du-17	腦戶	nǎo hù	Brain Door	noe ho 뇌호	nō ko?	Não hộ	
Du-18	強間	qiáng jiān	Rigid Space	gang gan 강간	kyō kan?	Cường gian	

Du-19	後頂	hòu dǐng	Back Vertex	hu jeong 후정	go chō?	Hậu đính	
Du-20	百會	bǎi huì	One Hundred Meetings	baek hoe 백회	hyaku e	Bách hội	
Du-21	前頂 (?)	qián dǐng(?)	Front Vertex	jeon jeong 전정	zen chō?	Tiền đính	
Du-22	囟會	xìn huì	Fontanelle Meeting	sin hoe 신회	shin e(?)	Tín hội	
Du-23	上星 (?)	shàng xīng(?)	Upper Star	sang seong 상성	jō sei?	Thượng tinh	
Du-24	神庭	shén tíng	Spirit Court-yard	sin jeong 신정	shin tei	Thần đình	
Du-25	素髎 (?)	sù liáo(?)	Plain Space	so ryo 소료	so ryō?	Tố liêu	
Du-26	人中	rén zhōng	Middle of the Person	in jung 인중/ su gu 수구	jin chu	Nhân trung (Thủy câu)	水溝 shuǐ gōu [Water Pit]
Du-27	兌端	duì duān	End Exchange	tae don 태단	da tan(?)	Đoài đoan	
Du-28	齦交	yín jiāo	Gum Union	eun gyo 은교	gin kō	Ngân giao	

Conception Vessel

Also known as Ren, abbreviated as CV and described in Chinese as 任脉穴 or 任脈 "The Conception Vessel".

Point		Pinyin	English	Han Geul 한글	Romaji	Vietnamese	Alternative names
Ren-1	會陰	huì yīn	Yin Meeting	hoe eum 회음	e in	Hội âm	
Ren-2	曲骨	qū gǔ	Crooked Bone	gok gol 곡골	kyok kotsu?	Khúc cốt	
Ren-3	中極	zhōng jí	Middle Ex-tremity	jung geuk 중극	chū kyo-ku?	Trung cực	
Ren-4	關元	guān yuán	Origin Pass	gwan won 관원	kan gen	Quan nguyên	
Ren-5	石門 (?)	shí mén(?)	Stone Gate	seong mun 석문	seki mon(?)	Thạch môn	
Ren-6	氣海	qì hǎi	Sea of Qi	gi hae 기해	ki kai	Khí hải	

Ren-7	陰交	yīn jiāo	Yin Intersection	eum gyo 음교	in kō	Âm giao	
Ren-8	神闕	shén què	Spirit Palace	sin gwol 신궐	shin ketsu(?)	Thần khuyết	
Ren-9	水分 (?)	shuǐ fēn(?)	Water Division	su bun 수분	sui bun(?)	Thủy phân	
Ren-10	下脘	xià wǎn [or xià guǎn]	Lower Epigastrium	ha wan 하완	ge kan	Hạ quản	
Ren-11	建里 (?)	jiàn lǐ(?)	Internal Foundation	geol li 건리	ken ri(?)	Kiến lý	健裡 jiàn lǐ
Ren-12	中脘	zhōng wǎn [or zhōng guǎn]	Middle Epigastrium	jung wan 중완	chū kan	Trung quản	
Ren-13	上脘	shàng wǎn [or shàng guǎn]	Upper Epigastrium	sang wan 상완	jo kan	Thượng quản	
Ren-14	巨闕 (?)	jù què(?)	Great Palace	geo gwol 거궐	ko ketsu(?)	Cự khuyết	
Ren-15	鳩尾 (?)	jiū wěi(?)	Bird Tail	gu mi 구미	kyū bi?	Cưu vĩ	
Ren-16	中庭 (?)	zhōng tíng(?)	Central Courtyard	jung jeong 중정	chū tei?	Trung đình	
Ren-17	膻中	shān zhōng	Middle of the Chest	dan jung 단중	dan chū	Đản trung	
Ren-18	玉堂 (?)	yù táng(?)	Jade Hall	ok dang 옥당	gyoku dō?	Ngọc đường	
Ren-19	紫宮 (?)	zǐ gōng(?)	Violet Palace	ja gung 자궁	shi kyū?	Tử cung	
Ren-20	華蓋	huá gài	Splendid Cover	hwa gae 화개	ko gai?	Hoa cái	ka gai
Ren-21	璇璣	xuán jī	Jade Rotator	seon gi 선기	sen ki	Toàn cơ	
Ren-22	天突	tiān tū	Heaven Projection	cheon dol 천돌	ten totsu	Thiên đột	
Ren-23	廉泉	lián quán	Lateral Spring	yeom cheon 염천	ren sen	Liêm tuyền	
Ren-24	承漿	chéng jiāng	Saliva Container	seung jang 승장	shō shō	Thừa tương	

Extra Points

There is no agreed-on naming scheme for extra points on the body; this table follows the numbering scheme of Peter Deadman.

Point		Pinyin	Romaji	Vietnamese	Location
M-LE-8	八風	bā fēng	?	Bát phong	Lower Extremity (Legs and feet)
M-UE-1	十宣	shí xuān	?	Thập tuyên	Upper Extremity (Arms and hands)
M-UE-9	八邪	bā xié	?	Bát tà	Upper Extremity (Arms and hands)
M-HN-3	印堂	yìn táng	?	Ấn đường	Head and neck
M-BW-35	華佗夾脊	huá túo jiā jǐ	?	Hoa đà giáp tích	Back and waist; often referred to as the 'jiā jǐ' points

Regulation of Acupuncture

Regulation of acupuncture is done by governmental bodies to ensure safe practice.

Japan

In Japan, acupuncture practitioners are licensed by the Minister of Health, Labour and Welfare after passing an examination and graduating from a technical school or university.

Australia

In 2000, the Chinese Medicine Registration Board of Victoria, Australia (CMBV) was established as an independent government agency to oversee the practice of Chinese Herbal Medicine and Acupuncture in the state. In 2005 the Parliamentary Committee on the Health Care Complaints Commission in the Australian state of New South Wales commissioned a report investigating Traditional Chinese medicine practice. They recommended the introduction of a government-appointed registration board that would regulate the profession by restricting use of the titles "acupuncturist", "Chinese herbal medicine practitioner" and "Chinese medicine practitioner". The aim of registration was to protect the public from the risks of acupuncture by ensuring a high baseline level of competency and education of registered acupuncturists, enforcing guidelines regarding continuing professional education and investigating complaints of practitioner conduct. Currently acupuncturists in NSW are bound by the guidelines in the Public Health (Skin Penetration) Regulation 2000 which is enforced at local council level. In 2012 the CMBV became the Chinese Medicine Board of Australia, and in 2013 established an interim accreditation standard for the profession in partnership with the Australian Health Practitioner Regulation Agency. The legislation put in place stipulates that only practitioners who are state-registered may use the following titles: Acupuncture, Chinese Medicine, Chinese Herbal Medicine, Registered Acupuncturist, Registered Chinese Medicine Practitioner, and Registered Chinese Herbal Medicine Practitioner.

Canada

In Canada the provinces of British Columbia, Ontario, Alberta and Quebec have acupuncture licensing programs. In many provinces that are not subject to government regulation, employers will require candidates qualify for membership at the local chapter of the Chinese Medicine and Acupuncture Association of Canada. The province of Ontario, Canada, created the Traditional Chinese Medicine Act in 2006, which created the College of Traditional Chinese Practitioners and Acupuncturists. To be licensed in Ontario, acupuncturists need to register with the college, pass a series of tests and demonstrate an experience-equivalent of having seen more than 2,000 patients over five years.

In Quebec, the practice of acupuncture has been regulated since 1995 by the Ordre des acupuncteurs du Québec (OAQ).

France

Since 1955, the French advisory body Académie Nationale de Médecine (*National Academy of Medicine*) has accepted acupuncture as part of medical practice. Acupuncture is also routinely reimbursed by social security when performed or prescribed by a doctor or practitioner.

Europe

At least 28 countries in Europe have professional associations for acupuncturists.

Germany

Following the German acupuncture trials from 2006 to 2007, the Federal Joint Committee (an agency similar to the National Institutes of Health in the United States) passed a law which allows the reimbursement of acupuncture treatment by the public health insurance system for the following ailments: chronic lower back pain and chronic knee pain caused by osteoarthritis. In 2006, German researchers published the results of one of the first and largest randomized controlled clinical trials. As a result of the trial's conclusions, some insurance corporations in Germany no longer reimburse acupuncture treatments. The trials also had a negative impact on acupuncture in the international community.

New Zealand

Traditional/lay acupuncture is not a regulated health profession. Osteopaths have a scope of practice for Western Medical Acupuncture and Related Needling Techniques. The state-owned Accident Compensation Corporation reimburses for acupuncture treatment by registered health care practitioners and some traditional/lay acupuncturists that belong to voluntary professional associations.

United Kingdom

Acupuncturists are not a nationally regulated profession in the United Kingdom. Acupuncture practice is regulated by law in England and Wales for health and safety criteria under The Local Government (Miscellaneous Provisions) Act 1982, which has been recently amended by the Local Government Act 2003. Each local authority implements its own policy in accordance with the Act. For example, the London boroughs use the London Local Authorities Act, 1991/2000. Premises and each practitioner offering acupuncture must be licensed. As there is no formal certification of acupuncture, practitioners are exempted from licensing by virtue of being current members of approved acupuncture associations such as the British Acupuncture Council. Physiotherapists are also required to be current members of an approved acupuncture association as body piercing is not part of the entry level curriculum for state registered physiotherapists regulated by the Health Professions Council. The approved acupuncture organisations have rigorous codes of practice and educational requirements and members are covered by the appropriate indemnity insurance. An estimated 7,500 practitioners practise acupuncture to some extent and belong to a relevant professional or regulatory body. About 2,400 are traditional acupuncturists who mostly belong to the British Acupuncture Council, which requires its members to be trained in both traditional acupuncture and relevant biomedical sciences. Approximately 2,200 registered doctors and other statutorily regulated health professionals belong to the British Medical Acupuncture Society. Some 2,650 physiotherapists belong to the Acupuncture Association of Chartered Physiotherapists and 250 nurses belong to the British Academy of Western Acupuncture. There are also practitioners of Traditional Chinese Medicine who belong to one or more associations.

The principal body for professional standards in traditional/lay acupuncture is the British Acupuncture Council, The British Medical Acupuncture Society an inter-disciplinary professional body for regulated health professional using acupuncture as a modality. The Acupuncture Association of Chartered Physiotherapists.

United States

In 1996, the Food and Drug Administration changed the status of acupuncture needles from Class III to Class II medical devices, meaning that needles are regarded as safe and effective when used appropriately by licensed practitioners.

As of 2004, nearly 50% of Americans who were enrolled in employer health insurance plans were covered for acupuncture treatments.

Acupuncturists in the United States are required to attend a three- or four-year graduate-level, accredited program to be licensed. While some schools are regionally accredited, most professional training programs are accredited by the Accreditation Commission for Acupuncture and Oriental Medicine (ACAOM). Forty-three states require certification, by the National Certification Commission for Acupuncture and Oriental Medicine (NCCAOM).

Acupuncture regulation in the US began in the 1970s, prompted by an article by New York Times reporter James Reston. Nevada was the first US state in the nation to declare traditional Chinese medicine, including acupuncture, a learned profession (Senate Bill No. 448); authorizing the practice of Chinese medicine and acupuncture was signed into law on April 20, 1973, and many states thereafter followed suit. This could not be done without the help of Dr. Yee Kung Lok, Nevada's first acupuncturist. https://www.leg.state.nv.us/Session/76th2011/Bills/ACR/ACR9.pdf

According to *The Way Forward for Chinese Medicine*, US licensing requirements vary dramatically from state to state, with some states being very stringent and others having looser regulations. The Food and Drug Administration first regulated acupuncture needles in 1972 as "investigational devices" and later recognized needles for acupuncture uses in 1996. Three trade associations were founded in 1981 to set standards of practice: the Accreditation Commission for Acupuncture and Oriental Medicine (ACAOM), the Council of Colleges of Acupuncture and Oriental Medicine (CCAOM) and the National Certification Commission for Acupuncture and Oriental Medicine (NCCAOM).

Electroacupuncture

Electroacupuncture is a form of acupuncture where a small electric current is passed between pairs of acupuncture needles. According to some acupuncturists, this practice augments the use of regular acupuncture, can restore health and well-being, and is particularly good for treating pain. There is evidence for some efficacy (when used in addition to antiemetics) in treating moderate post-chemotherapy vomiting, but not for acute vomiting or delayed nausea severity.

Use by Acupuncturists

According to *Acupuncture Today*, a trade journal for acupuncturists:

> "Electroacupuncture is quite similar to traditional acupuncture in that the same points are stimulated during treatment. As with traditional acupuncture, needles are inserted on specific points along the body. The needles are then attached to a device that generates continuous electric pulses using small clips. These devices are used to adjust the frequency and intensity of the impulse being delivered, depending on the condition being treated. Electroacupuncture uses two needles at time so that the impulses can pass from one needle to the other. Several pairs of needles can be stimulated simultaneously, usually for no more than 30 minutes at a time."

That article adds:

> "According to the principles of traditional Chinese medicine, illness is caused

when chi does not flow properly throughout the body. Acupuncturists determine whether chi is weak, stagnant or otherwise out of balance, which indicates the points to be stimulated. Electroacupuncture is considered to be especially useful for conditions in which there is an accumulation of chi, such as in chronic pain syndromes, or in cases where the chi is difficult to stimulate."

Electroacupuncture is also variously termed EA, electro-acupuncture or incorporated under the generic term electrotherapy.

Electroacupuncture according to Voll (EAV) claims to measure "energy" in acupuncture points and to diagnose ailments. Some devices are registered in FDA as galvanic skin response measuring devices; they may not be used in diagnosis and treatment. Units reportedly sell for around $15,000 and are promoted for diagnosis of conditions including "parasites, food and environmental sensitivities, candida, nutritional deficiencies and much more." It is promoted for diagnosis of allergies.

Scientific Research

The Cochrane Collaboration, a group of evidence-based medicine (EBM) reviewers, reviewed eleven randomized controlled trials on the use of electroacupuncture at the P6 acupuncture point to control chemotherapy-induced nausea or vomiting. The reviewers found that electroacupuncture applied along with anti-vomiting drugs reduced first-day vomiting after chemotherapy more effectively than anti-vomiting drugs alone. However, the drugs given were not the most modern drugs available, so the reviewers stated that further research with state-of-the-art drugs was needed to determine clinical relevance. The reviewers concluded:

> "This review complements data on post-operative nausea and vomiting suggesting a biologic effect of acupuncture-point stimulation. Electroacupuncture has demonstrated benefit for chemotherapy-induced acute vomiting, but studies combining electroacupuncture with state-of-the-art antiemetics and in patients with refractory symptoms are needed to determine clinical relevance. Self-administered acupressure appears to have a protective effect for acute nausea and can readily be taught to patients though studies did not involve placebo control.

The Cochrane Collaboration also reviewed acupuncture and electroacupuncture for the treatment of rheumatoid arthritis. Because of the small number and poor quality of studies, they found no evidence to recommend its use for this condition. The reviewers concluded:

> "Although the results of the study on electroacupuncture show that electroacupuncture may be beneficial to reduce symptomatic knee pain in patients with RA 24 hours and 4 months post treatment, the reviewers concluded that the poor quality of the trial, including the small sample size preclude its recommendation. The reviewers further conclude that acupuncture has no effect on ESR,

CRP, pain, patient's global assessment, number of swollen joints, number of tender joints, general health, disease activity and reduction of analgesics. These conclusions are limited by methodological considerations such as the type of acupuncture (acupuncture vs electroacupuncture), the site of intervention, the low number of clinical trials and the small sample size of the included studies."

A 2016 systematic review and meta-analysis found inconclusive evidence that electroacupuncture was effective for nausea and vomiting and hyperemesis gravidarum during pregnancy.

Regarding EAV devices, "results are not reproducible when subject to rigorous testing and do not correlate with clinical evidence of allergy". There is no credible evidence of diagnostic capability. The American Cancer Society has concluded that the evidence does not support the use of EAV "as a method that can diagnose, cure, or otherwise help people with cancer" or "as a reliable aid in diagnosis or treatment of .. other illness" In double-blind trials, "A wide variability of the measurements was found in most patients irrespective of their allergy status and of the substance tested. Allergic patients showed more negative skin electrical response at the second trial, compared to normal controls, independent of the tested substance. No significant difference in skin electrical response between allergens and negative controls could be detected."

Safety

Researchers at the U.S. Food and Drug Administration (FDA) Center for Devices and Radiological Health (Rockville, Maryland) evaluated three representative devices intended for electrostimulation of acupuncture needles. The abstract at PubMed summarizes their findings:

"Three representative electrostimulators were evaluated to determine whether they meet the manufacturers' labeled nominal output parameters and how the measured parameters compare with a safety standard written for implanted peripheral nerve stimulators. The pulsed outputs (pulse width, frequency, and voltage) of three devices were measured with an oscilloscope across a 500-ohm resistance, meant to simulate subdermal tissue stimulated during electroacupuncture. For each device, at least two measured parameters were not within 25% of the manufacturer's claimed values. The measured values were compared with the American National Standard ANSI/AAMI NS15 safety standard for implantable peripheral nerve stimulators. Although for two stimulators the pulse voltage at maximum intensity was above that specified by the standard, short-term clinical use may still be safe because the standard was written for long-term stimulation. Similarly, the net unbalanced DC current, which could lead to tissue damage, electrolysis, and electrolytic degradation of the acupuncture needle, was within the limits of the standard at 30 pulses per second, but not at higher frequencies. The primary conclusions are (1) that the outputs of electrostimulators must be calibrated and (2) that practitioners must be adequately trained to use these electrostimulators safely."

References

- Williams, WF (2013). Encyclopedia of Pseudoscience: From Alien Abductions to Zone Therapy. Encyclopedia of Pseudoscience. Routledge. pp. 3–4. ISBN 1135955220.

- Gwei-Djen Lu; Joseph Needham (October 25, 2002). Celestial Lancets: A History and Rationale of Acupuncture and Moxa. ISBN 0700714588.

- Porter, S.B. (2013). Tidy's Physiotherapy15: Tidy's Physiotherapy. Churchill Livingstone. Elsevier. p. 403. ISBN 978-0-7020-4344-4. Retrieved July 14, 2015.

- Jackson, M. (2011). The Oxford Handbook of the History of Medicine. Oxford Handbooks in History. OUP Oxford. p. 610. ISBN 978-0-19-954649-7. Retrieved July 14, 2015.

- Adrian White; Mike Cummings; Jacqueline Filshie (2008). "2". An Introduction to Western Medical Acupuncture. Churchill Livingstone. p. 7. ISBN 978-0-443-07177-5.

- Angela Hicks (2005). The Acupuncture Handbook: How Acupuncture Works and How It Can Help You (1 ed.). Piatkus Books. p. 41. ISBN 978-0749924720.

- Collinge, William J. (1996). The American Holistic Health Association Complete guide to alternative medicine. New York: Warner Books. ISBN 0-446-67258-0.

- Steven Aung; William Chen (10 January 2007). Clinical Introduction to Medical Acupuncture. Thieme. p. 116. ISBN 9781588902214. Retrieved 20 September 2012.

- Cui-lan Yan (January 1997). The Treatment of External Diseases with Acupuncture and Moxibustion. Blue Poppy Enterprises, Inc. pp. 112–. ISBN 978-0-936185-80-4.

- "Sonopuncture". American Cancer Society's Guide to complementary and alternative cancer methods. American Cancer Society. 2000. p. 158. ISBN 9780944235249.

- Alvarez, L. (2015). "Chapter 18: Acupuncture". In James S. Gaynor & William W. Muir III. Handbook of Veterinary Pain Management (3rd edition). Elsevier. ISBN 978-0323089357.

- Lee Goldman; Andrew I. Schafer (21 April 2015). Goldman-Cecil Medicine: Expert Consult - Online. Elsevier Health Sciences. pp. 98–. ISBN 978-0-323-32285-0.

- Aung & Chen Steven K. H. Aung; William Pai-Dei Chen (2007). Clinical Introduction to Medical Acupuncture. Thieme. pp. 11–12. ISBN 978-1-58890-221-4.

- Flaws, B; Finney, D (1996). A handbook of TCM patterns & their treatments (6 (2007) ed.). Blue Poppy Press. pp. 169–173. ISBN 9780936185705.

- Ulett, GA (2002). "Acupuncture". In Shermer, M. The Skeptic: Encyclopedia of Pseudoscience. ABC-CLIO. p. 283291. ISBN 1576076539.

- Taylor, K (2005). Chinese Medicine in Early Communist China, 1945–63: a Medicine of Revolution. RoutledgeCurzon. p. 109. ISBN 041534512X.

Important Therapeutic Approaches and Techniques

Cupping therapy, Chinese food therapy, Tui na and qigong are important therapeutic approaches and techniques discussed in this chapter. Tui na is a form of acupressure where instead of using oils, thumb presses or rubbing is involved whereas qigong is a form of exercise and meditation that combines breathing with focused awareness and helps in the balance of qi. This chapter closely examines all the therapeutic approaches to provide an extensive understanding of the subject.

Cupping Therapy

Cupping therapy is a form of alternative medicine in which a local suction is created on the skin. Cupping has been characterized as pseudoscience. There is no good evidence it has any benefit on health and there are some concerns it may be harmful.

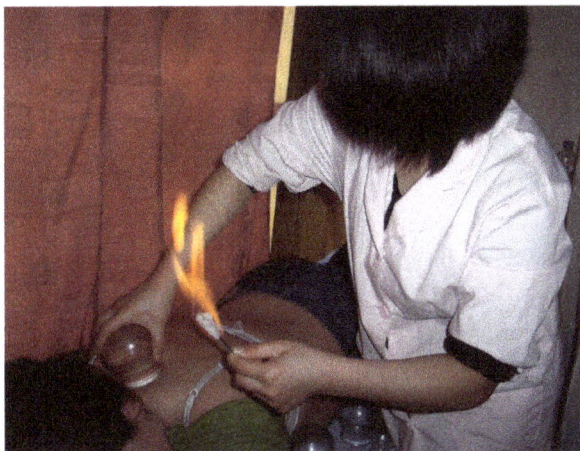

A person receiving fire cupping therapy

Description

Through suction, the skin is drawn into the cup by creating a vacuum in the cup placed on the skin over the targeted area. The vacuum can be created either by the heating and subsequent cooling of the air in the cup, or via a mechanical pump. The cup is usually left in place for somewhere between five and fifteen minutes. It is believed by some to help treat pain, deep scar tissues in the muscles and connective tissue, muscle knots, and swelling; however, the efficacy of this is unproven.

Effectiveness

Cupping as of 2015 is poorly supported by evidence. In their 2008 book *Trick or Treatment*, Simon Singh and Edzard Ernst write that no evidence exists of any beneficial effects of cupping for any medical condition. A 2011 review found tentative evidence for pain but nothing else. The way it works is unclear but might involve the placebo effect.. A 2015 review found it was useful, at least temporarily, for long term neck and low back pain.

The effectiveness of cupping is difficult to determine as it is difficult to construct a double blind or placebo-controlled clinical trial.

Some claim cupping is an alternative treatment for cancer. However, the American Cancer Society notes that "available scientific evidence does not support claims that cupping has any health benefits" and also that the treatment carries a small risk of burns.

Side Effects

Cupping is generally safe when done by trained health professionals on people who are otherwise healthy. It is not recommended in people with health problems due to side effects. Cupping is not recommended as a replacement for typical treatment. Cupping may result in bruising, burns, pain, or skin infection.

Research suggests that cupping is harmful, especially in people who are thin or obese. According to Jack Raso (1997), cupping results in capillary expansion, excessive fluid accumulation in tissues, and the rupture of blood vessels.

Reception

Individuals have been performing the action for over 3,000 years. The practice is typically performed unsupervised, without any medical background. Traditional Persian medicine in Iran uses wet cupping practices, with the belief that cupping with scarification may eliminate the scar tissue, and cupping without scarification would cleanse the body through the organs. Individuals with a profound interest in the practice are religious and seek purification.

Cupping has gained publicity due to its use by American sport celebrities including National Football League player DeMarcus Ware and Olympians Alexander Naddour, Natalie Coughlin, and Michael Phelps. Medical doctor Brad McKay wrote that Team USA was doing a great disservice to their fans who might "follow their lead", calling cupping an "ancient (but useless) traditional therapy." Practicing surgeon David Gorski claims, "it's all risk for no benefit. It has no place in modern medicine".

Critics of alternative medicine such as Harriet Hall, Mark Crislip, Simon Singh and Edzard Ernst call cupping "pseudoscience nonsense", "a celebrity fad", and "gibberish". They state that there is no evidence that cupping works any better than a placebo. Pharmacologist David Colquhoun writes that cupping is "laughable... and utterly implausible".

Methods

Broadly speaking there are two types of cupping: dry cupping and bleeding and/or wet cupping (controlled bleeding), with wet cupping being more common. Neither have any verifiable health benefit. Preference varies with practitioners and cultures.

Dry Cupping

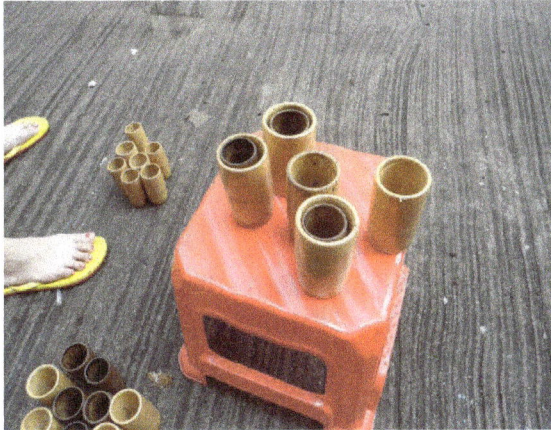

Bamboo cups

The cupping procedure commonly involves creating a small area of low air pressure next to the skin. However, there are varieties in the tools used, the methods of creating the low pressure, and the procedures followed during the treatment.

The cups can be various shapes including balls or bells, and may range in size from 1 to 3 inches (25 to 76 mm) across the opening. Plastic and glass are the most common materials used today, replacing the horn, pottery, bronze and bamboo cups used in earlier times. The low air pressure required may be created by heating the cup or the air inside it with an open flame or a bath in hot scented oils, then placing it against the skin. As the air inside the cup cools, it contracts and draws the skin slightly inside. More recently, vacuum can be created with a mechanical suction pump acting through a valve located at the top of the cup. Rubber cups are also available that squeeze the air out and adapt to uneven or bony surfaces.

In practice, cups are normally used only on softer tissue that can form a good seal with the edge of the cup. They may be used singly or with many to cover a larger area. They may be used by themselves or placed over an acupuncture needle. Skin may be lubricated, allowing the cup to move across the skin slowly.

Depending on the specific treatment, skin marking is common after the cups are removed. This may be a simple red ring that disappears quickly, the discolouration left by the cups is normally from bruising especially if dragging the cups while suctioned from one place to another to break down muscle fiber. Usually treatments are not painful.

Fire Cupping

Fire cupping involves soaking a cotton ball in 99% alcohol. The cotton is then clamped by a pair of forceps and lit via match or lighter. The flaming cotton ball is then, in one fluid motion, placed into the cup, quickly removed, and the cup is placed on the skin. Fire heats the inside of the cup and a small amount of suction is created by the air cooling down again and contracting. Massage oil may be applied to create a better seal as well as allow the cups to glide over muscle groups (e.g. trapezius, erectors, latisimus dorsi, etc.) in an act called "moving cupping". Dark circles may appear where the cups were placed because of rupture of the capillaries just under the skin, but are not the same as a bruise caused by blunt-force trauma. There are documented cases of burns caused by fire cupping.

Wet Cupping

Wet cupping is also known as Al-Hijamah or medicinal bleeding. The first documented uses are found in the teachings of the Islamic prophet Muhammad. According to Muhammad al-Bukhari, Muslim ibn al-Hajjaj Nishapuri and Ahmad ibn Hanbal, Muhammad approved of the Hijama (cupping) treatment.

A number of hadith support its recommendation and use by Muhammad. As a result, the practice of cupping therapy has survived in Muslim countries. Today, wet cupping is a popular remedy practiced in many parts of the Muslim world .

Alternatively, mild suction is created using a cup and a pump (or heat suction) on the selected area and left for about three minutes. The cup is then removed and small superficial skin incisions are made using a cupping scalpel. A second suction is used to carefully draw out a small quantity of blood.

In Finland, wet cupping has been done at least since the 15th century, and it is done traditionally in saunas. The cupping cups were made of cattle horns with a valve mechanism in it to create an partial vacuum by sucking the air out. Cupping is still used in Finland as an alternative medicine.

Traditional Chinese Medicine Cupping

According to traditional Chinese medicine (TCM) cupping is a method of creating a vacuum on the patient's skin to dispel stagnation — stagnant blood and lymph, thereby improving qi flow — to treat respiratory diseases such as the common cold, pneumonia and bronchitis. Cupping also is used on back, neck, shoulder and other musculoskeletal conditions. Its advocates say it has other applications, as well. Cupping is not advised over skin ulcers or to the abdominal or sacral regions of pregnant women.

History

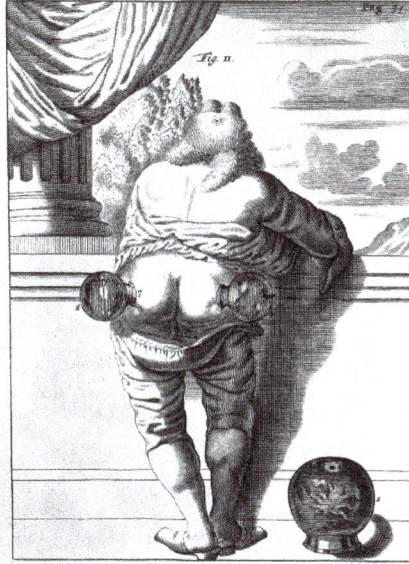

An illustration from a medical textbook "Exercitationes practicae" published in 1694 shows a man undergoing cupping on his buttocks.

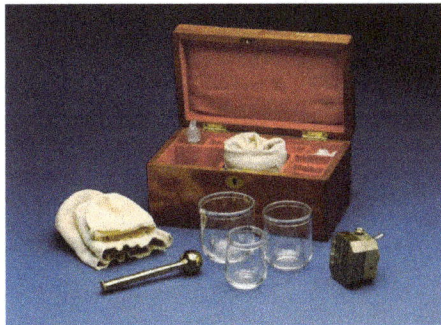

Cupping set, from London, England, 1860–1875.

There is reason to believe the practice dates from as early as 3000 BC. The Ebers Papyrus, written c. 1550 BC and one of the oldest medical textbooks in the Western world, describes the Egyptians' use of cupping, while mentioning similar practices employed by Saharan peoples. In ancient Greece, Hippocrates (c. 400 BC) used cupping for internal disease and structural problems. The method was highly recommended by Prophet Muhammed and hence well-practiced by Muslim scientist who elaborated and developed the method further. Consecutively, this method in its multiple forms spread into medicine throughout Asian and European civilizations. In China, the earliest use of cupping that is recorded is from the famous Taoist alchemist and herbalist, Ge Hong (281–341 A.D.). Cupping was also mentioned in Maimonides' book on health and was used within the Eastern European Jewish community. There is a description of cupping in George Orwell's essay "How the Poor Die", where he was surprised to find it practiced in a Paris hospital.

Chinese Food Therapy

Chinese food therapy (simplified Chinese: 食疗; traditional Chinese: 食療; pinyin: *shíliáo*; literally: "food therapy", also called nutrition therapy and dietary therapy) is a mode of dieting rooted in Chinese understandings of the effects of food on the human organism, and centred on concepts such as eating in moderation. Its basic precepts are a mix of folk views and concepts drawn from traditional Chinese medicine. It was the prescientific analog of modern medical nutrition therapy and now qualifies as alternative medicine.

Food therapy has long been a common approach to health among Chinese people both in China and overseas, and was popularized for western readers in the 1990s with the publication of books like *The Tao of Healthy Eating* (Flaws 1995a) and *The Wisdom of the Chinese Kitchen* (Young 1999), which also cites Flaws 1995b, Zhao & Ellis 1998, and Simonds 1999.

Origins

A number of ancient Chinese cookbooks and treatises on food (now lost) display an early Chinese interest in food, but no known focus on its medical value. The literature on "nourishing life" (养生; 養生; *yangsheng*) integrated advice on food within broader advice on how to attain immortality. Such books, however, are only precursors of "dietary therapy", because they did not systematically describe the effect of individual food items.

The earliest extant Chinese dietary text is a chapter of Sun Simiao's *Prescriptions Worth a Thousand Gold* (千金方; *Qiānjīn fāng*), which was completed in the 650s during the Tang dynasty. Sun's work contains the earliest known use of the term "food (or dietary) therapy" (食疗; 食療; *shíliáo*). Sun stated that he wanted to present current knowledge about food so that people would first turn to food rather than drugs when suffering from an ailment. His chapter contains 154 entries divided into four sections – on fruits, vegetables, cereals, and meat – in which Sun explains the properties of individual foodstuffs with concepts borrowed from the *Yellow Emperor's Inner Canon*: qi, the viscera, and vital essence (精; *jīng*), as well as correspondences between the Five Phases, the "five flavors" (sour, bitter, sweet, pungent, and salty), and the five grains. He also set a large number of "dietary interdictions" (食禁; *shíjìn*), some based on calendrical notions (no water chestnuts in the 7th month), others on purported interactions between foods (no clear wine with horse meat) or between different flavors.

Sun Simiao's disciple Meng Shen (孟诜; 孟詵; 621–713) compiled the first work entirely devoted to the therapeutic value of food: the *Materia Dietetica* (食疗本草; 食療本草; *Shíliáo běncǎo*; "food therapy *materia medica*"). This work has not survived, but it is quoted in later texts – like the 10th-century Japanese text Ishinpō – and a fragment of it has been found among the Dunhuang manuscripts. Surviving excerpts show that Meng gave less importance to dietary prohibitions than Sun, and that he provided information on how to prepare foodstuffs rather than just describe their properties. The works of Sun Simiao and Meng Shen established the genre of *materia dietetica* and shaped its development in the following centuries.

Precepts

Although the precepts of Chinese food therapy are neither systematic nor identical in all times and places, some basic concepts can be isolated. Food items are classified as "heating" (热; 熱; *rè*) or "cooling" (凉; 涼; *liáng*). "Heating" food is typically "high-calorie, subjected to high heat in cooking, spicy or bitter, or 'hot' in color (red, orange)", and includes red meat, innards, baked and deep-fried goods, and alcohol. They are to be avoided in the summer and can be used to treat "cold" illnesses like excessive pallor, watery feces, fatigue, chills, and low body temperature caused by a number of possible causes, including anemia. Green vegetables are the most typical cooling food, which is "low-calorie, watery, soothing or sour in taste, or 'cool' in color (whitish, green)". They are recommended for "hot" conditions: rashes, dryness or redness of skin, heartburns, and other "symptoms similar to those of a burn", but also sore throat, swollen gums, and constipation.

Auriculotherapy

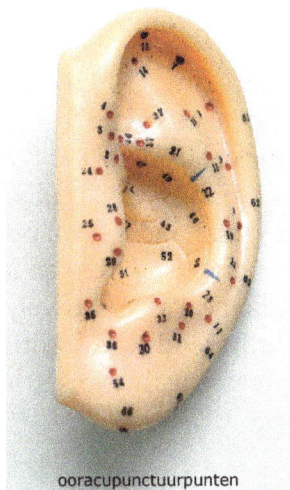

ooracupunctuurpunten

Acupuncture points in the ear.

Auriculotherapy, or auricular therapy, or ear acupuncture, or auriculoacupuncture is a form of alternative medicine based on the idea that the ear is a microsystem which reflects the entire body, represented on the auricle, the outer portion of the ear. Conditions affecting the physical, mental or emotional health of the patient are assumed to be treatable by stimulation of the surface of the ear exclusively. Similar mappings are used in many areas of the body, including the practices of reflexology and iridology. These mappings were not originally based on or supported by any medical or scientific evidence.

History

Auriculotherapy was first developed by the French neurologist Paul Nogier, who published his results in 1957 with his *Treatise of Auriculotherapy*. These developments were made by clinical trials based in a phrenological method of projection of a fetal Homunculus on the ear for reference of complaints and points for treatment. Nogier soon brought his discovery to the public, where members of the Chinese Army picked up the map and brought it back to the barefoot doctors. The ear map in China then was developed according to the theories of Traditional Chinese Medicine; however, Nogier is still known in China as the "Father of Auriculotherapy".

Nogier went on to publish what he called the Vascular Autonomic Signal, a distinct change in the amplitude of the pulse, easily felt with the tip of the thumb at the radial artery. This mechanism, Nogier said, would only produce a signal upon the introduction of new information to the patient's electromagnetic field. He was now working with the principle of matching resonance. He then said that he could use this signal to detect which points on the ear microsystem were active.

Mapping the Ear

The Chinese ear map, developed from the original discoveries of Nogier, is a map of points. Some of these points differ from Nogier's original map.

The developments made in Germany primarily by Frank Bahr and Beate Stritmatter have found the points on the ear to be consistently in the same location, regardless of the level of chronicity. German Auricular Medicine has developed into a system using frequencies to assess and treat conditions specifically. This form of the medicine has integrated the Chinese meridian system and has mapped each one on the ear. The use of low-level laser has been recently more widely used in the German form. Until 2002, the training in this form of the medicine was exclusively available to M.D.'s in Germany. Muriel Agnes of Vital Principle Institute in Nova Scotia brought Stritmatter to Canada in 2002 to train English-speaking massage therapists, homeopaths, and acupuncturists.

Effectiveness

Alternative medicine practitioners sometimes recommend auriculotherapy for treating insomnia, but there is no evidence it works. On the other hand no reports of harmful effects are known.

Qigong

Qigong, qi gong, chi kung, or chi gung (simplified Chinese: 气功; traditional Chinese: 氣功; pinyin: *qìgōng*; Wade–Giles: *chi gong*; literally: "Life Energy Cultivation") is a holistic system of coordinated body posture and movement, breathing, and meditation used for health, spirituality, and martial arts training. With roots in Chinese medicine, philosophy, and martial arts, qigong is traditionally viewed as a practice to cultivate and balance qi (chi), translated as "life energy".

According to Taoist, Buddhist, and Confucian philosophy, qigong allows access to higher realms of awareness, awakens one's "true nature", and helps develop human potential.

Qigong practice typically involves moving meditation, coordinating slow flowing movement, deep rhythmic breathing, and calm meditative state of mind. Qigong is now practiced throughout China and worldwide for recreation, exercise and relaxation, preventive medicine and self-healing, alternative medicine, meditation and self-cultivation, and training for martial arts.

Over the centuries, a diverse spectrum of qigong forms developed in different segments of Chinese society. Traditionally, qigong training has been esoteric and secretive, with knowledge passed from adept master to student in lineages that maintain their own unique interpretations and methods. Qigong practices were brought to the public beginning in the 1950s, when the Communist Party institutionalized and began research into traditional Chinese medicine. Although the practice of qigong was prohibited during the Cultural Revolution of the 1960s; it was once again allowed after 1976. On account of the political climate at the time, the emphasis of qigong practices shifted away from traditional philosophy and cultivation, and increasingly focused health benefits, medicine and martial arts applications, and a scientific perspective. Since a 1999 crackdown, practice of qigong in China has been restricted. Over the same period, interest in qigong has spread, with millions of practitioners worldwide.

Research concerning qigong has been conducted for a wide range of medical conditions, including hypertension, pain, and cancer treatment. Most systematic reviews of clinical trials have not been conclusive, and all have been based on poor quality clinical studies, such that no firm conclusions about the health effects of qigong can be drawn at this stage.

Etymology

Qigong (Pinyin), ch'i kung (Wade-Giles), and chi gung (Yale) are English words for two Chinese characters: *qì* (氣) and *gōng* (功).

Qi (or *chi*) is often translated as life energy, referring to energy circulating through the body; though a more general definition is universal energy, including heat, light, and electromagnetic energy; and definitions often involve breath, air, gas, or relationship between matter, energy, and spirit. Qi is the central underlying principle in traditional Chinese medicine and martial arts. *Gong* (or *kung*) is often translated as cultivation or work, and definitions include practice, skill, mastery, merit, achievement, service, result, or accomplishment, and is often used to mean gongfu (kung fu) in the traditional sense of achievement through great effort. The two words are combined to describe systems to cultivate and balance life energy, especially for health.

Although the term qigong (氣功) has been traced back to Daoist literature of the early Tang Dynasty (618-907 AD), the term *qigong* as currently used was promoted in the late 1940s through the 1950s to refer to a broad range of Chinese self-cultivation exercises, and to emphasize health and scientific approaches, while de-emphasizing spiritual practices, mysticism, and elite lineages.

History and Origins

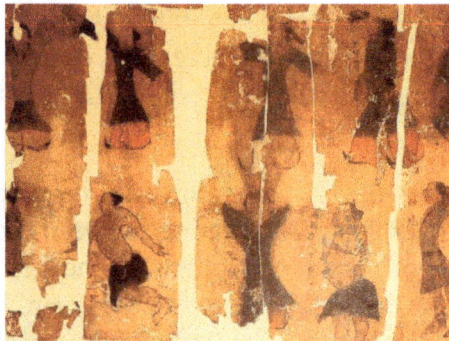

The physical exercise chart; a painting on silk depicting the practice of Qigong Taiji; unearthed in 1973 in Hunan Province, China, from the 2nd-century BC Western Han burial site of Mawangdui Han tombs site, Tomb Number 3.

With roots in ancient Chinese culture dating back more than 4,000 years, a wide variety of qigong forms have developed within different segments of Chinese society: in traditional Chinese medicine for preventive and curative functions, in Confucianism to promote longevity and improve moral character, in Daoism and Buddhism as part of meditative practice, and in Chinese martial arts to enhance fighting abilities. Contemporary qigong blends diverse and sometimes disparate traditions, in particular the Daoist meditative practice of "internal alchemy" (Neidan 內丹术), the ancient meditative practices of "circulating qi" (Xing qi 行氣) and "standing meditation" (Zhan zhuang 站桩), and the slow gymnastic breathing exercise of "guiding and pulling" (Dao yin 導引). Traditionally, knowledge about qigong was passed from adept master to student in elite unbroken lineages, typically with secretive and esoteric traditions of training and oral transmission, and with an emphasis on meditative practice by scholars and gymnastic or dynamic practice by the working masses.

Starting in the late 1940s and the 1950s, the mainland Chinese government tried to integrate disparate qigong approaches into one coherent system, with the intention of establishing a firm scientific basis for qigong practice. In 1949, Liu Guizhen established the name "Qigong" to refer to the system of life preserving practices that he and his associates developed based on Dao yin and other philosophical traditions. This attempt is considered by some sinologists as the start of the modern or scientific interpretation of qigong. During the Great Leap Forward (1958–1963) and the Cultural Revolution (1966–1976), qigong, along with other traditional Chinese medicine, was under tight control with limited access among the general public, but was encouraged in state-run rehabilitation centers and spread to universities and hospitals. After the Cultural Revolution, qigong, along with t'ai chi, was popularized as daily morning exercise practiced en masse throughout China.

Popularity of qigong grew rapidly during the Deng and Jiang eras after Mao Zedong's death in 1976 through the 1990s, with estimates of between 60 and 200 million practitioners throughout China. Along with popularity and state sanction came controversy and problems: claims of extraordinary abilities bordering on the supernatural, pseudoscience explanations to build credibility, a mental condition labeled qigong deviation, formation of cults, and exaggeration of claims by masters for personal benefit. In 1985, the state-run "National Qigong Science and Research Organization" was established to regulate the nation's qigong denominations. In 1999, in response to widespread revival of old traditions of spirituality, morality, and mysticism, and perceived challenges to State control, the Chinese government took measures to enforce control of public qigong practice, including shutting down qigong clinics and hospitals, and banning groups such as Zhong Gong and Falun Gong. Since the 1999 crackdown, qigong research and practice have only been officially supported in the context of health and traditional Chinese medicine. The Chinese Health Qigong Association, established in 2000, strictly regulates public qigong practice, with limitation of public gatherings, requirement of state approved training and certification of instructors, and restriction of practice to state-approved forms.

Through the forces of migration of the Chinese diaspora, tourism in China, and globalization, the practice of qigong spread from the Chinese community to the world. Today, millions of people around the world practice qigong and believe in the benefits of qigong to varying degrees. Similar to its historical origin, those interested in qigong come from diverse backgrounds and practice it for different reasons, including for recreation, exercise, relaxation, preventive medicine, self-healing, alternative medicine, self-cultivation, meditation, spirituality, and martial arts training.

Overview

Practices

Qigong comprises a diverse set of practices that coordinate body (調身), breath (調息), and mind (調心) based on Chinese philosophy. Practices include moving and still meditation, massage, chanting, sound meditation, and non-contact treatments, performed in a broad array of body postures. Qigong is commonly classified into two foundational categories: 1) dynamic or active qigong (dong gong), with slow flowing movement; and 2) meditative or passive qigong (jing gong), with still positions and inner movement of the breath. From a therapeutic perspective, qigong can be classified into two systems: 1) internal qigong, which focuses on self-care and self-cultivation, and; 2) external qigong, which involves treatment by a therapist who directs or transmits qi.

As moving meditation, qigong practice typically coordinates slow stylized movement, deep diaphragmatic breathing, and calm mental focus, with visualization of guiding qi through the body. While implementation details vary, generally qigong forms can be characterized as a mix of four types of practice: dynamic, static, meditative, and activities requiring external aids.

- Dynamic practice

    involves fluid movement, usually carefully choreographed, coordinated with breath and awareness. Examples include the slow stylized movements of T'ai chi ch'uan, Baguazhang, and Xing yi. Other examples include graceful movement that mimics the motion of animals in Five Animals (Wu Qin Xi qigong), White Crane, and Wild Goose (Dayan) Qigong. As a form of gentle exercise, qigong is composed of movements that are typically repeated, strengthening and stretching the body, increasing fluid movement (blood, synovial, and lymph), enhancing balance and proprioception, and improving the awareness of how the body moves through space.

- Static practice

    involves holding postures for sustained periods of time. In some cases this bears resemblance to the practice of Yoga and its continuation in the Buddhist tradition. For example Yiquan, a Chinese martial art derived from xingyiquan, emphasizes static stance training. In another example, the healing form Eight Pieces of Brocade (Baduanjin qigong) is based on a series of static postures.

- Meditative practice

    utilizes breath awareness, visualization, mantra, chanting, sound, and focus on philosophical concepts such as qi circulation, aesthetics, or moral values. In traditional Chinese medicine and Daoist practice, the meditative focus is commonly on cultivating qi in dantian energy centers and balancing qi flow in meridian and other pathways. In various Buddhist traditions, the aim is to still the mind, either through outward focus, for example on a place, or through inward focus on the breath, a mantra, a koan, emptiness, or the idea of the eternal. In the Confucius scholar tradition, meditation is focused on humanity and virtue, with the aim of self-enlightenment.

- Use of external agents

  Many systems of qigong practice include the use of external agents such as ingestion of herbs, massage, physical manipulation, or interaction with other living organisms. For example, specialized food and drinks are used in some medical and Daoist forms, whereas massage and body manipulation are sometimes used in martial arts forms. In some medical systems a qigong master uses non-contact treatment, purportedly guiding qi through his or her own body into the body of another person.

Forms

There are numerous qigong forms. 75 ancient forms that can be found in ancient literature and also 56 common or contemporary forms have been described in a qigong compendium. The list is by no means exhaustive. Many contemporary forms were developed by people who had recovered from their illness after qigong practice.

In 2003, the Chinese Health Qigong Association officially recognized four health qigong forms:

- Muscle-Tendon Change Classic (Yì Jīn Jīng 易筋经).

- Five Animals (Wu Qin Xi 五禽戲).

- Six Healing Sounds (Liu Zi Jue 六字訣).

- Eight Pieces of Brocade (Ba Duan Jin 八段錦).

In 2010, the Chinese Health Qigong Association officially recognized five additional health qigong forms:

- Tai Chi Yang Sheng Zhang (太极养生杖): a tai chi form from the stick tradition.

- Shi Er Duan Jin (十二段锦): seated exercises to strengthen the neck, shoulders, waist, and legs.

- Daoyin Yang Sheng Gong Shi Er Fa (导引养生功十二法): 12 routines from Daoyin tradition of guiding and pulling qi.

- Mawangdui Daoyin (马王堆导引术): guiding qi along the meridians with synchronous movement and awareness.

- Da Wu (大舞): choreographed exercises to lubricate joints and guide qi.

Other commonly practiced qigong styles and forms include:

- Soaring Crane Qigong

- Wisdom Healing Qigong

- Pan Gu Mystical Qigong

- Wild Goose (Dayan) Qigong

- Dragon and Tiger Qigong

- Primordial Qigong (Wujigong)

Techniques

Whether viewed from the perspective of exercise, health, philosophy, or martial arts training, several main principles emerge concerning the practice of qigong:

- Intentional movement: careful, flowing balanced style

- Rhythmic breathing: slow, deep, coordinated with fluid movement

- Awareness: calm, focused meditative state

- Visualization: of qi flow, philosophical tenets, aesthetics

- Chanting/Sound: use of sound as a focal point

Additional principles:

- Softness: soft gaze, expressionless face

- Solid Stance: firm footing, erect spine

- Relaxation: relaxed muscles, slightly bent joints

- Balance and Counterbalance: motion over the center of gravity

Advanced goals:

- Equanimity: more fluid, more relaxed

- Tranquility: empty mind, high awareness

- Stillness: smaller and smaller movements, eventually to complete stillness

The most advanced practice is generally considered to be with little or no motion.

Traditional and Classical Theory

Over time, five distinct traditions or schools of qigong developed in China, each with its own theories and characteristics: Chinese Medical Qigong, Daoist Qigong, Buddhist Qigong, Confucian Qigong, and martial arts qigong. All of these qigong traditions include practices intended to cultivate and balance qi.

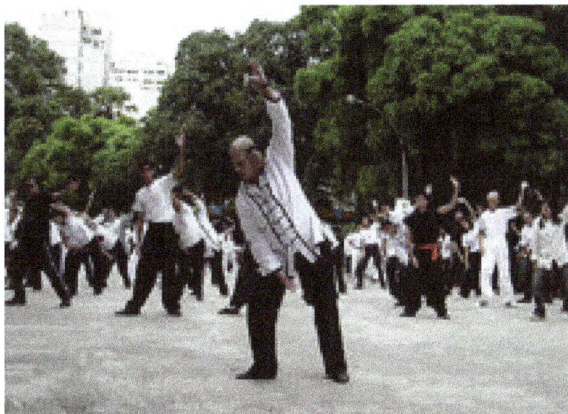

Qigong practitioners in Brazil

Traditional Chinese Medicine

The theories of ancient Chinese Medical Qigong include the Yin-Yang and Five Phases Theory, Essence-Qi-Spirit Theory, Zang-Xiang Theory, and Meridians and Qi-Blood Theory, which have been synthesized as part of Traditional Chinese Medicine (TCM).[45-57] TCM focuses on tracing and correcting underlying disharmony, in terms of deficiency and excess, using the complementary and opposing forces of yin and yang (陰陽), to create a balanced flow of qi. Qi is believed to be cultivated and stored in three main dantian energy centers and to travel through the body along twelve main meridians (Jīng Luò 經絡), with numerous smaller branches and tributaries. The main meridians correspond to twelve main organs (Zàng fǔ 臟腑)). Qi is balanced in terms of yin and yang in the context of the traditional system of Five Phases (Wu xing 五行). A person is believed to become ill or die when qi becomes diminished or unbalanced. Health is believed to be returned by rebuilding qi, eliminating qi blockages, and correcting qi imbalances. These TCM concepts do not translate readily to modern science and medicine.

Daoism

In Daoism various practices now known as Daoist Qigong are claimed to provide a way to achieve longevity and spiritual enlightenment, as well as a closer connection with the natural world.

Buddhism

In Buddhism meditative practices now known as Buddhist Qigong are part of a spiritual path that leads to spiritual enlightenment or Buddhahood.

Confucianism

In Confucianism practices now known as Confucian Qigong provide a means to become a Junzi (君子) through awareness of morality.

Contemporary Qigong

In contemporary China, the emphasis of qigong practice has shifted away from traditional philosophy, spiritual attainment, and folklore, and increasingly to health benefits, traditional medicine and martial arts applications, and a scientific perspective. Qigong is now practiced by millions worldwide, primarily for its health benefits, though many practitioners have also adopted traditional philosophical, medical, or martial arts perspectives, and even use the long history of qigong as evidence of its effectiveness.

Contemporary Chinese Medical Qigong

Qigong has been recognized as a "standard medical technique" in China since 1989, and is sometimes included in the medical curriculum of major universities in China. The 2013 English translation of the official Chinese Medical Qigong textbook used in China defines CMQ as "the skill of body-mind exercise that integrates body, breath, and mind adjustments into one" and emphasizes that qigong is based on "adjustment" (tiao 調, also translated as "regulation", "tuning", or "alignment.") of body, breath, and mind. As such, qigong is viewed by practitioners as being more than common physical exercise, because qigong combines postural, breathing, and mental training in one to produce a particular psychophysiological state of being.[15] While CMQ is still based on traditional and classical theory, modern practitioners also emphasize the importance of a strong scientific basis. According to the 2013 CMQ textbook, physiological effects of qigong are numerous, and include improvement of respiratory and cardiovascular function, as well as possible beneficial effects on neurophysiology.

Conventional Medicine

Conventional or mainstream medicine includes specific practices and techniques based on the best available evidence demonstrating effectiveness and safety. Qigong is not generally considered to be part of mainstream medicine because clinical research concerning effectiveness of qigong for specific medical conditions is inconclusive at this stage, and because at present there is no medical consensus concerning effectiveness of qigong.

Integrative, Complementary, and Alternative Medicine

Integrative medicine (IM) refers to "the blending of conventional and complementary medicines and therapies with the aim of using the most appropriate of either or both modalities to care for the patient as a whole", whereas complementary generally refers to "using a non-mainstream approach together with conventional medicine", and alternative refers to "using a non-mainstream approach in place of conventional medicine". Qigong is used by integrative medicine practitioners to complement conventional medical treatment, based on complementary and alternative medicine (CAM) interpretations of the effectiveness and safety of qigong.

Scientific Basis

Scientists interested in qigong have sought to describe or verify the effects of qigong, to explore mechanisms of effects, to form scientific theory with respect to Qigong, and to identify appropriate research methodology for further study. In terms of traditional theory, the existence of qi has not been independently verified in an experimental setting, and the scientific basis for much of TCM and CAM has not been demonstrated.

Health Applications

Recreation and Popular Use

People practice qigong for many different reasons, including for recreation, exercise and relaxation, preventive medicine and self-healing, meditation and self-cultivation, and training for martial arts. In recent years a large number of books and videos have been published that focus primarily on qigong as exercise and associated health benefits. Practitioners range from athletes to the physically challenged. Because it is low impact and can be done lying, sitting, or standing, qigong is accessible for disabled persons, seniors, and people recovering from injuries.

Therapeutic Use

Therapeutic use of qigong is directed by TCM, CAM, integrative medicine, and other health practitioners. In China, where it is considered a "standard medical technique",[34] qigong is commonly prescribed to treat a wide variety of conditions, and clinical applications include hypertension, coronary artery disease, peptic ulcers, chronic liver diseases, diabetes mellitus, obesity, menopause syndrome, chronic fatigue syndrome, insomnia, tumors and cancer, lower back and leg pain, cervical spondylosis, and myopia. Outside China qigong is used in integrative medicine to complement or supplement accepted medical treatments, including for relaxation, fitness, rehabilitation, and treatment of specific conditions.

Effectiveness

Based on systematic reviews of clinical research, it is not advisable to draw conclusions concerning effectiveness of qigong for specific medical conditions at this stage.

Safety and cost

Qigong is generally viewed as safe. No adverse effects have been observed in clinical trials, such that qigong is considered safe for use across diverse populations. Cost for self-care is minimal, and cost efficiencies are high for group delivered care. Typically the cautions associated with qigong are the same as those associated with any physical activity, including risk of muscle strains or sprains, advisability of stretching to prevent injury, general safety for use alongside conventional medical treatments, and consulting with a physician when combining with conventional treatment.

Research

Overview of Clinical Research

Although clinical research examining health effects of qigong is increasing, there is little financial or medical incentive to support research, and still only a limited number of studies meet accepted medical and scientific standards of randomized controlled trials (RCTs). Clinical research concerning qigong has been conducted for a wide range of medical conditions, including bone density, cardiopulmonary effects, physical function, falls and related risk factors, quality of life, immune function, inflammation, hypertension, pain, and cancer treatment. A 2011 overview of systematic reviews of clinical trials concluded that "the effectiveness of qigong is based mostly on poor quality research" and "therefore, it would be unwise to draw firm conclusions at this stage". Although a 2010 comprehensive literature review found 77 peer-reviewed RCTs; systematic reviews for particular health conditions show that most clinical research is of poor quality, typically because of small sample size and lack of proper control groups, with lack of blinding associated with high risk of bias.

Systematic Reviews of Clinical Research

A systematic review of the effect of qigong exercises on hypertension found that the available studies were encouraging for the exercises to lower systolic blood pressure. However, an analysis of the studies that found these results showed that they were of relatively poor quality, with the lack of blinding raising the possibility of bias in the results, so no definitive conclusions could be reached. Another systematic review found that qigong exercises improved blood pressure compared to doing nothing, but was not superior to standard treatment such as medications or conventional exercise.

A 2007 systematic review of the effect of qigong exercises on diabetes mellitus management concluded that there may be beneficial effects, but that no firm conclusions could be drawn due to the methodological problems with the underlying clinical trials studies, especially the lack of a control group. A more recent 2009 systematic review found that due to the underlying methodological problems, "the evidence is insufficient to suggest that qigong is an effective treatment for type 2 diabetes".

A systematic review on the effect of qigong exercises on reducing pain concluded that "the existing trial evidence is not convincing enough to suggest that internal qigong is an effective modality for pain management." Another systematic review, which focused on external qigong and its effect on pain, concluded "that evidence for the effectiveness of external qigong is encouraging, though further studies are warranted" due to the small number of studies and participants involved which precluded any firm conclusions about the specific effects of qigong on pain.

A systematic review of the effect of qigong exercises on cancer treatment concluded "the effectiveness of qigong in cancer care is not yet supported by the evidence from rigorous clinical trials." A separate systematic review that looked at the effects of qigong exercises on various physiological or psychological outcomes found that the available studies were poorly designed, with a high of bias in the results. Therefore, the authors concluded, "Due to limited number of RCTs in the field and methodological problems and high risk of bias in the included studies, it is still too early to reach a conclusion about the efficacy and the effectiveness of qigong exercise as a form of health practice adopted by the cancer patients during their curative, palliative, and rehabilitative phases of the cancer journey."

A systematic review of the effect of qigong exercises on movement disorders found that the evidence was insufficient to recommend its use for this purpose.

Mental Health Research

Many claims have been made that qigong can benefit or ameliorate mental health conditions, including improved mood, decreased stress reaction, and decreased anxiety and depression. Most medical studies have only examined psychological factors as secondary goals, although various studies have shown significant benefits such as decrease in cortisol levels, a chemical hormone produced by the body in response to stress.

Research in China

Basic and clinical research in China during the 1980s was mostly descriptive, and few results were reported in peer-reviewed English-language journals. A 1996 review of selected Chinese research concluded that there are many potential medical applications of qigong. Qigong became known outside China in the 1990s, and clinical randomized controlled trials (RTCs) investigating the effectiveness of qigong on health and mental conditions began to be published worldwide, along with systematic reviews.

Challenges for Research

The White House Commission on Complementary and Alternative Medicine (CAM) Policy recognized challenges and complexities to rigorous research concerning effectiveness and safety of CAM therapies such as qigong; emphasized that research must adhere to the same standards as conventional research, including statistically significant sample sizes, adequate controls, definition of response specificity, and reproducibility of results; and recommended substantial increases in funding to for rigorous research. Most existing clinical trials have small sample sizes and many have inadequate controls. Of particular concern is the impracticality of double blinding using appropriate sham treatments, and the difficulty of placebo control, such that benefits often cannot be distinguished from the placebo effect. Also of concern is the choice of which qigong form to use and how to standardize the treatment or dose with respect to the skill of the practitioner leading or administering treatment, the tradition of individualization of treatments, and the treatment length, intensity, and frequency.

Meditation and Self-cultivation Applications

Qigong is practiced for meditation and self-cultivation as part of various philosophical and spiritual traditions. As meditation, qigong is a means to still the mind and enter a state of consciousness that brings serenity, clarity, and bliss. Many practitioners find qigong, with its gentle focused movement, to be more accessible than seated meditation.

Qigong for self-cultivation can be classified in terms of traditional Chinese philosophy: Daoist, Buddhist, and Confucian.

Martial Arts Applications

The practice of qigong is an important component in both internal and external style Chinese martial arts. Focus on qi is considered to be a source of power as well as the foundation of the internal style of martial arts (Neijia). T'ai chi ch'uan, Xing yi, and Baguazhang are representative of the types of Chinese martial arts that rely on the concept of qi as the foundation. Extraordinary feats of martial arts prowess, such as the ability to withstand heavy strikes (Iron Shirt, 鐵衫) and the ability to break hard objects (Iron Palm, 铁掌) are abilities attributed to qigong training.

T'ai Chi Ch'uan and Qigong

T'ai chi ch'uan (Taijiquan) is a widely practiced Chinese internal martial style based on the theory of taiji ("grand ultimate"), closely associated with qigong, and typically involving more complex choreographed movement coordinated with breath, done slowly for health and training, or quickly for self-defense. Many scholars consider t'ai chi ch'uan to be a type of qigong, traced back to an origin in the seventeenth century. In modern practice, qigong typically focuses more on health and meditation rather than martial applications, and plays an important role in training for t'ai chi ch'uan, in particular used to build strength, develop breath control, and increase vitality ("life energy").

Tui Na

Tui na or tuina (/ˌtwiː ˈnɑː/, Chinese: 推拿; pinyin: *tuī ná*), is a form of Chinese manipulative therapy often used in conjunction with acupuncture, moxibustion, fire cupping, Chinese herbalism, t'ai chi, and qigong. Tui na is a hands-on body treatment that uses Chinese taoist principles in an effort to bring the eight principles of Traditional Chinese

Medicine (TCM) into balance. The practitioner may brush, knead, roll, press, and rub the areas between each of the joints, known as the eight gates, to attempt to open the body's defensive chi (Wei Qi) and get the energy moving in the meridians and the muscles. Techniques may be gentle or quite firm. The name comes from two of the actions: *tui* means "to push" and *na* means "to lift and squeeze." Other strokes include shaking and tapotement. The practitioner can then use range of motion, traction, with the stimulation of acupressure points. These techniques are claimed to aid in the treatment of both acute and chronic musculoskeletal conditions, as well as many non-musculoskeletal conditions. As with many other traditional Chinese medical practices, there are different schools which vary in their approach to the discipline. It is related also to Japanese massage or *anma* (按摩).

In ancient China, medical therapy was often classified as either "external" or "internal" treatment. Tui na was one of the external methods, thought to be especially suitable for use on the elderly population and on infants. In modern China, many hospitals include tui na as a standard aspect of treatment, with specialization for infants, adults, orthopedics, traumatology, cosmetology, rehabilitation, and sports medicine. In the West, tui na is taught as a part of the curriculum at some acupuncture schools.

- Tui na treatment

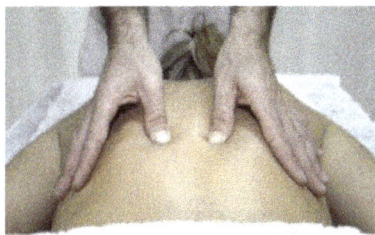

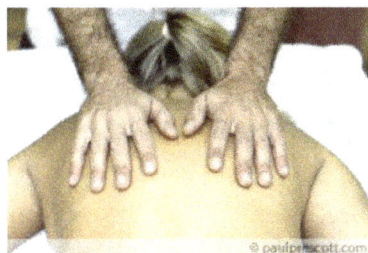

Moxibustion

Moxibustion (Chinese: 灸; pinyin: *jiǔ*) is a traditional Chinese medicine therapy which consists of burning dried mugwort (*moxa*) on particular points on the body. It plays an important role in the traditional medical systems of China (including Tibet), Japan, Korea, Vietnam, and Mongolia. Suppliers usually age the mugwort and grind it up to a fluff; practitioners burn the fluff or process it further into a cigar-shaped stick. They can use it indirectly, with acupuncture needles, or burn it on the patient's skin.

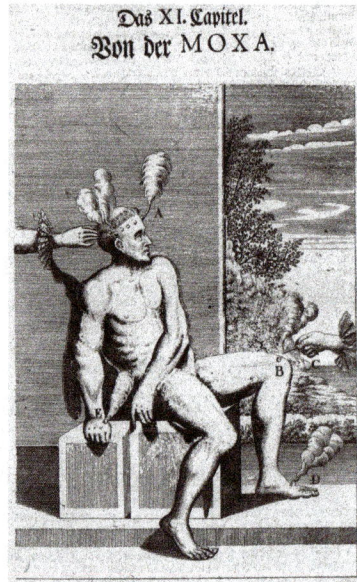

Moxibustion in Michael Bernhard Valentini's *Museum Museorum* (Frankfurt am Main, 1714)

Terminology

The first Western remarks on moxibustion can be found in letters and reports written by Portuguese missionaries in 16th-century Japan. They called it "botão de fogo" (fire button), a term originally used for round-headed Western cautery irons. Hermann Buschoff, who published the first Western book on this matter in 1674 (English edition 1676), used the Japanese word *mogusa*. As the u is not very strongly enunciated, he spelled it "Moxa". Later authors blended "Moxa" with the Latin word combustio (burning).

The name of the herb Artemisia (mugwort) species used to produce Moxa is *yomogi* (蓬) in Japan and *ài* or *àicǎo* (艾, 艾草) in Chinese.

The Chinese names for moxibustion are *jiǔ* (灸) or *jiǔshù* (灸術); Japanese use the same characters and pronounce them as *kyū* and *kyūjutsu*. In Korean the reading is *tteum* (뜸). Korean folklore attributes the development of moxibustion to the legendary emperor Dangun.

Theory and Practice

Practitioners use moxa to warm regions and meridian points with the intention of stimulating circulation through the points and inducing a smoother flow of blood and qi. Some believe it can treat conditions associated with the "cold" or "yang deficiencies" in Chinese Medicine. It is claimed that moxibustion mitigates against cold and dampness in the body, and can serve to turn breech babies.

Practitioners claim moxibustion to be especially effective in the treatment of chronic problems, "deficient conditions" (weakness), and gerontology. Bian Que (*fl. circa* 500 BCE), one of the most famous semi-legendary doctors of Chinese antiquity and the first specialist in moxibustion, discussed the benefits of moxa over acupuncture in his classic work *Bian Que Neijing*. He asserted that moxa could add new energy to the body and could treat both excess and deficient conditions.

Practitioners may use acupuncture needles made of various materials in combination with moxa, depending on the direction of *qi* flow they wish to stimulate.

There are several methods of moxibustion. Three of them are direct scarring, direct non-scarring, and indirect moxibustion. Direct scarring moxibustion places a small cone of moxa on the skin at an acupuncture point and burns it until the skin blisters, which then scars after it heals. Direct non-scarring moxibustion removes the burning moxa before the skin burns enough to scar, unless the burning moxa is left on the skin too long. Indirect moxibustion holds a cigar made of moxa near the acupuncture point to heat the skin, or holds it on an acupuncture needle inserted in the skin to heat the needle. There is also stick-on moxa.

Medical Research

The first modern scientific publication on moxibustion was written by the Japanese physician Hara Shimetarō who conducted intensive research about the hematological effects of moxibustion in 1927. Two years later his doctoral dissertation on that matter was accepted by the Medical Faculty of the Kyūshū Imperial University. Hara's last publication appeared in 1981.

A Cochrane Review found limited evidence for the use of moxibustion in correcting breech presentation of babies, and called for more experimental trials. Moxibustion has also been studied for the treatment of pain, cancer, stroke, ulcerative colitis, constipation, and hypertension. Systematic reviews have found that these studies are of low quality and positive findings could be due to publication bias.

Parallel Uses of Mugwort

Mugwort amongst other herbs was often bound into smudge sticks. The Chumash people from southern California have a similar ritual. Europeans placed sprigs of mugwort under pillows to provoke dreams; and the herb had associations with the practice of magic in Anglo-Saxon times.

References

- Russell J; Rovere A, eds. (2009). "Cupping". American Cancer Society Complete Guide to Complementary and Alternative Cancer Therapies (2nd ed.). American Cancer Society. pp. 189–191. ISBN 9780944235713.

- Cohen, K. S. (1999). The Way of Qigong: The Art and Science of Chinese Energy Healing. Random House of Canada. ISBN 0-345-42109-4.

- Liang, Shou-Yu; Wu, Wen-Ching; Breiter-Wu, Denise (1997). Qigong Empowerment: A Guide to Medical, Taoist, Buddhist, and Wushu Energy Cultivation. Way of the Dragon Pub. ISBN 1-889659-02-9.

- Ho, Peng Yoke (Oct 2000). Li, Qi, and Shu: An Introduction to Science and Civilization in China. Dover Publications. ISBN 0-486-41445-0.

- Yang, Jwing-Ming. (1989). The root of Chinese Chi kung: the secrets of Chi kung training. Yang's Martial Arts Association. ISBN 0-940871-07-6.

- Holland, Alex (2000). Voices of Qi: An Introductory Guide to Traditional Chinese Medicine. North Atlantic Books. ISBN 1-55643-326-3.

- Yang, Jwing-Ming (1998). Qigong for health and martial arts: exercises and meditation. YMAA Publication Center. ISBN 1-886969-57-4.

- Chen, Nancy N. (2003). Breathing Spaces: Qigong, Psychiatry, and Healing in China. Columbia University Press. ISBN 0-231-12804-5.

- Wanjek, Christopher (2003). Bad medicine: misconceptions and misuses revealed, from distance healing to vitamin O. John Wiley and Sons. pp. 182–187. ISBN 0-471-43499-X.

- Scheid, Volker (2002). Chinese medicine in contemporary China: plurality and synthesis. Durham, NC: Duke University Press. ISBN 0-8223-2872-0.

- Zhang, Hong-Chao (2000). Wild Goose Qigong: Natural Movement for Healthy Living. YMAA Publication Center. ISBN 978-1-886969-78-0.

- Connor, Danny; Tse, Michael (1992). Qigong: Chinese movement meditation for health. York Beach, Me.: S. Weiser. ISBN 978-0-87728-758-2.

- Frantzis, Bruce Kumar (2008). The Chi Revolution: Harnessing the Healing Power of Your Life Force. Blue Snake Books. ISBN 1-58394-193-2.

- Diepersloot, Ja (2000). The Tao of Yiquan: The Method of Awareness in the Martial Arts. Center For Healing & The Arts. ISBN 0-9649976-1-4.

- Dong, Paul; Raffill, Thomas. Empty Force: The Power of Chi for Self-Defense and Energy Healing. Blue Snake Books/Frog, Ltd. ISBN 978-1-58394-134-8.

Anatomical Perspective of Traditional Chinese Medicine

This chapter explains to the reader the significance of the body in traditional Chinese medicine. Qi, meridian, zang-fu and other principles are the functional entities used by the Chinese tradition. Such methods of treatment evolved much before the Enlightenment and scientific medical practice and are still practiced in many parts of the world.

The Body in Traditional Chinese Medicine

The model of the body in traditional Chinese medicine (TCM) has the following elements:

- the Fundamental Substances;
- Qi, Blood, Jing (Essence), Shen (Mind) that nourish and protect the Zang-Fu organs;
- and the meridians (*jing-luo*) which connect and unify the body.

Every diagnosis is a "Pattern of disharmony" that affects one or more organs, such as "Spleen Qi Deficiency" or "Liver Fire Blazing" or "Invasion of the Stomach by Cold", and every treatment is centered on correcting the disharmony.

The traditional Chinese model is concerned with function. Thus, the TCM Spleen is not a specific piece of flesh, but an aspect of function related to transformation and transportation within the body, and of the mental functions of thinking and studying. Indeed, the San Jiao or Triple Burner has no anatomical correspondent at all, and is said to be completely a functional entity.

Chinese Medicine and The Model of the Body is founded on the balance of the five elements: Earth, Metal, Water, Wood, and Fire.

The elements are infinitely linked, consuming and influencing each other.

Each element corresponds to different organs in the body.

The organs act as representatives of the qualities of different elements, which impact the physical and mental body in respective ways.

Each organ is categorized as either Yin or Yang.

The energies of Yin and Yang are conflicting yet inter-reliant.

When the two(Yin+Yang) forces are united they create a divine energy, which supports the flow of all life.

Yin organs represent femininity, coldness, compression, darkness, and submission.

Yang organs represent masculinity, expansion, heat, motion, and action.

This duality must be in balance or else disease of the mind and body will occur.

Each organ governs energy channels, which distribute chi and connect all parts of the body to one another. These channels are called meridians.

Wood

Wood is an element of growth, originality, creativity, and evolution.

The Liver(1) and the Gallbladder(2) are the two wood governed organs in the body.

(1) The Liver, a Yin organ, influences emotional flexibility and the flow of energy on a cellular level.

The organ has a strong impact on the efficiency and effectiveness of the immune system along with storing the body's blood, a physical manifestation of one's true self.

The Liver rules one's direction, vision, sense of self-purpose and opens into the eyes.

Last, the Liver absorbs what is not digested and regulates blood sugar. Imbalance in the Liver can lead to great problems.

Moodiness, anger, pain, poor self-esteem, lack of direction, addiction, and indecision are all associated with the Liver organ.

Muscle spasms, numbness, tremors, eye diseases, hypertension, allergies, arthritis, and multiple sclerosis are also a result of Liver imbalances.

The Liver Meridian begins on the big toe, runs along the inner leg through the genitals and ends on the chest.

(2) The Gallbladder, a wood controlled Yang organ, governs decisiveness.

The Gallbladder also stores bile. Imbalance of the Gallbladder can lead to indecisiveness along with obesity.

The Gallbladder meridian begins at the outer edge of the eye, moves to the side of the head and trunk, and ends on the outside of the fourth toe.

Fire

Fire is an element of transformation, demolition, primal power, and divinity.

(1) The Heart, (2) Small Intestine, (3) Heart Protector, and (4) Triple Heater are the organs that fire controls.

(1) The Heart, a Yin organ, regulates the pulse, manifests in the face and tongue, and bridges the connection between the human and the celestial.

Dysfunction of the Heart leads to insomnia, disturbance of the spirit, and an irregular pulse.

The Heart Meridian begins in the chest moves to the inner aspect of the arm down to the palm of the hand and ends on the pinky.

(2) The Small Intestine, a Yang organ, separates pure food and fluid essences from the polluted.

The pure essences are distributed to the spleen while the polluted are sent to the bladder and the large intestine.

Dysfunction of the Small Intestine can lead to bowl problems and a sense of distrust of one's self.

The Small Intestine Meridian begins on the pinky, moves to the underside of the arm, up to the top of the shoulder blade, the neck, and ends on the front of the ear.

(3) The Heart Protector, a Yin organ, shields the heart. It filters psychic inclinations and stabilizes emotions.

A problem with the Heart Protector can lead to anxiety and heart palpitations.

The Heart Protector Meridian begins on the chest, travels through the armpit to the arm and ends on the top of the middle finger.

(4)The Triple Heater, a Yang organ, disperses fluids throughout the body and regulates the relationship between all organs.

The Triple Heater Meridian begins on the ring finger, moves up the back of the arm to the side of the neck, goes around the ear and ends of the eyebrow.

Earth

Earth is an element of fertility, cultivation, femininity, and wrath.

Earth governs the Spleen (1) and the Stomach (2).

(1) The Spleen, a Yin organ, regulates digestion and the metabolism.

It also holds the flesh and organs in their proper place while directing the movement of ascending fluids and essences.

Mentally, the Spleen aids in concentration.

Imbalance of the Spleen leads to chi deficiencies, diarrhea, organ prolapses, and headaches.

The Spleen Meridian begins at the big toe, moves to the inner aspect of the leg, up to the front of the torso, and ends on the side of the trunk.

(2) The Stomach, the most active yang organ, breaks down food and controls the descending movement of chi.

Imbalance of the stomach leads to vomiting and belching.

The Stomach Meridian begins below the eye, moves down the front of the face, torso, to the outer part of the leg, and ends on the third toe.

Metal

Metal is an element of purity, treasure, and masculinity.

Metal controls the Lungs(1) and the Large Intestine(2).

(1) The Lungs, a Yin organ, draws in pure chi by inhalation and eliminates impurities by exhalation.

The lungs also disperse bodily fluids, defend the body from a cold or flu, govern the sense of smell, and open in the nose.

Dysfunction of the Lungs leads to colds, the flu, phlegm, and asthma.

The Lung Meridian begins at the chest moves to the inner arm, palm, and ends on the thumb.

(2) The Large Intestine, a Yang organ, controls the removal of waste and feces.

Imbalance in the Large Intestine leads to constipation, diarrhea and the inability to emotionally detach and let go.

The Large Intestine Meridian begins on the forefinger, moves to the back of the arm, shoulder, side of the neck, cheek, and ends beside the opposite nostril.

Water

Water is an element of life and death.

Water governs the Kidneys (1) and the Bladder (2).

(1) The Kidneys, a Yin organ, are the source of all the Yin and Yang energy in the body.

The Kidneys also govern the endocrine system, receive air from the lungs, govern bones, govern teeth, control water in the body, and store essence.

Dysfunction of the Kidneys leads to deficiencies of Yin or Yang.

It also leads to imbalanced hormones, weak bones, an impaired sex drive, and dizziness.

Water in excess leads to bipolar disorder.

Depressive episodes are characterized by Kidney Yin excess while manic episodes are characterized by Kidney Yang excess.

The Kidney Meridian begins on the sole, moves up the inner leg to the groin, up the trunk, and ends under the collarbone.

(2) The Bladder, a Yang organ, stores and removes fluid from the body by receiving Kidney chi.

Imbalance of the Bladder leads to frequent or uncontrolled urination.

The Bladder Meridian begins in the corner of the eye, moves down the back, and ends on the back of the knee.

The Bladder also has another line, which starts alongside the previous line, moves down to the outer edge of the foot and ends on the small toe.

Qi

In traditional Chinese culture, *qì* or *ch'i* (qì, also known as *khí* in Vietnamese culture, 기 or *ki* in Korean culture, *ki* in Japanese culture, хийг or ᠬᠡᠢ or *khiig* in Mongolian culture, *qi* in Filipino culture, *chi* in Malay culture, ลมปราณ or *lmprā* in Thai culture, *chi* in Indonesian culture, or *aasaat* in Burmese culture, ຊີວິດ or *sivid* in Lao culture, ឈី or *chhi* in Khmer culture and *qi* in Timorese culture) is an active principle forming part of any living thing. *Qi* literally translates as "breath", "air", or "gas", and figuratively as "material energy", "life force", or "energy flow". *Qi* is the central underlying principle in traditional Chinese medicine and martial arts.

Concepts similar to *qi* can be found in many cultures: *prana* in Hinduism (and elsewhere in Indian culture), *chi* in the Igbo religion, *pneuma* in ancient Greece, *mana* in Hawaiian culture, *lüng* in Tibetan Buddhism, *manitou* in the culture of the indigenous peoples of the Americas, *ruah* in Jewish culture, and vital energy in Western philosophy.

Some elements of the concept of *qi* can be found in the term energy when used in the context of various esoteric forms of spirituality and alternative medicine. Elements of the concept can also be found in Western popular culture, for example "The Force" in *Star Wars* and the related Jediism, a religion based on the Jedi and even in Eastern popular culture like *Dragon Ball* and *One-Punch Man*. Notions in the West of *energeia*, *élan vital*, or vitalism are purported to be similar.

Despite widespread belief in the reality of Qi, it is a non-scientific, unverifiable concept.

Linguistic Aspects

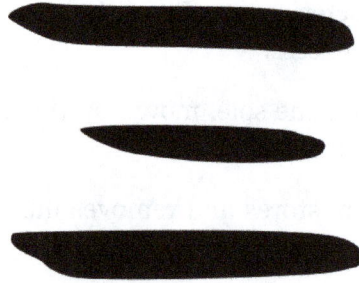

Oracle bone script for *qì* 气

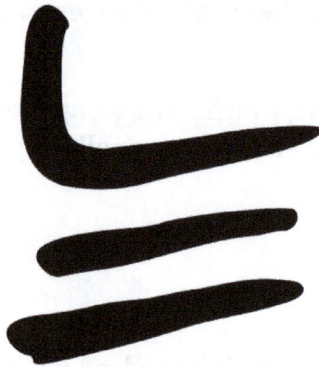

Bronzeware script for *qì* 气

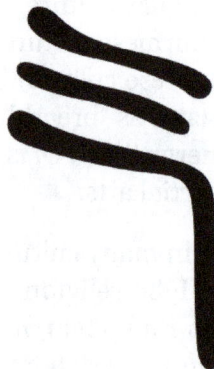

Large seal script for *qì* 气

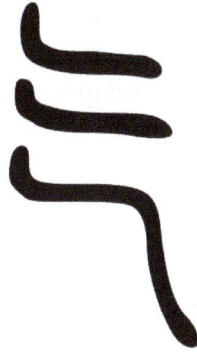

Small seal script for *qì* 气

This cultural keyword *qì* is analyzable in terms of Chinese and Sino-Xenic pronunciations, possible etymologies, the logographs 氣, 气, and 気, various meanings ranging from "vapor" to "anger", and the English loanword *qi* or *ch'i*.

Pronunciations and Etymologies

The logograph 氣 is read with two Chinese pronunciations, the usual *qì* 氣 "air; vital energy" and the rare archaic *xì* 氣 "to present food" (later disambiguated with 餼).

Pronunciations of 氣 in modern varieties of Chinese, from the infobox with standardized IPA equivalents, include: Standard Chinese *qì* /tɕʰi⁵¹/, Wu Chinese *qi* /tɕʰi³⁴/, Southern Min *khì* /kʰi²¹/, Eastern Min *ké* /kʰɛi²¹³/, Standard Cantonese *hei³* /hei̯³³/, and Hakka Chinese *hi* /hi⁵⁵/.

Pronunciations of 氣 in Sino-Xenic borrowings include: Japanese language *ki*, Korean language *gi*, and Vietnamese language *khi*.

Reconstructions of the Middle Chinese pronunciation of 氣, standardized to IPA transcription, include: /kʰei̯ᴴ/ (Bernard Karlgren), /kʰiəi̯ᴴ/ (Wang Li), /kʰiəi̯ᴴ/ (Li Rong), /kʰɨjᴴ/ (Edwin Pulleyblank), and /kʰɨiᴴ/ (Zhengzhang Shangfang).

Reconstructions of the Old Chinese pronunciation of 氣, standardized to IPA transcription, include: /*kʰɯds/ (Zhengzhang Shangfang), and /*C.qʰəp-s/ (William H. Baxter and Laurent Sagart).

The etymology of *qì* (reconstructed as Middle Chinese *kʰjeiᶜ* and Old Chinese **kə(t)s* 氣 "air; breath; vapor; vital principle", as well as its cognate *kài* (MC *kʰâiᶜ* and OC **khə ˆ(t) s*) 愾 "sigh; angry", interconnects with Kharia *kʰis* "anger", Sora *kissa* "move with great effort", Khmer *kʰɛs* "strive after; endeavor", and Gyalrongic *kʰɐs* "anger".

Characters

In East Asian languages, Chinese *qì* "air; breath" has three logographs: 氣 is the traditional Chinese character, Korean *hanja*, and Japanese *kyūjitai* "old character form" *kanji*; 気 is the Japanese *shinjitai* "new character form" *kanji*, and 气 is the simplified Chinese character. In addition, *qì* 炁 is an uncommon character especially used in writing Daoist talismans. Historically, the word *qì* was generally written as 气 until the Han dynasty (206 BCE-220 CE), when it was replaced by the 氣 graph clarified with *mǐ* 米 "rice" indicating "steam (rising from rice as it cooks)".

This primary graph 气 corresponds to the earliest written characters for *qì*, which consisted of three wavy horizontal lines seen in Shang dynasty (c. 1600–1046 BCE) oracle bone script, Zhou dynasty (1046 BCE- 256 BCE) bronzeware script and large seal script, and Qin dynasty (221-206 BCE) small seal script. These oracle, bronze, and seal scripts graphs for *qì* 气 "air; breath; etc." were anciently used as a phonetic loan character to write *qǐ* 乞 "plead for; beg; ask", which did not have an early character.

The vast majority of Chinese characters are classified as radical-phonetic characters, which combine a semantically suggestive "radical" or "signific" with a "phonetic" element approximating ancient pronunciation. For example, the widely known word *dào* 道 "the Dao; the way" graphically combines the "walk" radical 辶 with a *shǒu* 首 "head" phonetic—although the modern *dào* and *shǒu* pronunciations are dissimilar, the Old Chinese *lˤuʔ-s 道 and *l̥uʔ-s 首 were alike. The regular script character *qì* 氣 is unusual because *qì* 气 is both the "air radical" and the phonetic, with *mǐ* 米 "rice" semantically indicating "steam; vapor".

This *qì* 气 "air/gas radical", which was only used in a few native Chinese characters like *yīnyūn* 氤氲 "thick mist/smoke", was used to create new scientific characters for gaseous chemical elements. Some examples are based on pronunciations in European languages: *fú* 氟 (with a *fú* 弗 phonetic) "fluorine" and *nǎi* 氖 (with a *nǎi* 乃 phonetic) "neon"; others are based on semantics: *qīng* 氢 (with a *jīng* 巠 phonetic, abbreviating *qīng* 輕 "light-weight") "hydrogen (the lightest element)" and *lǜ* 氯 (with a *lù* 彔 phonetic, abbreviating *lǜ* 綠 "green") "(greenish-yellow) chlorine".

Qì 氣 is the phonetic element in a few characters such as *kài* 愾 "hate" with the "heart-mind radical" 忄 or 心, *xì* 熸 "set fire to weeds" with the "fire radical" 火, and *xì* 餼 "to present food" with the "food radical" 食.

The first Chinese dictionary of characters, the (121 CE) *Shuowen Jiezi* notes that the primary *qì* 气 is a pictographic character depicting 雲气 "cloudy vapors", and that the full 氣 combines 米 "rice" with the phonetic *qi* 气, meaning 饋客芻米 "present provisions to guests" (later disambiguated as *xì* 餼).

Meanings

Qi is a polysemous word; the unabridged Chinese-Chinese character dictionary *Hanyu Da Zidian* lists one meaning "present food or provisions" for the *xì* pronunciation and 23 meanings for the *qì* pronunciation. The modern *ABC Chinese-English Comprehensive Dictionary*, which enters *xì* 餼 "grain; animal feed; make a present of food" but not classical *xì* 氣, has a *qì* 氣 entry giving seven translation equivalents for the noun, two for bound morphemes, and three for the verb.

n. ① air; gas ② smell ③ spirit; vigor; morale ④ vital/material energy (in Ch[inese] metaphysics) ⑤ tone; atmosphere; attitude ⑥ anger ⑦ breath; respiration b.f. ① weather 天氣 *tiānqì* ② [linguistics] aspiration 送氣 *sòngqì* v. ① anger ② get angry ③ bully; insult.

English Borrowing

Qi was an early Chinese loanword in English, romanized as: *k'i* in Church Romanization in the early-19th century, *ch'i* in Wade–Giles in the mid-19th century (sometimes misspelled *chi* omitting the apostrophe indicating aspirated consonant stops, e.g., spelling the martial art *ch'i kung* as "*chi kung*"), and *qi* in Pinyin in the mid-20th century. The *Oxford English Dictionary* entry for *qi* gives the pronunciation as IPA (tʃi), the etymology from Chinese *qì* "air; breath", and a definition of "The physical life-force postulated by certain Chinese philosophers; the material principle." The *OED* gives eight usage examples, with the first recorded example of *k'i* in 1850 (*The Chinese Repository*), of *ch'i* in 1917 (*The Encyclopaedia Sinica*), and *qi* in 1971 (Felix Mann's *Acupuncture*)

Concept

References to concepts analogous to the *qi* taken to be the life-process or flow of energy that sustains living beings are found in many belief systems, especially in Asia. Philosophical conceptions of *qi* from the earliest records of Chinese philosophy (5th century BCE) correspond to Western notions of humours, the ancient Hindu yogic concept of *prana* ("life force" in Sanskrit) and traditional Jewish sources refer to as the Nefesh level of soul within the body. An early form of the idea comes from the writings of the Chinese philosopher Mencius (4th century BCE). Historically, the *Huangdi Neijing/"The Yellow Emperor's Classic of Medicine"* (circa 2nd century BCE) is credited with first establishing the pathways through which *qi* circulates in the human body.

Within the framework of Chinese thought, no notion may attain such a degree of abstraction from empirical data as to correspond perfectly to one of our modern universal concepts. Nevertheless, the term *qi* comes as close as possible to constituting a generic designation equivalent to our word "energy". When Chinese thinkers are unwilling or unable to fix the quality of an energetic phenomenon, the character *qi* (氣) inevitably flows from their brushes.

—Manfred Porkert

The ancient Chinese described it as "life force". They believed *qi* permeated everything and linked their surroundings together. They likened it to the flow of energy around and through the body, forming a cohesive and functioning unit. By understanding its rhythm and flow they believed they could guide exercises and treatments to provide stability and longevity.

Traditional Chinese character *qì*, also used in Korean hanja. In Japanese kanji, this character was used until 1946, when it was changed to 気.

Although the concept of *qi* has been important within many Chinese philosophies, over the centuries the descriptions of *qi* have varied and have sometimes been in conflict. Until China came into contact with Western scientific and philosophical ideas, they had not categorized all things in terms of matter and energy. *Qi* and *li* (理: "pattern") were 'fundamental' categories similar to matter and energy.

Fairly early on, some Chinese thinkers began to believe that there were different fractions of *qi* and that the coarsest and heaviest fractions of *qi* formed solids, lighter fractions formed liquids, and the most ethereal fractions were the "lifebreath" that animates living beings.

Yuán qì is a notion of innate or pre-natal *qi* to distinguish it from acquired *qi* that a person may develop over the course of their lifetime.

Philosophical Roots

The earliest texts that speak of *qi* give some indications of how the concept developed. The philosopher Mo Di used the word *qi* to refer to noxious vapors that would in due time arise from a corpse were it not buried at a sufficient depth. He reported that early civilized humans learned how to live in houses to protect their *qi* from the moisture that had troubled them when they lived in caves. He also associated maintaining one's *qi* with providing oneself adequate nutrition. In regard to another kind of *qi*, he recorded how some people performed a kind of prognostication by observing the *qi* (clouds) in the sky.

In the Analects of Confucius, compiled from the notes of his students sometime after his death in 479 B.C., *qi* could mean "breath", and combining it with the Chinese word for blood (making 血氣, *xue-qi*, blood and breath), the concept could be used to account for motivational characteristics.

The [morally] noble man guards himself against 3 things. When he is young, his *xue-qi* has not yet stabilized, so he guards himself against sexual passion. When he reaches his prime, his *xue-qi* is not easily subdued, so he guards himself against combativeness. When he reaches old age, his *xue-qi* is already depleted, so he guards himself against acquisitiveness.

—Confucius, Analects, 16:7

Mencius described a kind of *qi* that might be characterized as an individual's vital energies. This *qi* was necessary to activity and it could be controlled by a well-integrated willpower. When properly nurtured, this *qi* was said to be capable of extending beyond the human body to reach throughout the universe. It could also be augmented by means of careful exercise of one's moral capacities. On the other hand, the *qi* of an individual could be degraded by adverse external forces that succeed in operating on that individual.

Not only human beings and animals were believed to have *qi*. Zhuangzi indicated that wind is the *qi* of the Earth. Moreover, cosmic yin and yang "are the greatest of *qi*." He described *qi* as "issuing forth" and creating profound effects. He said "Human beings are born [because of] the accumulation of *qi*. When it accumulates there is life. When it dissipates there is death... There is one *qi* that connects and pervades everything in the world."

Another passage traces life to intercourse between Heaven and Earth: "The highest Yin is the most restrained. The highest Yang is the most exuberant. The restrained comes forth from Heaven. The exuberant issues forth from Earth. The two intertwine and penetrate forming a harmony, and [as a result] things are born."

"The Guanzi essay Neiye 內業 (Inward training) is the oldest received writing on the subject of the cultivation of vapor *[qi]* and meditation techniques. The essay was probably composed at the Jixia Academy in Qi in the late fourth century B.C."

Xun Zi, another Confucian scholar of the Jixia Academy, followed in later years. At 9:69/127, Xun Zi says, "Fire and water have *qi* but do not have life. Grasses and trees have life but do not have perceptivity. Fowl and beasts have perceptivity but do not have *yi* (sense of right and wrong, duty, justice). Men have *qi*, life, perceptivity, and *yi*." Chinese people at such an early time had no concept of radiant energy, but they were aware that one can be heated by a campfire from a distance away from the fire. They accounted for this phenomenon by claiming "*qi*" radiated from fire. At 18:62/122, he also uses "*qi*" to refer to the vital forces of the body that decline with advanced age.

Among the animals, the gibbon and the crane were considered experts at inhaling the *qi*. The Confucian scholar Dong Zhongshu (ca. 150 BC) wrote in Luxuriant Dew of the Spring and Autumn Annals: "The gibbon resembles a macaque, but he is larger, and his color is black. His forearms being long, he lives eight hundred years, because he is expert in controlling his breathing." ("猿似猴。大而黑。長前臂。所以壽八百。好引氣也。")

Later, the syncretic text assembled under the direction of Liu An, the Huai Nan Zi, or "Masters of Huainan", has a passage that presages most of what is given greater detail by the Neo-Confucians:

Heaven (seen here as the ultimate source of all being) falls (*duo* 墮, i.e., descends into proto-immanence) as the formless. Fleeting, fluttering, penetrating, amorphous it is, and so it is called the Supreme Luminary. The *dao* begins in the Void Brightening. The Void Brightening produces the universe (*yu-zhou*). The universe produces *qi*. *Qi* has bounds. The clear, yang [*qi*] was ethereal and so formed heaven. The heavy, turbid [*qi*] was congealed and impeded and so formed earth. The conjunction of the clear, yang [*qi*] was fluid and easy. The conjunction of the heavy, turbid [*qi*] was strained and difficult. So heaven was formed first and earth was made fast later. The pervading essence (*xi-jing*) of heaven and earth becomes yin and yang. The concentrated (*zhuan*) essences of yin and yang become the four seasons. The dispersed (*san*) essences of the four seasons become the myriad creatures. The hot *qi* of yang in accumulating produces fire. The essence (*jing*) of the fire-*qi* becomes the sun. The cold *qi* of yin in accumulating produces water. The essence of the water-*qi* becomes the moon. The essences produced by coitus (yin) of the sun and moon become the stars and celestial markpoints (*chen*, planets).

—Huai-nan-zi, 3:1a/19

Role in Traditional Chinese Medicine

Traditional Chinese medicine (TCM) asserts that the body has natural patterns of *qi* that circulate in channels called meridians. In TCM, symptoms of various illnesses are believed to be the product of disrupted, blocked, or unbalanced *qi* movement through the body's meridians, as well as deficiencies or imbalances of *qi* in the *Zang Fu* organs. Traditional Chinese medicine often seeks to relieve these imbalances by adjusting the circulation of *qi* using a variety of techniques including herbology, food therapy, physical training regimens (qigong, t'ai chi ch'uan, and other martial arts training), moxibustion, *tui na*, and acupuncture.

Qi Field

A *qi* field (*chu-chong*) refers to the cultivation of an energy field by a group, typically for healing or other benevolent purposes. A *qi* field is believed to be produced by visualization and affirmation, and is an important component of Wisdom Healing *Qigong* (*Zhineng Qigong*), founded by Grandmaster Ming Pang.

Scientific View

Qi is a non-scientific, unverifiable concept.

A United States National Institutes of Health consensus statement on acupuncture in 1997 noted that concepts such as *qi* "are difficult to reconcile with contemporary bio-medical information."

The April 22, 2014 Skeptoid podcast episode titled "Your Body's Alleged Energy Fields" relates a Reiki practitioner's report of what was happening as she passed her hands over a subject's body:

What we'll be looking for here, within John's auric field, is any areas of intense heat, unusual coldness, a repelling energy, a dense energy, a magnetizing energy, tingling sensations, or actually the body attracting the hands into that area where it needs the reiki energy, and balancing of John's qi.

Evaluating these claims scientific skeptic author Brian Dunning reported:

...his aura, his qi, his reiki energy. None of these have any counterpart in the physical world. Although she attempted to describe their properties as heat or magnetism, those properties are already taken by - well, heat and magnetism. There are no properties attributable to the mysterious field she describes, thus it cannot be authoritatively said to exist."

Practices Involving Qi

Feng Shui

The traditional Chinese art of geomancy, the placement and arrangement of space called feng shui, is based on calculating the balance of *qi*, interactions between the five elements, yin and yang, and other factors. The retention or dissipation of *qi* is believed to affect the health, wealth, energy level, luck and many other aspects of the occupants of the space. Attributes of each item in a space affect the flow of *qi* by slowing it down, redirecting it or accelerating it, which is said to influence the energy level of the occupants.

One use for a *luopan* is to detect the flow of *qi*. The quality of *qi* may rise and fall over time, feng shui with a compass might be considered a form of divination that assesses the quality of the local environment.

Qigong

Qìgōng (气功 or 氣功) is a practice involving coordinated breathing, movement, and awareness, traditionally viewed as a practice to cultivate and balance *qi*. With roots in traditional Chinese medicine, philosophy, and martial arts, *qigong* is now practiced worldwide for exercise, healing, meditation, and training for martial arts. Typically a *qigong* practice involves rhythmic breathing coordinated with slow stylized movement, a calm mindful state, and visualization of guiding *qi*.

Martial Arts

Qi is a didactic concept in many Chinese, Korean and Japanese martial arts. Martial *qigong* is a feature of both internal and external training systems in China and other East Asian cultures. The most notable of the *qi*-focused "internal" force (jin) martial arts are Baguazhang, Xing Yi Quan, T'ai Chi Ch'uan, Southern Praying Mantis, Snake Kung Fu, Southern Dragon Kung Fu, Aikido, Kendo, Aikijujutsu, Luohan Quan and Liu He Ba Fa.

Demonstrations of *qi* or *ki* are popular in some martial arts and may include the immovable body, the unraisable body, the unbendable arm, and other feats of power. Some of these feats can alternatively be explained using biomechanics and physics.

Acupuncture and Moxibustion

Acupuncture is a part of traditional Chinese medicine that involves insertion of needles into superficial structures of the body (skin, subcutaneous tissue, muscles) at acupuncture points to balance the flow of *qi*. Acupuncture is often accompanied by moxibustion, a treatment that involves burning mugwort on or near the skin at an acupuncture point.

Meridian (Chinese Medicine)

Meridian system

The meridian system (simplified Chinese: 经络; traditional Chinese: 經絡; pinyin: *jīngluò*, also called channel network) is a traditional Chinese medicine (TCM) belief about a path through which the life-energy known as "qi" flows.

Acupuncture points and meridians have not been proven. Much of the research exploring acupuncture points and potential benefits are newly emerging. Larger and more diverse randomized control trials (RCT) are needed.

Main Concepts

The meridian network is typically divided into 2 categories, the *jingmai* (經脈) or meridian channels and the *luomai* (絡脈) or associated vessels (sometimes called "collaterals"). The jingmai contain the 12 tendinomuscular meridians, the 12 divergent meridians, the 12 principal meridians, the 8 extraordinary vessels as well as the Huato channel, a set of bilateral points on the lower back whose discovery is attributed to the famous physician in ancient China. The collaterals contain 15 major arteries that connect the 12 principal meridians in various ways, in addition to the interaction with their associated internal organs and other related internal structures. The collateral system also incorporates a branching expanse of capillary-like vessels which spread throughout the body, namely in the 12 cutaneous regions as well as emanating from each point on the principal meridians. If one counts the number of unique points on each meridian, the total comes to 361, although 365 is usually used since it coincides with the number of days in a year. Note that this method ignores the fact that the bulk of acupoints are bilateral, making the actual total 670.

There are about 400 acupuncture points (not counting bilateral points twice) most of which are situated along the major 20 pathways (i.e. 12 primary and 8 extraordinary channels). However, by the 2nd Century AD, 649 acupuncture points were recognized in China (reckoned by counting bilateral points twice). There are "Twelve Principal Meridians" where each meridian corresponds to either a hollow or solid organ; interacting with it and extending along a particular extremity (i.e. arm or leg). There are also "Eight Extraordinary Channels", two of which have their own sets of points, and the remaining ones connecting points on other channels.

Twelve Standard Meridians

The twelve standard meridians, also called Principal Meridians, are divided into Yin and Yang groups. The Yin meridians of the arm are Lung, Heart, and Pericardium. The Yang meridians of the arm are Large Intestine, Small Intestine, and Triple Burner. The Yin Meridians of the leg are Spleen, Kidney, and Liver. The Yang meridians of the leg are Stomach, Bladder, and Gall Bladder.

The table below gives a more systematic list of the twelve standard meridians:

Meridian name (Chinese)	Quality of Yin or Yang	Extremity	Five Elements	Organ	Time of Day
Taiyin Lung Channel of Hand (手太阴肺经) or Hand's Major Yin Lung Meridian	Greater Yin (taiyin, 太阴)	Hand (手)	Metal (金)	Lung (肺)	寅 [yín] 3 a.m. to 5 a.m.
Shaoyin Heart Channel of Hand (手少阴心经) or Hand's Minor Yin Heart Meridian	Lesser Yin (shaoyin, 少阴)	Hand (手)	Fire (火)`	Heart (心)	午 [wǔ] 11 a.m. to 1 p.m.
Jueyin Pericardium Channel of Hand (手厥阴心包经) or Hand's Absolute Yin Heart Protector Meridian	Faint Yin (jueyin - 厥阴)	Hand (手)	Fire (火)	Pericardium (心包)	戌 [xū] 7 p.m. to 9 p.m.
Shaoyang Sanjiao Channel of Hand (手少阳三焦经) or Hand's Minor Yang Triple Burner Meridian	Lesser Yang (shaoyang, 少阳)	Hand (手)	Fire (火)	Triple Burner (三焦)	亥 [hài] 9 p.m. to 11 p.m.
Taiyang Small Intestine Channel of Hand (手太阳小肠经) or Hand's Major Yang Small Intestine Meridian	Greater Yang (taiyang, 太阳)	Hand (手)	Fire (火)	Small Intestine (小肠)	未 [wèi] 1 p.m. to 3 p.m.
Yangming Large Intestine Channel of Hand (手阳明大肠经) or Hand's Yang Supreme Large Intestine Meridian	Yang Bright (yangming, 阳明)	Hand (手)	Metal (金)	Large Intestine (大腸)	卯 [mǎo] 5 a.m. to 7 a.m.
Taiyin Spleen Channel of Foot (足太阴脾经) or Foot's Major Yin Spleen Meridian	Greater Yin (taiyin, 太阴)	Foot (足)	Earth (土)	Spleen (脾)	巳 [sì] 9 a.m. to 11 a.m.
Shaoyin Kidney Channel of Foot (足少阴肾经) or Foot's Minor Yin Kidney Meridian	Lesser Yin (shaoyin, 少阴)	Foot (足)	Water (水)	Kidney (腎)	酉 [yǒu] 5 p.m. to 7 p.m.
Jueyin Liver Channel of Foot (足厥阴肝经) or Foot's Absolute Yin Liver Meridian	Faint Yin (jueyin, 厥阴)	Foot (足)	Wood (木)	Liver (肝)	丑 [chǒu] 1 a.m. to 3 a.m.
Shaoyang Gallbladder Channel of Foot (足少阳胆经) or Foot's Minor Yang Gallbladder Meridian	Lesser Yang (shaoyang, 少阳)	Foot (足)	Wood (木)	Gall Bladder (膽)	子 [zǐ] 11 p.m. to 1 a.m.
Taiyang Bladder Channel of Foot (足太阳膀胱经) or Foot's Major Yang Urinary Bladder Meridian	Greater Yang (taiyang, 太阳)	Foot (足)	Water (水)	Urinary bladder (膀胱)	申 [shēn] 3 p.m. to 5 p.m.
Yangming Stomach Channel of Foot (足阳明胃经) or Foot's Yang Supreme Stomach Meridian	Yang Bright (yangming, 阳明)	Foot (足)	Earth (土)	Stomach (胃)	辰 [chén] 7 a.m. to 9 a.m.

Eight Extraordinary Meridians

The eight extraordinary meridians are of pivotal importance in the study of Qigong, T'ai chi ch'uan and Chinese alchemy. These eight extra meridians are different to the standard twelve organ meridians in that they are considered to be storage vessels or reservoirs of energy and are not associated directly with the Zang Fu, i.e. internal organs. These channels were first systematically referred to in the "Spiritual Axis" chapters 17, 21 and 62, the "Classic of Difficulties" chapters 27, 28 and 29 and the "Study of the 8 Extraordinary vessels" (Qi Jing Ba Mai Kao) by Li Shi Zhen 1578.

The eight extraordinary vessels are (奇經八脈; qí jīng bā mài):

1. Conception Vessel (Ren Mai) - 任脈 [rèn mài]

2. Governing Vessel (Du Mai) - 督脈 [dū mài]

3. Penetrating Vessel (Chong Mai) - 衝脈 [chōng mài]

4. Girdle Vessel (Dai Mai) - 帶脈 [dài mài]

5. Yin linking vessel (Yin Wei Mai) - 陰維脈 [yīn wéi mài]

6. Yang linking vessel (Yang Wei Mai) - 陽維脈 [yáng wéi mài]

7. Yin Heel Vessel (Yin Qiao Mai) - 陰蹻脈 [yīn qiāo mài]

8. Yang Heel Vessel (Yang Qiao Mai) - 陽蹻脈 [yáng qiāo mài]

Scientific View of Traditional Chinese Meridian Theory

According to evidence-based medicine, "TCM is a pre-scientific superstitious view of biology and illness, similar to the humoral theory of Galen, or the notions of any pre-scientific culture. It is strange and unscientific to treat TCM as anything else. Any individual diagnostic or treatment method within TCM should be evaluated according to standard principles of science and science-based medicine, and not given special treatment."

The National Council Against Health Fraud concluded that,

The World Health Organization has listed forty conditions for which claims of effectiveness have been made. They include acute and chronic pain, rheumatoid and osteoarthritis, muscle and nerve "difficulties", depression, smoking, eating disorders, drug "behavior problems", migraine, acne, ulcers, cancer, and constipation. Some chiropractors and psychologists have made unsubstantiated claims to improve dyslexia and learning disorders by acupressure. However, scientific evidence supporting these claims is either inadequate or nonexistent.

Zang-Fu

The zàng-**fǔ** (simplified Chinese: 脏腑; traditional Chinese: 臟腑) organs are functional entities stipulated by Traditional Chinese medicine (TCM). They constitute the centre piece of TCM's general concept of how the human body works. The term zàng (脏) refers to the organs considered to be yin in nature – Heart, Liver, Spleen, Lung, Kidney – while fǔ (腑) refers to the yang organs – Small Intestine, Large Intestine, Gall Bladder, Urinary Bladder, Stomach and Sānjiaō.

Each zàng is paired with a fǔ, and each pair is assigned to one of the Wǔ Xíng. The zàng-fǔ are also connected to the twelve standard meridians – each yang meridian is attached to a fǔ organ and each yin meridian is attached to a zàng. They are five systems of Heart, Liver, Spleen, Lung, Kidney.

To highlight the fact that the zàng-fǔ are not equivalent to the anatomical organs, their names are often capitalized.

Anatomical Organs

To understand the zàng-fǔ it is important to realize that their concept did not primarily develop out of anatomical considerations. The need to describe and systematize the bodily *functions* was more significant to ancient Chinese physicians than opening up a dead body and seeing what morphological structures there actually were. Thus, the zàng-fǔ are *functional entities* first and foremost, and only loosely tied to (rudimentary) anatomical assumptions.

Yin/Yang and the Five Elements

Each zàng-fǔ organ has a yin and a yang aspect, but overall, the zàng organs are considered to be yin, and the fǔ organs yang.

Since the concept of the zàng-fǔ was developed on the basis of Wǔ Xíng philosophy, they're incorporated into a system of allocation to one of five elemental qualities (i.e., the Five Elements or Five Phases). The zàng-fǔ share their respective element's allocations (e.g., regarding colour, taste, season, emotion etc.) and interact with each other cyclically in the same way the Five Elements do: each zàng organ has one corresponding zàng organ that it enfeebles, and one that it reinforces.

The correspondence between zàng-fǔ and Five Elements are stipulated as:

- Fire (火) = Heart (心) and Small Intestine (小肠) (and, secondarily, Sānjiaō [三焦, "Triple Burner"] and Pericardium [心包])

- Earth (土) = Spleen (脾) and Stomach (胃)

- Metal (金) = Lung (肺) and Large Intestine (大肠)

- Water (水) = Kidney (肾) and Bladder (膀胱)

- Wood (木) = Liver (肝) and Gall Bladder (胆)

Details

The zàng organs' essential functions consist in manufacturing and storing qì and blood (and, in the case of the Kidney, essence). The fǔ organs' main purpose is to transmit and digest (传化, pinyin: *chuán-huà*) substances (like waste, food, etc.).

Zang

Each zàng has a corresponding "orifice" it "opens" into. This means the functional entity of a given zàng includes the corresponding orifice's functions (e.g. blurry vision is primarily seen as a dysfunction of the Liver zàng as the Liver "opens" into the eyes).

In listing the functions of the zàng organs, TCM regularly uses the term "governing" (主, pinyin: *zhǔ*) – indicating that the main responsibility of regulating something (e.g. blood, qì, water metabolism etc.) lies with a certain zàng.

Although the zàng are functional entities in the first place, TCM gives vague locations for them – namely, the general area where the anatomical organ of the same name would be found. One could argue that this (or any) positioning of the zàng is irrelevant for the TCM system; there is some relevance, however, in whether a certain zàng would be attributed to the upper, middle or lower jiāo.

Heart

The Heart:

- "Stores" (藏, pinyin: *cáng*) the *shén* (神, "Aggregate Soul", usually translated as *mind*)

- Governs xuě (blood) and vessels/meridians

- Opens into the tongue

- Reflects in facial complexion

Pericardium

Since there are only five zàng organs but six yin channels, the remaining meridian is assigned to the Pericardium. Its concept is closely related to the Heart, and its stipulated main function is to protect the Heart from attacks by Exterior Pathogenic Factors. Like the Heart, the Pericardium governs blood and stores the mind. The Pericardium's corresponding yang channel is assigned to the Sānjiāo ("Triple Burner").

Spleen

The Spleen:

- Governs "transportation and absorption" (运化, pinyin: *yùn-huà*), i.e. the extraction of jīng weī (精微, lit. "essence bits", usually translated with *food essence*, sometimes also called jīng qì [精气, *essence qi*]) – and water – from food and drink, and the successive distribution of it to the other zàng organs.

- Is the source of "production and mutual transformation" (生化, pinyin: *shēng-huà*) of qì and xuě (blood)

- "Contains" (统, pinyin: *tǒng*) the blood inside the vessels

- Opens into the lips (and mouth)

- Governs muscles and limbs

Liver

The Liver:

- Governs "unclogging and deflation" (疏泄, pinyin: *shū-xiè*) primarily of qì. The free flow of qì in turn will ensure the free flow of emotions, blood, and water.

- "Stores" (藏, pinyin: *cáng*) blood

- Opens into the eyes

- Governs the tendons

- Reflects in the nails

Lung

Metal. Home of the *Po* (魄, Corporeal Soul), paired with the *Large intestine*.

The function of the Lung is to descend and disperse qi throughout the body. It receives qi through the breath, and exhales the waste. The Lung governs the skin and hair and also governs the exterior (one part of immunity). A properly functioning Lung organ will ensure the skin and hair are of good quality and that the immune system is strong and able to fight disease. The normal direction of the Lung is downwards, when Lung qi "rebels" it goes upwards, causing coughing and wheezing. When the Lung is weak, there can be skin conditions such as eczema, thin or brittle hair, and a propensity to catching colds and flu. The Lung is weakened by dryness and the emotion of grief or sadness.

Kidney

Water. Home of the *Zhi* (志, Will), paired with the *bladder*.

The Kidneys store Essence, govern birth, growth, reproduction and development. They also produce the Marrow which fills the brain and control the bones. The Kidneys are often referred to as the "Root of Life" or the "Root of the Pre-Heaven Qi". Kidneys house the Will Power (Zhi).

Criticism

The concept of the zàng-fǔ is not scientific – the underlying assumptions and theory have not been (and are not expected to be) verified or falsified by experiment. Probably because of this, the concept (and TCM as a whole) has been criticized as pseudoscientific.

References

- Ho, Peng Yoke (Oct 2000). Li, Qi, and Shu: An Introduction to Science and Civilization in China. Dover Publications. ISBN 0-486-41445-0.

- Frantzis, Bruce Kumar (2008). The Chi Revolution: Harnessing the Healing Power of Your Life Force. Blue Snake Books. ISBN 1-58394-193-2.

- Porkert, Manfred (1974). The Theoretical Foundations of Chinese Medicine: Systems of Correspondence. MIT Press. ISBN 0-262-16058-7. OCLC 123145357.

- Ooi, Kean Hin (2010). . Zhineng Qigong: The science, theory and practice. CreateSpace Independent Publishing Platform. ISBN 978-1453867600.

- Cohen, K. S. (1999). The Way of Qigong: The Art and Science of Chinese Energy Healing. Random House of Canada. ISBN 0-345-42109-4.

- Liang, Shou-Yu; Wen-Ching Wu, Denise Breiter-Wu (1997). Qigong Empowerment: A Guide to Medical, Taoist, Buddhist, and Wushu Energy Cultivation. Way of the Dragon Pub. ISBN 1-889659-02-9.

- Yang, Jwing-Ming (1998). Qigong for health and martial arts: exercises and meditation. YMAA Publication Center. ISBN 1-886969-57-4.

- Wile, Douglas (1995). Lost T'ai-chi Classics from the Late Ch'ing Dynasty (Chinese Philosophy and Culture). State University of New York Press. ISBN 978-0-7914-2654-8. OCLC 34546989.

- Bishop, Mark (1989). Okinawan Karate: Teachers, Styles and Secret Techniques. A&C Black, London. ISBN 0-7136-5666-2. OCLC 19262983.

- Dillman, George and Chris, Thomas. Advanced Pressute Point Fighting of Ryukyu Kempo. A Dillman Karate International Book, 1994. ISBN 0-9631996-3-3

- Peter Deadman and Mazin Al-Khafaji with Kevin Baker. "A Manuel of Acupuncture" Journal of Chinese Medicine, 2007. ISBN 978-0-9510546-5-9

- Agnes Fatrai, Stefan Uhrig (eds.): Chinese Ophthalmology – Acupuncture, Herbal Therapy, Dietary Therapy, Tuina and Qigong. Tipani-Verlag, Wiesbaden 2015, ISBN 978-3-9815471-1-5.

Philosophical Background of Traditional Chinese Medicine

Chinese traditional medicine has a strong philosophical background. Some of the philosophical beliefs are yin and yang, wu xing, deng shui, the eight principles and the three treasures. Disease is perceived as an imbalance in the functions of yin and yang, qui, meridians or an imbalance in the interaction between the human body and the environment. The aspects elucidated in this chapter are of vital importance, and provide a better understanding of traditional Chinese medicine.

Yin and Yang

In Chinese philosophy, yin and yang (also *yin-yang* or *yin yang*, 陰陽 *yīnyáng* "dark—bright") describe how seemingly opposite or contrary forces may actually be complementary, interconnected, and interdependent in the natural world, and how they may give rise to each other as they interrelate to one another. Many tangible dualities (such as light and dark, fire and water, expanding and contracting) are thought of as physical manifestations of the duality symbolized by yin and yang. This duality lies at the origins of many branches of classical Chinese science and philosophy, as well as being a primary guideline of traditional Chinese medicine, and a central principle of different forms of Chinese martial arts and exercise, such as baguazhang, taijiquan (t'ai chi), and qigong (Chi Kung), as well as appearing in the pages of the *I Ching*.

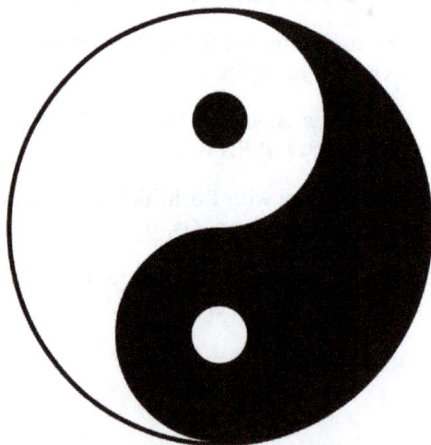

The modern "yin and yang symbol" (*taijitu*).

Duality is found in many belief systems, but Yin and Yang are parts of a Oneness that is also equated with the Tao. A term has been coined dualistic-monism or dialectical monism. Yin and yang can be thought of as complementary (rather than opposing) forces that interact to form a dynamic system in which the whole is greater than the assembled parts. Everything has both yin and yang aspects, (for instance shadow cannot exist without light). Either of the two major aspects may manifest more strongly in a particular object, depending on the criterion of the observation. The yin yang (i.e. taijitu symbol) shows a balance between two opposites with a portion of the opposite element in each section.

In Taoist metaphysics, distinctions between good and bad, along with other dichotomous moral judgments, are perceptual, not real; so, the duality of yin and yang is an indivisible whole. In the ethics of Confucianism on the other hand, most notably in the philosophy of Dong Zhongshu (c. 2nd century BC), a moral dimension is attached to the idea of yin and yang.

Linguistic Aspects

The Chinese terms *yīn* 陰 or 阴 "shady side" and *yáng* 陽 or 阳 "sunny side" are linguistically analyzable in terms of Chinese characters, pronunciations and etymology, meanings, topography, and loanwords.

Characters

The Traditional Chinese characters 陰 and 陽 for the words *yīn* and *yáng* are both classified as radical-phonetic characters, combining the semantically significant "mound; hill" radical 阝 or 阜 with the phonetic indicators *yīn* 侌 and *yáng* 昜. The first phonetic *yīn* 侌 "cloudy" ideographically combines *jīn* 今 "now; present" and *yún* 云 "cloud", denoting the "今 presence of 云 clouds". The second phonetic *yáng* 昜 "bright" originally pictured 日 the "sun" with 勿 "rays coming down". This phonetic is expanded with the "sun" radical into *yáng* 暘 "rising sun; sunshine". The "mound; hill" radical 阝 full forms semantically specify *yīn* 陰 "shady/dark side of a hill" and *yáng* 陽 "sunny/light side of a hill".

The Simplified Chinese characters 阴 and 阳 for *yīn* and *yáng* combine the same "hill" radical 阝 with the non-phonetic *yuè* 月 "moon" and *rì* 日 "sun", graphically denoting "shady side of a hill" and "sunny side of a hill". Compare the Classical Chinese names (which contain *tài* 太 "great") for these two heavenly bodies: *Tàiyīn* 太陰 "moon" and *Tàiyáng* 太陽 "sun".

Pronunciations and Etymologies

The Modern Standard Chinese pronunciation of 陰 or 阴 is usually level first tone *yīn* "shady; cloudy" or sometimes falling fourth tone *yìn* "to shelter; shade", and 陽 or 9"sunny" is always pronounced with rising second tone *yáng*.

Sinologists and historical linguists have reconstructed Middle Chinese pronunciations from data in the (7th century CE) *Qieyun* rime dictionary and later rime tables, which was subsequently used to reconstruct Old Chinese phonology from rimes in the (11th-7th centuries BCE) *Shijing* and phonological components of Chinese characters. Reconstructions of Old Chinese have illuminated the etymology of modern Chinese words.

Compare these Middle Chinese and Old Chinese (with asterisk) reconstructions of *yīn* 陰 and *yáng* 陽:

- ·*iəm* < *·*iəm* and *iang* < *diang* (Bernhard Karlgren)

- *jəm* and *raŋ* (Li Fang-Kuei)

- *(r)jum* and *ljang* (William H. Baxter),

- *jəm* < *ʔəm* and *jiaŋ* < *laŋ* (Axel Schuessler)

- '*im* < *qrum* and *yang* < *laŋ* (William H. Baxter and Laurent Sagart)

Schuessler gives probable Sino-Tibetan etymologies for both Chinese words.

Yin < *əm* compares with Burmese *ʔum^C* "overcast; cloudy", Adi *muk-jum* "shade", and Lepcha *so'yŭm* "shade"; and is probably cognate with Chinese *àn* < *ə^m 黯 "dim; gloomy" and *qīn* < *khəm* 衾 "blanket"

Yang < *laŋ* compares with Lepcha *a-lóŋ* "reflecting light", Burmese *laŋ^B* "be bright" and *ə-laŋ^B* "light", and Tai *plaŋ^A1* "bright"; and is perhaps cognate with Chinese *chāng* < *k-hlaŋ* 昌 "prosperous; bright" (cf. Proto-Viet-Mong *hlaŋ^B* "bright"), and *bǐng* < *braŋ* 炳 "bright".

Meanings

Yin and *yang* are semantically complex words.

A reliable Chinese-English dictionary gives the following translation equivalents.

Yin 陰 or 阴 Noun ① [philosophy] negative/passive/female principle in nature ② Surname Bound morpheme ① the moon ② shaded orientation ③ covert; concealed; hidden ④ ⑦ negative ⑧ north side of a hill ⑨ south bank of a river ⑩ reverse side of a stele in intaglio Stative verb ① overcast ② sinister; treacherous

Yang 陽 or 阳 Bound morpheme ① [Chinese philosophy] positive/active/male principle in nature ②the sun ④ in relief ⑤ open; overt ⑥ belonging to this world ⑦ [linguistics] masculine ⑧ south side of a hill ⑨ north bank of a river

The compound *yinyang* 陰陽 or 阴阳 means "yin and yang; opposites; ancient Chinese astronomy; occult arts; astrologer; geomancer; etc.".

The sinologist Rolf Stein etymologically translates Chinese *yin* 陰 "shady side (of a mountain)" and *yang* 陽 "sunny side (of a mountain)" with the uncommon English geographic terms *ubac* "shady side of a mountain" and *adret* "sunny side of a mountain" (which are of French origin).

Toponymy

Many Chinese place names or toponyms contain the word *yang* "sunny side" and a few contain *yin* "shady side". In China, as elsewhere in the Northern Hemisphere, sunlight comes predominantly from the south, and thus the south face of a mountain or the north bank of a river will receive more direct sunlight than the opposite side.

Yang refers to the "south side of a hill" in Hengyang 衡陽, which is south of Mount Heng 衡山 in Hunan province, and to the "north bank of a river" in Luoyang 洛陽, which is located north of the Luo River 洛河 in Henan.

Similarly, *yin* refers to "north side of a hill" in Huayin 華陰, which is north of Mount Hua 華山 in Shaanxi province.

Loanwords

English *yin*, *yang*, and *yin-yang* are familiar loanwords of Chinese origin.

The *Oxford English Dictionary* defines:

yin Also Yin, Yn. [Chinese *yīn* shade, feminine; the moon.]

a. In Chinese philosophy, the feminine or negative principle (characterized by dark, wetness, cold, passivity, disintegration, etc.) of the two opposing cosmic forces into which creative energy divides and whose fusion in physical matter brings the phenomenal world into being. Also *attrib.* or as *adj.*, and *transf.* Cf. yang.

b. *Comb.*, as yin-yang, the combination or fusion of the two cosmic forces; freq. attrib., esp. as yin-yang symbol, a circle divided by an S-shaped line into a dark and a light segment, representing respectively *yin* and *yang*, each containing a 'seed' of the other.

yang (jæŋ) Also Yang. [Chinese *yáng* yang, sun, positive, male genitals.]

a. In Chinese philosophy, the masculine or positive principle (characterized by light, warmth, dryness, activity, etc.) of the two opposing cosmic forces into which creative energy divides and whose fusion in physical matter brings the phenomenal world into being. Also *attrib.* or as *adj.* Cf. yin.

b. *Comb.*: yang-yin = *yin-yang* s.v. yin b.

For the earliest recorded "yin and yang" usages, the *OED* cites 1671 for *yin* and *yang*, 1850 for *yin-yang*, and 1959 for *yang-yin*.

In English, *yang-yin* (like *ying-yang*) occasionally occurs as a mistake or typographical error for the Chinese loanword *yin-yang*— yet they are not equivalents. Chinese does have some *yangyin* collocations, such as 洋銀 (lit. "foreign silver") "silver coin/dollar", but not even the most comprehensive dictionaries (e.g., the *Hanyu Da Cidian*) enter *yangyin* *陽陰. While *yang* and *yin* can occur together in context, *yangyin* is not synonymous with *yinyang*. The linguistic term "irreversible binomial" refers to a collocation of two words A-B that cannot normally be reversed as B-A, for example, English *cat and mouse* (not *mouse and cat) and *friend or foe* (not *foe or friend). Similarly, the usual pattern among Chinese binomial compounds is for positive A and negative B, where the A word is dominant or privileged over B, for example, *tiandi* 天地 "heaven and earth" and *nannü* 男女 "men and women". *Yinyang* meaning "dark and light; female and male; moon and sun", however, is an exception. Scholars have proposed various explanations for why *yinyang* violates this pattern, including "linguistic convenience" (it is easier to say *yinyang* than *yangyin*), the idea that "proto-Chinese society was matriarchal", or perhaps, since *yinyang* first became prominent during the late Warring States period, this term was "purposely directed at challenging persistent cultural assumptions".

History

Needham discusses Yin and Yang together with Five Elements as part of the School of Naturalists. He says that it would be proper to begin with Yin and Yang before Five Elements because the former: "lay, as it were, at a deeper level in Nature, and were the most ultimate principles of which the ancient Chinese could conceive. But it so happens that we know a good deal more about the historical origin of the Five-Element theory than about that of the Yin and the Yang, and it will therefore be more convenient to deal with it first." He then discusses Zou Yan (□□; 305 – 240 BC) who is most associated with these theories. Although Yin and Yang are not mentioned in any of the surviving documents of Zou Yan, his school was known as the Yin Yang Jia (Yin and Yang School) Needham concludes "There can be very little doubt that the philosophical use of the terms began about the beginning of the -4th century, and that the passages in older texts which mention this use are interpolations made later than that time."

Nature

In Daoist philosophy, dark and light, yin and yang, arrive in the Tao Te Ching at chapter 42. It becomes sensible from an initial quiescence or emptiness (wuji, sometimes symbolized by an empty circle), and continues moving until quiescence is reached again. For instance, dropping a stone in a calm pool of water will simultaneously raise waves and lower troughs between them, and this alternation of high and low points in the water will radiate outward until the movement dissipates and the pool is calm once more. Yin and yang thus are always opposite and equal qualities. Further, whenever one quality reaches its peak, it will naturally begin to transform into the opposite quality: for example, grain that reaches its full height in summer (fully yang) will produce seeds and die back in winter (fully yin) in an endless cycle.

It is impossible to talk about yin or yang without some reference to the opposite, since yin and yang are bound together as parts of a mutual whole (for example, there cannot be the bottom of the foot without the top). A way to illustrate this idea is to postulate the notion of a race with only men or only women; this race would disappear in a single generation. Yet, men and women together create new generations that allow the race they mutually create (and mutually come from) to survive. The interaction of the two gives birth to things, like manhood. Yin and yang transform each other: like an undertow in the ocean, every advance is complemented by a retreat, and every rise transforms into a fall. Thus, a seed will sprout from the earth and grow upwards towards the sky—an intrinsically yang movement. Then, when it reaches its full potential height, it will fall. Also, the growth of the top seeks light, while roots grow in darkness.

Certain catchphrases have been used to express yin and yang complementarity:

- The bigger the front, the bigger the back.

- Illness is the doorway to health.

- Tragedy turns to comedy.

- Disasters turn out to be blessings.

Symbolism and Importance

Yin is the black side with the white dot in it, and yang is the white side with the black dot in it. The relationship between yin and yang is often described in terms of sunlight playing over a mountain and a valley. Yin (literally the 'shady place' or 'north slope') is the dark area occluded by the mountain's bulk, while yang (literally the 'sunny place' or 'south slope') is the brightly lit portion. As the sun moves across the sky, yin and yang gradually trade places with each other, revealing what was obscured and obscuring what was revealed.

Yin is characterized as slow, soft, yielding, diffuse, cold, wet, and passive; and is associated with water, earth, the moon, femininity, and nighttime.

Yang, by contrast, is fast, hard, solid, focused, hot, dry, and active; and is associated with fire, sky, the sun, masculinity and daytime.

Yin and yang applies to the human body. In traditional Chinese medicine good health is directly related to the balance between yin and yang qualities within oneself. If yin and yang become unbalanced, one of the qualities is considered deficient or has vacuity.

I Ching

In the *I Ching*, originally a divination manual of the Western Zhou period (c. 1000–750

BC), yin and yang are represented by broken and solid lines: yin is broken (□) and yang is solid (□). These are then combined into trigrams, which are more yang (*e.g.* ☳) or more yin (*e.g.* ☶) depending on the number of broken and solid lines (*e.g.*, ☰ is heavily yang, while ☷ is heavily yin), and trigrams are combined into hexagrams (*e.g.* □ and □). The relative positions and numbers of yin and yang lines within the trigrams determines the meaning of a trigram, and in hexagrams the upper trigram is considered yang with respect to the lower trigram, yin, which allows for complex depictions of interrelations.

Taijitu

The principle of yin and yang is represented in Taoism by the Taijitu (literally "Diagram of the Supreme Ultimate"). The term is commonly used to mean the simple "divided circle" form, but may refer to any of several schematic diagrams representing these principles, such as the swastika, common to Hinduism, Buddhism, and Jainism. Similar symbols have also appeared in other cultures, such as in Celtic art and Roman shield markings.

Taijiquan

Taijiquan (Chinese: 太极拳), a form of martial art, is often described as the principles of yin and yang applied to the human body and an animal body. Wu Jianquan, a famous Chinese martial arts teacher, described Taijiquan as follows:

Various people have offered different explanations for the name *Taijiquan*. Some have said: – 'In terms of self-cultivation, one must train from a state of movement towards a state of stillness. *Taiji* comes about through the balance of *yin* and *yang*. In terms of the art of attack and defense then, in the context of the changes of full and empty, one is constantly internally latent, to not outwardly expressive, as if the *yin* and *yang* of *Taiji* have not yet divided apart.' Others say: 'Every movement of *Taijiquan* is based on circles, just like the shape of a *Taijitu*. Therefore, it is called *Taijiquan*.

— *Wu Jianquan, The International Magazine of T'ai Chi Ch'uan*

Wu Xing

The Wu Xing (Chinese: 五行; pinyin: *Wǔ Xíng*), also known as the Five Elements, Five Phases, the Five Agents, the Five Movements, Five Processes, the Five Steps/Stages and the Five Planets is the short form of "Wǔ zhǒng liúxíng zhī qì" (五種流行之氣) or "the five types of chi dominating at different times". It is a fivefold conceptual scheme that many traditional Chinese fields used to explain a wide array of phenomena, from cosmic cycles to the interaction between internal organs, and from the succession of political regimes to the properties of medicinal drugs. The "Five Phases" are Wood (木 *mù*), Fire (火 *huǒ*), Earth (土 *tǔ*), Metal (金 *jīn*), and Water (水 *shuǐ*). This order of presentation is known as the "mutual generation" (相生 *xiāngshēng*) sequence. In the order of "mutual overcoming" (相剋/相克 *xiāngkè*), they are Wood, Earth, Water, Fire, and Metal.

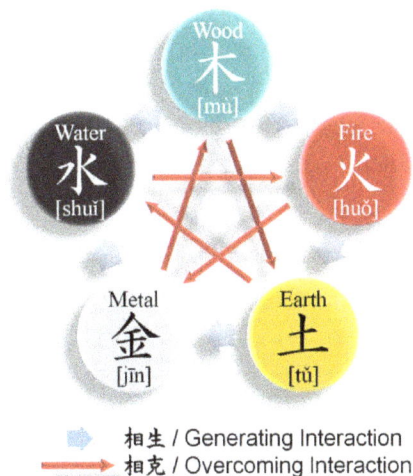

相生 / Generating Interaction
相克 / Overcoming Interaction

Diagram of the interactions between the Wu Xing. The "generative" cycle is illustrated by grey arrows running clockwise on the outside of the circle, while the "destructive" or "conquering" cycle is represented by red arrows inside the circle.

The system of five phases was used for describing interactions and relationships between phenomena. After it came to maturity in the second or first century BCE during the Han dynasty, this device was employed in many fields of early Chinese thought, including seemingly disparate fields such as geomancy or Feng shui, astrology, traditional Chinese medicine, music, military strategy, and martial arts. The system is still used as a reference in some forms of complementary and alternative medicine and martial arts.

Names

Xing (Chinese: 行) of 'Wu Xing' means moving; a planet is called a 'moving star'(Chinese: 行星) in Chinese. Wu Xing (Chinese: 五行) originally refers to the five major planets (Jupiter, Saturn, Mercury, Venus, Mars) that create five dimensions of earth life. "Wu Xing" is also widely translated as Five Elements and this is used extensively by many including practitioners of Five Element acupuncture. This translation arose by false analogy with the Western system of the four elements. Whereas the classical Greek elements were concerned with substances or natural qualities, the Chinese *xíng* are "primarily concerned with process and change," hence the common translation as "phases" or "agents". By the same token, *Mù* is thought of as "Tree" rather than "Wood". The word 'element' is thus used within the context of Chinese medicine with a different meaning to its usual meaning.

It should be recognized that the word *phase*, although commonly preferred, is not perfect. *Phase* is a better translation for the five *seasons* (五運 Wǔ Yùn) mentioned below, and so *agents* or *processes* might be preferred for the primary term *xíng*. Manfred Porkert attempts to resolve this by using *Evolutive Phase* for 五行 *Wǔ Xíng* and *Circuit Phase* for 五運 *Wǔ Yùn*, but these terms are unwieldy.

Some of the Mawangdui Silk Texts (no later than 168 BC) also present the Wu Xing as "five virtues" or types of activities. Within Chinese medicine texts the Wu Xing are also referred to as Wu Yun (五運 wǔ yùn) or a combination of the two characters (Wu Xing-Yun) these emphasise the correspondence of five elements to five ‹seasons› (four seasons plus one). Another tradition refers to the *Wǔ Xíng* as *Wǔ Dé* (五德), the Five Virtues (zh:五德終始說).

The Phases

The five phases are usually used to describe the state in nature:

- Wood/Spring=(72 days) a period of growth, which generates abundant wood and vitality

- Fire/Summer=(72 days) a period of swelling, flowering, brimming with fire and energy

- Earth=(72 days=4x18days (4 transitional seasons x 18days each) the in-between transitional seasonal periods, or a separate ‘season’ known as Late Summer or Long Summer - in the latter case associated with leveling and dampening (moderation) and fruition

- Metal/Autumn=(72 days) a period of harvesting and collecting

- Water/Winter=(72 days) a period of retreat, where stillness and storage pervades

Cycles

The doctrine of five phases describes two cycles, a generating or creation (生, *shēng*) cycle, also known as "mother-son", and an overcoming or destruction (剋/克, *kè*) cycle, also known as "grandfather-nephew", of interactions between the phases. Within Chinese medicine the effects of these two main relations are further elaborated:

- Inter-promoting (mother/son)

- Inter-acting (grandmother/grandson)

- Over-acting (*kè* cycle)

- Counter-acting (reverse *kè*)

Generating

The common memory jogs, which help to remind in what order the phases are:

- Wood feeds Fire

- Fire creates Earth (ash)

- Earth bears Metal

- Metal collects Water

- Water nourishes Wood

Other common words for this cycle include "begets", "engenders" and "mothers".

Overcoming

- Wood parts Earth (such as roots or trees can prevent soil erosion)

- Earth dams (or muddles or absorbs) Water

- Water extinguishes Fire

- Fire melts Metal

- Metal chops Wood

This cycle might also be called "controls", "restrains" or "fathers".

Cosmology and Feng Shui

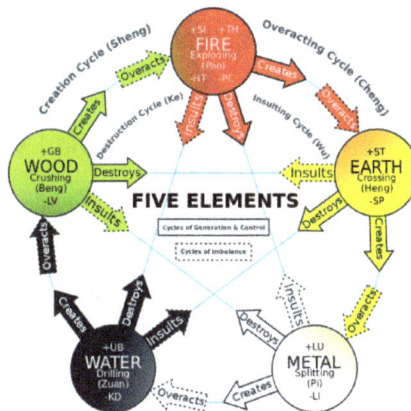

Another illustration of the cycle.

According to Wu Xing theory, the structure of the cosmos mirrors the five phases. Each phase has a complex series of associations with different aspects of nature, as can be seen in the following table. In the ancient Chinese form of geomancy known as Feng Shui practitioners all based their art and system on the five phases (Wu Xing). All of these phases are represented within the trigrams. Associated with these phases are colors, seasons and shapes; all of which are interacting with each other.

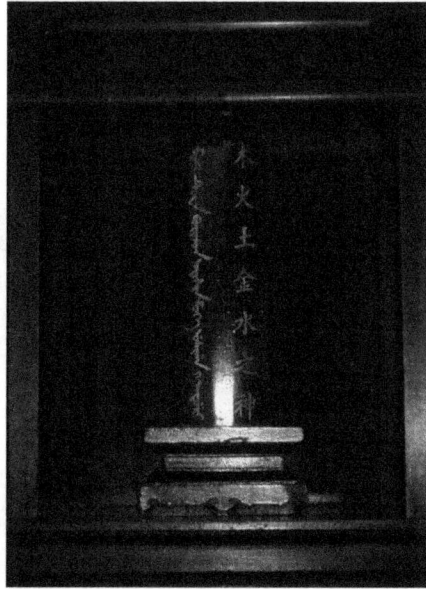

Tablet, in Chinese and Manchu, for the gods of the five elements in the Temple of Heaven. The Manchu word "usiha", meaning star, explains that this tablet is dedicated to the five basic planets, Jupiter, Mars, Saturn, Venus & Mercury rather than their respect element itself.

Based on a particular directional energy flow from one phase to the next, the interaction can be expansive, destructive, or exhaustive. A proper knowledge of each aspect of energy flow will enable the Feng Shui practitioner to apply certain cures or rearrangement of energy in a way they believe to be beneficial for the receiver of the Feng Shui Treatment.

Movement	Metal	Metal	Fire	Wood	Wood	Water	Earth	Earth
Trigram hanzi	乾	兌	離	震	巽	坎	艮	坤
Trigram pinyin	qián	duì	lí	zhèn	xùn	kǎn	gèn	kūn
Trigrams	☰	☱	☲	☳	☴	☵	☶	☷
I Ching	Heaven	Lake	Fire	Thunder	Wind	Water	Mountain	Earth
Color	Silver	White	Red	Green	Purple	Black	Blue	Yellow
Season	Fall	Fall	Summer	Spring	Spring	Winter	Intermediate	Intermediate
Cardinal direction	West	West	South	East	East	North	Center	Center

Chinese Medicine

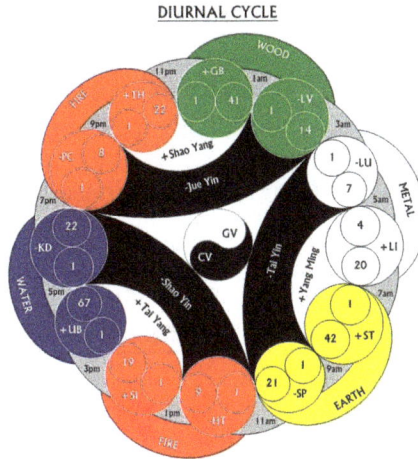

Five Chinese Elements - Diurnal Cycle

The interdependence of Zang Fu networks in the body was said to be a circle of five things, and so mapped by the Chinese doctors onto the five phases.

The Liver (Wood phase) is said to be the "mother" of the Heart (Fire phase).

The Kidneys (Water phase) the mother of the Liver.

The key observation was things like Kidney deficiency affecting the function of the Liver. In this case, the "mother" is weak, and cannot support the child.

However, the Kidneys control the Heart along the Kè cycle, so the Kidneys are claimed to restrain the Heart.

The citation order of the Five Phases, i.e., the order in which they are cited in the *Bo hu tong* 白虎通 and other Han dynasty texts, is Metal, Wood, Water, Fire, and Earth.

The organs are most effectively treated, according to theory, in the following 4-hour(2h-Yin + 2h-Yang) periods throughout the day, beginning with the 3 a.m. to 7 a. m. period:

Metal organs= Lung[Yin] 3am-5am /\ Large intestine[Yang] 5am-7am

Earth organs= Stomach[Yang] 7am-9am /\ Spleen[Yin] 9am-11am

$Fire_1$ organs= Heart[Yin] 11am-1pm /\ Small Intestine[Yang] 1pm-3pm

Water organs= Bladder[Yang] 3pm-5pm /\ Kidney[Yin] 5pm-7pm

$Fire_2$=Ministerial Fire=Lifegate Fire (the "non-empirical" Pericardium and Triple Burner organs)= Pericard[Yin] 7pm-9pm /\ Triple Burner[Yang] 9pm-11pm

Wood organs which is the reverse of the citation order (plus an extra use of Fire and the non-empirical organs to take care of the sixth four-hour period of the day) = Gallbladder[Yang] 11pm-1am /\ Liver[Yin] 1am-3am

These two orders are further related to the sequence of the planets going outward from the sun (Mercury, Venus, Mars, Jupiter, Saturn, or Water, Metal, Fire, Wood, and Earth) by a star diagram similar to the one shown above.

The sequence of the five elements (Traditional Chinese medicine)：promotion, inhibition, Wu (insult).

Movement	Wood	Fire	Earth	Metal	Water
Planet	Jupiter	Mars	Saturn	Venus	Mercury
Mental Quality	idealism, spontaneity, curiosity	passion, intensity	agreeableness, honesty	intuition, rationality, mind	erudition, resourcefulness, wit
Emotion	anger, determination	hatred, love	anxiety, joy	grief, bravery	fear, gentleness
Zang (yin organs)	liver	heart/pericardium	spleen/pancreas	lung	kidney
Fu (yang organs)	gall bladder	small intestine/San Jiao	stomach	large intestine	urinary bladder
Sensory organ	eyes	tongue	mouth	nose	ears
Body Part	tendons	pulse	muscles	skin	bones
Body Fluid	tears	sweat	saliva	mucus	urine
Finger	index finger	middle finger	thumb	ring finger	pinky finger
Sense	sight	taste	touch	smell	hearing
Taste	sour	bitter	sweet	pungent, umami	salty
Smell	rancid	scorched	fragrant	rotten	putrid
Life	birth	youth	adulthood	old age	death, conception
Animal	scaly	feathered	human	furred	shelled

Celestial Stem

Movement	Wood	Fire	Earth	Metal	Water
Heavenly Stem	Jia 甲 Yi 乙	Bing 丙 Ding 丁	Wu 戊 Ji 己	Geng 庚 Xin 辛	Ren 壬 Gui 癸
Year ends with	4, 5	6, 7	8, 9	0, 1	2, 3

Music

The *Yuèlìng* chapter (月令篇) of the *Lǐjì* (禮記) and the *Huáinánzǐ* (淮南子) make the following correlations:

Movement	Wood	Fire	Earth	Metal	Water
Colour	Green	Red	Yellow	White	Black
Arctic Direction	east	south	center	west	north
Basic Pentatonic Scale pitch	角	徵	宮	商	羽
Basic Pentatonic Scale pitch pinyin	*jué*	*zhǐ*	*gōng*	*shāng*	*yǔ*
solfege	mi or E	sol or G	do or C	re or D	la or A

- The Chinese word 青 *qīng*, has many meanings, including green, azure, cyan, and black. It refers to green in Wu Xing.

- In most modern music, various seven note or five note scales (e.g., the major scale) are defined by selecting seven or five frequencies from the set of twelve semi-tones in the Equal tempered tuning. The Chinese "lǜ" tuning is closest to the ancient Greek tuning of Pythagoras.

Martial Arts

T'ai chi ch'uan uses the five elements to designate different directions, positions or footwork patterns. Either forward, backward, left, right and centre, or three steps forward (attack) and two steps back (retreat).

The Five Steps (五步 wǔ bù):

- *Jìn bù* (進步) Forward step

- *Tùi bù* (退步) Backward step

- *Zǔo gù* (左顧, in simplified characters 左顾) Left step

- *Yòu pàn* (右盼) Right step

- *Zhōng dìng* (中定) Central position, balance, equilibrium.

Xingyiquan uses the five elements metaphorically to represent five different states of combat.

Movement	Fist	Chinese	Pinyin	Description
Metal	Splitting	劈	Pī	To split like an axe chopping up and over.
Water	Drilling	鑽	Zuān	Drilling forward horizontally like a geyser.
Wood	Crushing	崩	Bēng	To collapse, as a building collapsing in on itself.
Fire	Pounding	炮	Pào	Exploding outward like a cannon while blocking.
Earth	Crossing	橫	Héng	Crossing across the line of attack while turning over.

Tea Ceremony

There are spring, summer, fall, and winter teas. The perennial tea ceremony ("perennial", literally means four steps or sequences that are linked together, each representing a season of the year) includes four tea settings (茶席) and a tea master (司茶). The tea settings are:

- earth, (Incense), yellow, center, up and down

- wood, 春風 (Spring Wind), green, east

- fire, 夏露 (Summer Dew), red, south

- metal, 秋籟 (Fall Sounds), white, west

- water, 冬陽 (Winter Sunshine) black/blue, north

Each tea setting is arranged and stands for the four directions (north, south, east, and west). A vase of the seasons' flowers is put on tea table. Sometimes if four tea masters are included then five chairs are arranged per tea setting, making a total of twenty plus the 4 tea masters equalling 24, which symbolizes the 24 solar terms of the Chinese calendar, and represents that nature continues or is perennial.

Taijitu

A taijitu (Traditional Chinese: 太極圖; Simplified Chinese: 太极图; Pinyin: tàijítú; Wade-Giles: t'ai⁴chi²t'u²) is a symbol or diagram (图 *tú*) in Chinese philosophy representing Taiji (太极 *tàijí* "great pole" or "supreme ultimate") representing both its monist (*wuji*) and its dualist (yin and yang) aspects. Such a diagram was first introduced by Song Dynasty philosopher Zhou Dunyi (周敦頤 1017–1073) in his *Taijitu shuo* 太極圖說.

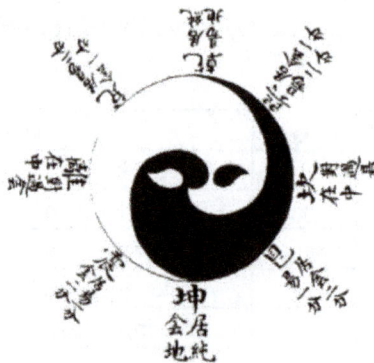

18th-century representation of the *taijitu* of Zhao Huiqian (1370s)

The modern Daoist canon, compiled during the Ming era, has at least half a dozen variants of such *taijitu*. The two most similar are the "Taiji Primal Heaven" (太極先天

圖 *tàijí xiāntiān tú*) and the "wuji" (無極圖 *wújí tú*) diagrams, both of which have been extensively studied during the Qing period for their possible connection with Zhou Dunyi's *taijitu*.

Ming period author Lai Zhide (1525–1604) simplified the *taijitu* to a design of two interlocking spirals. In the Ming era, the combination of the two interlocking spirals of the *taijitu* with two black-and-white dots superimposed on them became identified with the *He tu* or "Yellow River diagram" (河圖). This version was reported in Western literature of the late 19th century as the "Great Monad", and has been widely popularised in Western popular culture as the "yin-yang symbol" since the 1960s. The contemporary Chinese term for the modern symbol is 太极两仪图 "two-part Taiji diagram".

Unicode features the "yin-yang symbol" in the Miscellaneous Symbols block, at code point U+262F (YIN YANG ☯). The related "double body symbol" is included at U+0F-CA (TIBETAN SYMBOL NOR BU NYIS -KHYIL ࿊), in the Tibetan block.

Ornamental patterns with visual similarity to the "yin-yang symbol" are found in archaeological artefacts of European prehistory; such designs are sometimes descriptively dubbed "yin yang symbols" in archaeological literature by modern scholars.

Structure

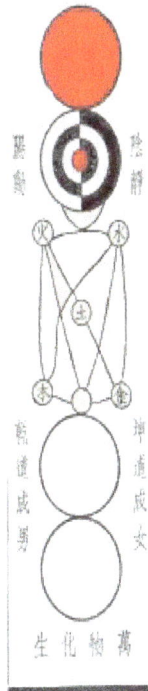

Ming-era Daoist *Taijitu*

The *taijitu* consists of five parts. Strictly speaking the "yin and yang symbol", itself popularly called *taijitu*, represents the second of these five parts of the diagram.

- At the top, an empty circle depicts the absolute (*Wuji*)

- A second circle represents the Taiji as harboring Dualism, yin and yang, represented by filling the circle in a black-and-white pattern. In some diagrams, there is a smaller empty circle at the center of this, representing Emptiness as the foundation of duality.

- Below this second circle is a five-part diagram representing the Five Agents (*Wuxing*), representing a further stage in the differentiation of Unity into Multiplicity. The Five Agents are connected by lines indicating their proper sequence, Wood (木) → Fire (火) → Earth (土) → Metal (金) → Water (水).

- The circle below the Five Agents represents the conjunction of Heaven and Earth, which in turn gives rise to the "ten thousand things". This stage is also represented by the Eight Trigrams (*Bagua*).

- The final circle represents the state of multiplicity, glossed "The ten thousand things are born by transformation" (生化物萬; modern 化生万物)

History

The term *taijitu* in modern Chinese is commonly used to mean the simple "divided circle" form (☯), but it may refer to any of several schematic diagrams that contain at least one circle with an inner pattern of symmetry representing yin and yang.

Song Era

While the concept of yin and yang dates to Chinese antiquity, the interest in "diagrams" (圖 *tú*) is an intellectual fashion of Neo-Confucianism during the Song period (11th century), and it declined again in the Ming period, by the 16th century.

The original description of a *taijitu* is due to Song era philosopher Zhou Dunyi (1017–1073), author of the *Taijitu shuo* 太極圖說 "Explanation of the Diagram of the Supreme Ultimate", which became the cornerstone of Neo-Confucianist cosmology. His brief text synthesized aspects of Chinese Buddhism and Taoism with metaphysical discussions in the *Yijing*.

Zhou's key terms Wuji and Taiji appear in the opening line 無極而太極, which Adler notes could also be translated "The Supreme Polarity that is Non-Polar".

Non-polar (*wuji*) and yet Supreme Polarity (*taiji*)! The Supreme Polarity in activity generates *yang*; yet at the limit of activity it is still. In stillness it generates *yin*; yet at the limit of stillness it is also active. Activity and stillness alternate; each is the basis of the other. In distinguishing *yin* and *yang*, the Two Modes are thereby established. The alternation and combination of *yang* and *yin* generate water, fire, wood, metal, and earth. With these five [phases of] *qi* harmoniously arranged, the Four Seasons proceed through them. The Five Phases are simply *yin* and *yang*; *yin* and *yang* are simply the Supreme Polarity; the Supreme Polarity is fundamentally Non-polar. [Yet] in the generation of the Five Phases, each one has its nature.

Instead of usual *Taiji* translations "Supreme Ultimate" or "Supreme Pole", Adler uses "Supreme Polarity" because Zhu Xi describes it as the alternating principle of *yin* and *yang*, and ...

insists that *taiji* is not a thing (hence "Supreme Pole" will not do). Thus, for both Zhou and Zhu, *taiji* is the *yin-yang* principle of bipolarity, which is the most fundamental ordering principle, the cosmic "first principle." *Wuji* as "non-polar" follows from this.

Since the 12th century, there has been a vigorous discussion in Chinese philosophy regarding the ultimate origin of Zhou Dunyi's diagram. Zhu Xi (12th century) insists that Zhou Dunyi had composed the diagram himself, against the prevailing view that he had received it from Daoist sources. Zhu Xi could not accept a Daoist origin of the design, because it would have undermined the claim of uniqueness attached to the Neo-Confucian concept of *dao*.

Ming Era

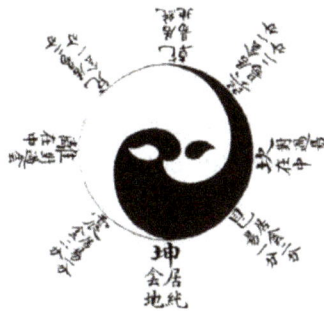

Diagram from of Zhao Huiqian's *Liushu benyi* (1370s) as represented in the *Siku Quanshu* edition (1751).

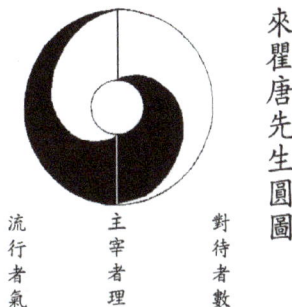

Simplified form of Lai Zhide's "*Taiji* River Diagram" (1599).

While Zhou Dunyi (1017–1073) popularized the circular diagram, the introduction of "swirling" patterns first appears in the Ming period.

Zhao Huiqian (趙撝謙, 1351–1395) was the first to introduce the "swirling" variant of the *taijitu* in his *Liushu benyi* (六書本義, 1370s). The diagram is combined with the eight trigrams (*bagua*) and called the "River Chart spontaneously generated by Heaven and Earth". By the end of the Ming period, this diagram had become a widespread representation of Chinese cosmology. The dots are introduced in the later Ming period (replacing the droplet-shapes used earlier, in the 16th century) and are encountered more frequently in the Qing period.

Lai Zhide's design is similar to the *gakyil* (*dga' 'khyil* or "wheel of joy") symbols of Tibetan Buddhism; but while the Tibetan designs have three or four swirls (representing the Three Jewels or the Four Noble Truths, i.e. as a triskele and a tetraskele design), Lai Zhide's taijitu has two swirls, terminating in a central circle.

Modern Yin-yang Symbol

The Ming-era design of the taijitu of two interlocking spirals has been reported as "yin-yang symbol" in the first half of the 20th century. The flag of South Korea, originally introduced as the flag of Joseon era Korea in 1882, shows this symbol in red and blue. This was a modernisation of the older (early 19th century) form of the Bat Quai Do used as the Joseon royal standard.

Since the 1960s, "yin-yang symbol" is most widely applied to the *He tu* symbol which combines the two interlocking spirals with two dots. In the standard form of the contemporary "yin-yang symbol", one draws on the diameter of a circle two non-overlapping circles each of which has a diameter equal to the radius of the outer circle. One keeps the line that forms an "S," and one erases or obscures the other line. The design is also described "pair of fishes nestling head to tail against each other".

The modern symbol has also been widely used in martial arts, particularly t'ai chi ch'uan (Taijiquan), and Jeet Kune Do, since the 1970s. In this context, it is generally used to represent the interplay between hard and soft techniques.

The dots in the modern "yin-yang symbol" have been given the additional interpretation of "intense interaction" between the complementary principles.

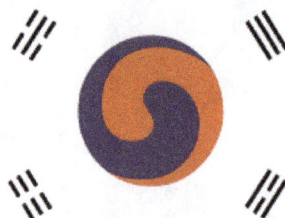

The 1882 flag of Korea (since 1949 the flag of South Korea)

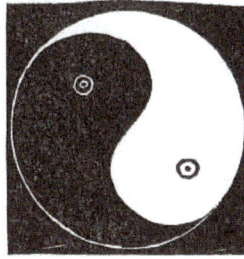

"The Great Monad" from Edna Kenton's *Book of Earths* (1928),
after the design shown by Hampden Coit DuBose (1887)

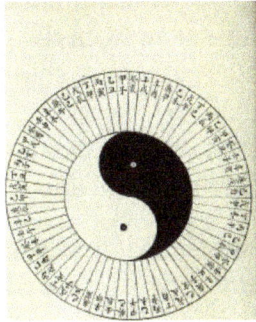

The "cycle of Cathay" as depicted by William Alexander Parsons Martin in 1897.

Comparison with Prehistoric Symbols

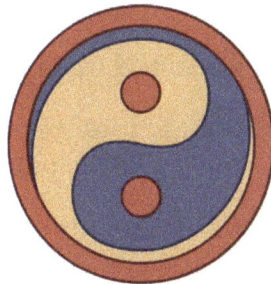

Shield pattern of the Western Roman infantry unit *armigeri defensores seniores* (ca. AD 430).

As discussed above, a modern form of the "yin yang symbol" is by no means representative of graphical representations of *tajitu* prior to the 19th century, but it has become widely recognizable, and the term is also used for unrelated designs dividing a circle by an "S"-shape. Such unrelated designs are widespread, and are found, for example, in artefacts of the European Neolithic. Such similarities have notably been used to illustrate a supposed "similarity of Tripilja culture and the culture of ancient China" in the Ukraine pavilion at the Expo 2010 in Shanghai, China. The "interlocking comma" design is also found in artefacts of the European Iron Age, popularly dubbed "Celtic yin-yang". While the design appears to become a standard ornamental motif in the La Tène culture by the 3rd century BC, found on a wide variety of artefacts, it is not clear what symbolic value, if any, was attached to it. Unlike the classic Taoist symbol, the

"Celtic yin-yang" whorls consistently lack the element of mutual penetration, and the two halves are not always portrayed in different colors. Comparable designs are also found in Etruscan art.

Feng Shui

Feng Shui (pinyin: *fēng shuǐ*, pronounced [fɤˊ ŋ ʂwèi] (listen) *FUNG shway*) is a Chinese philosophical system of harmonizing everyone with the surrounding environment. It is closely linked to Taoism. The term *feng shui* literally translates as "wind-water" in English. This is a cultural shorthand taken from the passage of the now-lost *Classic of Burial* recorded in Guo Pu's commentary: Feng shui is one of the Five Arts of Chinese Metaphysics, classified as physiognomy (observation of appearances through formulas and calculations). The feng shui practice discusses architecture in metaphoric terms of "invisible forces" that bind the universe, earth, and humanity together, known as *qi*.

There is no replicable scientific evidence that feng shui's mystical claims are real, and it is considered by the scientific community to be pseudoscience.

Historically, feng shui was widely used to orient buildings—often spiritually significant structures such as tombs, but also dwellings and other structures—in an auspicious manner. Depending on the particular style of feng shui being used, an auspicious site could be determined by reference to local features such as bodies of water, stars, or a compass.

Qi rides the wind and scatters, but is retained when encountering water.

Feng shui was suppressed in mainland China during the state-imposed Cultural Revolution of the 1960s but has since then regained popularity.

The Skeptic Encyclopedia of Pseudoscience briefly summarizes the history and practice of feng shui. It states that the principles of feng shui related to living harmoniously with nature are "quite rational," but does not otherwise lend credibility to the nonscientific claims. After a comprehensive 2016 evaluation of the subject by scientific skeptic author Brian Dunning, he concluded that there is nothing demonstrably real at all about the practice and stated that:

There's no real science behind feng shui... It's also a simple matter to dismiss the mystical energies said to be at its core; they simply don't exist.

History

Origins

As of 2013 the Yangshao and Hongshan cultures provide the earliest known evidence for the use of feng shui. Until the invention of the magnetic compass, feng shui apparently relied on astronomy to find correlations between humans and the universe. In 4000 BC, the doors of Banpo dwellings aligned with the asterism *Yingshi* just after the winter solstice—this sited the homes for solar gain. During the Zhou era, *Yingshi* was known as *Ding* and used to indicate the appropriate time to build a capital city, according to the *Shijing*. The late Yangshao site at Dadiwan (c. 3500-3000 BC) includes a palace-like building (F901) at the center. The building faces south and borders a large plaza. It stands on a north-south axis with another building that apparently housed communal activities. Regional communities may have used the complex.

A grave at Puyang (around 4000 BC) that contains mosaics— actually a Chinese star map of the Dragon and Tiger asterisms and Beidou (the Big Dipper, Ladle or Bushel)— is oriented along a north-south axis. The presence of both round and square shapes in the Puyang tomb, at Hongshan ceremonial centers and at the late Longshan settlement at Lutaigang, suggests that *gaitian* cosmography (heaven-round, earth-square) existed in Chinese society long before it appeared in the *Zhou Bi Suan Jing*.

Cosmography that bears a striking resemblance to modern feng shui devices and formulas appears on a piece of jade unearthed at Hanshan and dated around 3000 BC. Archaeologist Li Xueqin links the design to the *liuren* astrolabe, *zhinan zhen*, and luopan.

Beginning with palatial structures at Erlitou, all capital cities of China followed rules of feng shui for their design and layout. During the Zhou era, the *Kaogong ji* (simplified Chinese: 考工记; traditional Chinese: 考工記; "Manual of Crafts") codified these rules. The carpenter's manual *Lu ban jing* (simplified Chinese: 鲁班经; traditional Chinese: 鲁班經; "Lu ban's manuscript") codified rules for builders. Graves and tombs also followed rules of feng shui, from Puyang to Mawangdui and beyond. From the earliest records, the structures of the graves and dwellings seem to have followed the same rules.

Early Instruments and Techniques

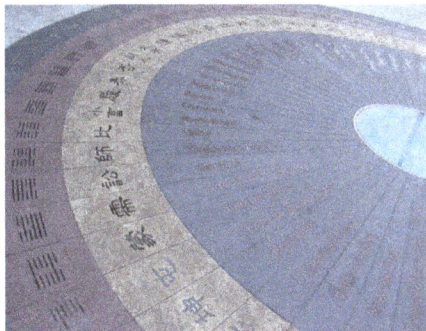

A feng shui spiral at LA Chinatown's Metro station

The history of feng shui covers 3,500+ years before the invention of the magnetic compass. It originated in Chinese astronomy. Some current techniques can be traced to Neolithic China, while others were added later (most notably the Han dynasty, the Tang, the Song, and the Ming).

The astronomical history of feng shui is evident in the development of instruments and techniques. According to the *Zhouli*, the original feng shui instrument may have been a *gnomon*. Chinese used circumpolar stars to determine the north-south axis of settlements. This technique explains why Shang palaces at Xiaotun lie 10° east of due north. In some cases, as Paul Wheatley observed, they bisected the angle between the directions of the rising and setting sun to find north. This technique provided the more precise alignments of the Shang walls at Yanshi and Zhengzhou. Rituals for using a feng shui instrument required a diviner to examine current sky phenomena to set the device and adjust their position in relation to the device.

The oldest examples of instruments used for feng shui are *liuren* astrolabes, also known as *shi*. These consist of a lacquered, two-sided board with astronomical sightlines. The earliest examples of liuren astrolabes have been unearthed from tombs that date between 278 BC and 209 BC. Along with divination for Da Liu Ren the boards were commonly used to chart the motion of Taiyi through the nine palaces. The markings on a *liuren/shi* and the first magnetic compasses are virtually identical.

The magnetic compass was invented for feng shui and has been in use since its invention. Traditional feng shui instrumentation consists of the Luopan or the earlier south-pointing spoon (指南針 *zhinan zhen*)—though a conventional compass could suffice if one understood the differences. A feng shui ruler (a later invention) may also be employed.

Foundation Theories

The goal of feng shui as practiced today is to situate the human-built environment on spots with good *qi*. The "perfect spot" is a location and an axis in time.

Qi (Ch'i)

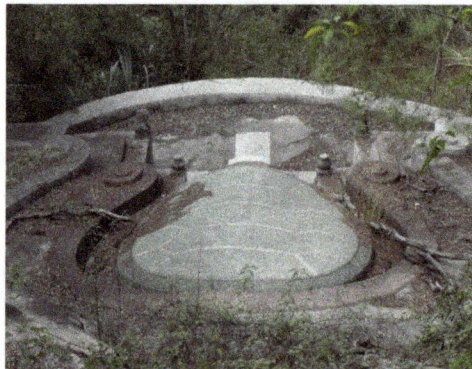

A traditional turtle-back tomb of southern Fujian, surrounded by an omega-shaped
ridge protecting it from the "noxious winds" from the three sides

Qi（氣）(pronounced "chee" in English) is a movable positive or negative life force which plays an essential role in feng shui. In feng shui as in Chinese martial arts, it refers to 'energy', in the sense of 'life force' or *élan vital*. A traditional explanation of *qi* as it relates to feng shui would include the orientation of a structure, its age, and its interaction with the surrounding environment, including the local microclimates, the slope of the land, vegetation, and soil quality.

The *Book of Burial* says that burial takes advantage of "vital *qi*". Wu Yuanyin (Qing dynasty) said that vital *qi* was "congealed *qi*", which is the state of *qi* that engenders life. The goal of feng shui is to take advantage of vital *qi* by appropriate siting of graves and structures. Some people destroyed graveyards of their enemies to weaken their qi.

One use for a *loupan* is to detect the flow of *qi*. Magnetic compasses reflect local geomagnetism which includes geomagnetically induced currents caused by space weather. Professor Max Knoll suggested in a 1951 lecture that qi is a form of solar radiation. As space weather changes over time, and the quality of *qi* rises and falls over time, feng shui with a compass might be considered a form of divination that assesses the quality of the local environment—including the effects of space weather. Often people with good karma live in land with good qi.

Polarity

Polarity is expressed in feng shui as *yin* and *yang* theory. Polarity expressed through *yin* and *yang* is similar to a magnetic dipole. That is, it is of two parts: one creating an exertion and one receiving the exertion. *Yang* acting and *yin* receiving could be considered an early understanding of chirality. The development of this theory and its corollary, five phase theory (five element theory), have also been linked with astronomical observations of sunspots.

The Five Elements or Forces (*wu xing*) – which, according to the Chinese, are metal, earth, fire, water, and wood – are first mentioned in Chinese literature in a chapter of the classic *Book of History*. They play a very important part in Chinese thought: 'elements' meaning generally not so much the actual substances as the forces essential to human life. Earth is a buffer, or an equilibrium achieved when the polarities cancel each other. While the goal of Chinese medicine is to balance yin and yang in the body, the goal of feng shui has been described as aligning a city, site, building, or object with yin-yang force fields.

Bagua (Eight Trigrams)

Two diagrams known as *bagua* (or *pa kua*) loom large in feng shui, and both predate their mentions in the *Yijing* (or *I Ching*). The *Lo (River) Chart* (*Luoshu*) was developed first, and is sometimes associated with *Later Heaven* arrangement of the bagua. This and the *Yellow River Chart* (*Hetu*, sometimes associated with the *Earlier Heaven bagua*) are linked to astronomical events of the sixth millennium BC, and with the Turtle Calendar from the time of Yao. The Turtle Calendar of Yao (found in the *Yaodian* section of the *Shangshu* or *Book of Documents*) dates to 2300 BC, plus or minus 250 years.

In *Yaodian*, the cardinal directions are determined by the marker-stars of the mega-constellations known as the Four Celestial Animals:

East

> The Azure Dragon (Spring equinox)—*Niao* (Bird 鳥), α Scorpionis

South

> The Vermilion Bird (Summer solstice)—*Huo* (Fire 火), α Hydrae

West

> The White Tiger (Autumn equinox)—*Măo* (Hair 毛), η Tauri (the Pleiades)

North

> The Black Tortoise (Winter solstice)—*Xū* (Emptiness, Void 虛), α Aquarii, β Aquarii

The diagrams are also linked with the *sifang* (four directions) method of divination used during the Shang dynasty. The *sifang* is much older, however. It was used at Niuheliang, and figured large in Hongshan culture's astronomy. And it is this area of China that is linked to Yellow Emperor (Huangdi) who allegedly invented the south-pointing spoon.

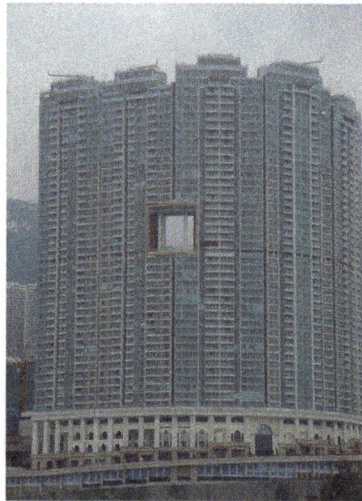

A building in Hong Kong with a hollow middle hole, utilizing feng shui benefits

Traditional Feng Shui

Traditional feng shui is an ancient system based upon the observation of heavenly time and earthly space. The literature of ancient China, as well as archaeological evidence, provide some idea of the origins and nature of the original feng shui techniques.

Form School

The Form School is the oldest school of feng shui. Qing Wuzi in the Han dynasty describes it in the "Book of the Tomb" and Guo Pu of the Jin dynasty follows up with a more complete description in *The Book of Burial*

The Form School was originally concerned with the location and orientation of tombs (Yin House feng shui), which was of great importance. The school then progressed to the consideration of homes and other buildings (Yang House feng shui).

The "form" in Form School refers to the shape of the environment, such as mountains, rivers, plateaus, buildings, and general surroundings. It considers the five celestial animals (phoenix, green dragon, white tiger, black turtle, and the yellow snake), the yin-yang concept and the traditional five elements (Wu Xing: wood, fire, earth, metal, and water).

The Form School analyses the shape of the land and flow of the wind and water to find a place with ideal qi. It also considers the time of important events such as the birth of the resident and the building of the structure.

Compass School

The Compass School is a collection of more recent feng shui techniques based on the eight cardinal directions, each of which is said to have unique qi. It uses the Luopan, a disc marked with formulas in concentric rings around a magnetic compass.

The Compass School includes techniques such as Flying Star and Eight Mansions.

Transmission of Traditional Feng Shui Techniques

Aside from the books written throughout history by feng shui masters and students, there is also a strong oral history. In many cases, masters have passed on their techniques only to selected students or relatives.

Current Usage of Traditional Schools

There is no contemporary agreement that one of the traditional schools is most correct. Therefore, modern practitioners of feng shui generally draw from multiple schools in their own practices.

Western Forms of Feng Shui

More recent forms of feng shui simplify principles that come from the traditional schools, and focus mainly on the use of the bagua.

Aspirations Method

The Eight Life Aspirations style of feng shui is a simple system which coordinates each of the eight cardinal directions with a specific life aspiration or station such as family, wealth, fame, etc., which come from the Bagua government of the eight aspirations. Life Aspirations is not otherwise a geomantic system.

Black Sect

Thomas Lin Yun introduced Black Sect Tantric Buddhism Feng Shui to America in the 1970s. Black Sect is a religion that goes beyond feng shui to include elements of transcendentalism, Taoism and Tibetan Buddhism. Black Sect is concerned mainly with the interior of a building. Instead of orienting the bagua to the compass, it is oriented to the entryway. Each of the eight sectors represent a particular area of one's life.

List of Specific Feng Shui Schools

Ti Li (Form School)

Popular Xingshi Pai (形势派) "forms" methods

- Luan Tou Pai, 巒頭派, Pinyin: luán tóu pài, (environmental analysis without using a compass)

- Xing Xiang Pai, 形象派 or 形像派, Pinyin: xíng xiàng pài, (Imaging forms)

- Xingfa Pai, 形法派, Pinyin: xíng fǎ pài

Liiqi Pai (Compass School)

Popular Liiqi Pai (理气派) "Compass" methods

San Yuan Method, 三元派 (Pinyin: sān yuán pài)

- Dragon Gate Eight Formation, 龍門八法 (Pinyin: lóng mén bā fǎ)

- Xuan Kong, 玄空 (time and space methods)

- Xuan Kong Fei Xing 玄空飛星 (Flying Stars methods of time and directions)

- Xuan Kong Da Gua, 玄空大卦 ("Secret Decree" or 64 gua relationships)

- Xuan Kong Mi Zi, 玄空秘旨 (Mysterious Space Secret Decree)

- Xuan Kong Liu Fa, 玄空六法 (Mysterious Space Six Techniques)

- Zi Bai Jue, 紫白訣 (Purple White Scroll)

San He Method, 三合派 (environmental analysis using a compass)

- Accessing Dragon Methods

- Ba Zhai, 八宅 (Eight Mansions)

- Yang Gong Feng Shui, 杨公风水

- Water Methods, 河洛水法

- Local Embrace

Others

- Yin House Feng Shui, 阴宅风水 (Feng Shui for the deceased)

- Four Pillars of Destiny, 四柱命理 (a form of hemerology)

- Zi Wei Dou Shu, 紫微斗数 (Purple Star Astrology)

- I-Ching, 易经 (Book of Changes)

- Qi Men Dun Jia, 奇门遁甲 (Mysterious Door Escaping Techniques)

- Da Liu Ren, 大六壬 (Divination: Big Six Heavenly Yang Water Qi)

- Tai Yi Shen Shu, 太乙神数 (Divination: Tai Yi Magical Calculation Method)

- Date Selection, 择日 (Selection of auspicious dates and times for important events)

- Chinese Palmistry, 掌相学 (Destiny reading by palm reading)

- Chinese Face Reading, 面相学 (Destiny reading by face reading)

- Major & Minor Wandering Stars (Constellations)

- Five phases, 五行 (relationship of the five phases or *wuxing*)

- BTB Black (Hat) Tantric Buddhist Sect (Westernised or Modern methods not based on Classical teachings)

- Symbolic Feng Shui, (new-age Feng Shui methods that advocate substitution with symbolic (spiritual, appropriate representation of five elements) objects if natural environment or object/s is/are not available or viable)

- Pierce Method of Feng Shui (Sometimes Pronounced : Von Shway) The practice of melding striking with soothing furniture arrangements to promote peace and prosperity

Contemporary Uses of Traditional Feng Shui

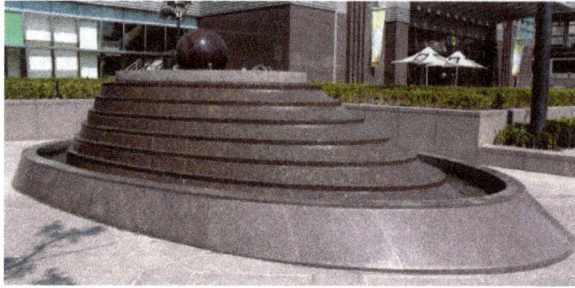

A modern "feng shui fountain" at Taipei 101, Taiwan

- Landscape ecologists often find traditional feng shui an interesting study. In many cases, the only remaining patches of old forest in Asia are "feng shui woods", associated with cultural heritage, historical continuity, and the preservation of various flora and fauna species. Some researchers interpret the presence of these woods as indicators that the "healthy homes", sustainability and environmental components of *ancient* feng shui should not be easily dismissed.

- Environmental scientists and landscape architects have researched traditional feng shui and its methodologies.

- Architects study feng shui as an ancient and uniquely Asian architectural tradition.

- Geographers have analyzed the techniques and methods to help locate historical sites in Victoria, British Columbia, Canada, and archaeological sites in the American Southwest, concluding that ancient Native Americans also considered astronomy and landscape features.

Criticisms

Traditional Feng Shui

Traditional feng shui relies upon the compass to give accurate readings. However, critics point out that the compass degrees are often inaccurate as fluctuations caused by solar winds have the ability to greatly disturb the electromagnetic field of the earth. Determining a property or site location based upon Magnetic North will result in inaccuracies because true magnetic north fluctuates.

Matteo Ricci (1552–1610), one of the founding fathers of Jesuit China missions, may have been the first European to write about feng shui practices. His account in *De Christiana expeditione apud Sinas...* tells about feng shui masters (*geologi*, in Latin) studying prospective construction sites or grave sites "with reference to the head and the tail and the feet of the particular dragons which are supposed to dwell beneath that spot". As a Catholic missionary, Ricci strongly criticized the "recondite science" of geomancy along with astrology as yet another *superstitio absurdissima* of the heathens: "What could be more absurd than their imagining that the safety of a family, honors, and their entire existence must depend upon such trifles as a door being opened from one side or another, as rain falling into a courtyard from the right or from the left, a window opened here or there, or one roof being higher than another?".

Victorian-era commentators on feng shui were generally ethnocentric, and as such skeptical and derogatory of what they knew of feng shui. In 1896, at a meeting of the Educational Association of China, Rev. P.W. Pitcher railed at the "rottenness of the whole scheme of Chinese architecture," and urged fellow missionaries "to erect unabashedly Western edifices of several stories and with towering spires in order to destroy nonsense about *fung-shuy*".

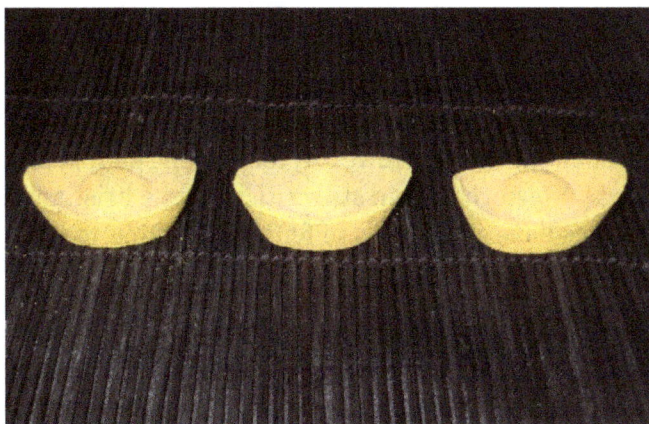

Sycee-shaped incense used in feng shui

After the founding of the People's Republic of China in 1949, feng shui was officially considered a "feudalistic superstitious practice" and a "social evil" according to the state's ideology and was discouraged and even banned outright at times. Feng shui remained popular in Hong Kong, and also in the Republic of China (Taiwan), where traditional culture was not suppressed.

Persecution was the most severe during the Cultural Revolution, when feng shui was classified as a custom under the so-called Four Olds to be wiped out. Feng shui practitioners were beaten and abused by Red Guards and their works burned. After the death of Mao Zedong and the end of the Cultural Revolution, the official attitude became more tolerant but restrictions on feng shui practice are still in place in today's China. It is illegal in the PRC today to register feng shui consultation as a business and similarly advertising feng shui practice is banned. There have been frequent crackdowns on feng shui practitioners on the grounds of "promoting feudalistic superstitions" such as one in Qingdao in early 2006 when the city's business and industrial administration office shut down an art gallery converted into a feng shui practice. Some communist officials who had previously consulted feng shui were terminated and expelled from the Communist Party.

Partly because of the Cultural Revolution, in today's mainland China less than one-third of the population believe in feng shui, and the proportion of believers among young urban Chinese is said to be much lower Learning feng shui is still somewhat considered taboo in today's China. Nevertheless, it is reported that feng shui has gained adherents among Communist Party officials according to a BBC Chinese news commentary in 2006, and since the beginning of Chinese economic reforms the number of feng shui practitioners is increasing. A number of Chinese academics permitted to research on the subject of feng shui are anthropologists or architects by profession, studying the history of feng shui or historical feng shui theories behind the design of heritage buildings, such as Cao Dafeng, the Vice-President of Fudan University, and Liu Shenghuan of Tongji University.

Contemporary Feng Shui

Westerners were criticized at the start of the anti-Western Boxer Rebellion for violating the basic principles of feng shui in the construction of railroads and other conspicuous public structures throughout China. However, today, feng shui is practiced not only by the Chinese, but also by Westerners and still criticized by Christians around the world. Many modern Christians have an opinion of feng shui similar to that of their predecessors:

It is entirely inconsistent with Christianity to believe that harmony and balance result from the manipulation and channeling of nonphysical forces or energies, or that such can be done by means of the proper placement of physical objects. Such techniques, in fact, belong to the world of sorcery.

Still others are simply skeptical of feng shui. Evidence for its effectiveness is based primarily upon anecdote and users are often offered conflicting advice from different practitioners. Feng shui practitioners use these differences as evidence of variations in practice or different schools of thought. Critical analysts have described it thus: "Feng shui has always been based upon mere guesswork". Some are skeptical of feng shui's lasting impact Mark Johnson:

This present state of affairs is ludicrous and confusing. Do we really believe that mirrors and flutes are going to change people's tendencies in any lasting and meaningful way? ... There is a lot of investigation that needs to be done or we will all go down the tubes because of our inability to match our exaggerated claims with lasting changes.

Nonetheless, after Richard Nixon journeyed to the People's Republic of China in 1972, feng shui became marketable in the United States and has since been reinvented by New Age entrepreneurs for Western consumption. Critics of contemporary feng shui are concerned that with the passage of time much of the theory behind it has been lost in translation, not paid proper consideration, frowned upon, or even scorned. Robert T. Carroll sums up what feng shui has become in some instances:

...feng shui has become an aspect of interior decorating in the Western world and alleged masters of feng shui now hire themselves out for hefty sums to tell people such as Donald Trump which way his doors and other things should hang. Feng shui has also become another New Age "energy" scam with arrays of metaphysical products...offered for sale to help you improve your health, maximize your potential, and guarantee fulfillment of some fortune cookie philosophy.

Others have noted how, when feng shui is not applied properly, it can even harm the environment, such as was the case of people planting "lucky bamboo" in ecosystems that could not handle them.

Feng shui practitioners in China find superstitious and corrupt officials easy prey, despite official disapproval. In one instance, in 2009, feng shui practitioners gulled county officials in Gansu into hauling a 369-ton "spirit rock" to the county seat to ward off "bad luck."

The stage magician duo Penn and Teller dedicated an episode of their *Bullshit!* television show to criticise the construal of contemporary practice of Feng Shui in the Western World as science. In this episode, they devised a test in which the same dwelling was visited by five different Feng Shui consultants, all five producing different opinions about said dwelling, by which means it was attempted to show there is no consistency in the professional practice of Feng Shui.

Feng Shui Practice Today

Apart from any mystical implications, Feng Shui may be simply understood as a traditional test of architectural goodness using a collection of metaphors. The test may be static or a simulation. Simulations may involve moving an imaginary person or organic creature, such as a dragon of a certain size and flexibility, through a floor plan to uncover awkward turns and cramped spaces before actual construction. This is entirely analogous to imagining how a wheelchair might pass through a building, and is a plausible exercise for architects, who are expected to have exceptional spatial visualization talents. A static test might try to measure comfort in architecture through a 'hills and valleys' metaphor. The big hill at your back is a metaphor for security, the open valley and stream represents air and light, and the circle of low hills in front represents both invitation to visitors and your control of your immediate environment. The various Feng Shui tenets represent a set of metaphors that suggest architectural qualities that the average human finds comfortable.

Many Asians, especially people of Chinese descent, believe it is important to live a prosperous and healthy life as evident by the popularity of Fu Lu Shou in the Chinese communities. Many of the higher-level forms of feng shui are not easily practiced without having connections in the community or a certain amount of wealth because hiring an expert, altering architecture or design, and moving from place to place requires a significant financial output. This leads some people of the lower classes to lose faith in feng shui, saying that it is only a game for the wealthy. Others, however, practice less expensive forms of feng shui, including hanging special (but cheap) mirrors, forks, or woks in doorways to deflect negative energy.

In recent years,a new brand of easier-to-implement DIY Feng Shui known as *Symbolic Feng Shui*, which is popularized by Grandmaster Lillian Too, is being practised by Feng Shui enthusiasts. It entails placements of auspicious (and preferably aesthetically pleasing) Five Element objects, such as *Money God* and *tortoise*, at various locations of the house so as to achieve a pleasing and substitute-alternative *Productive-Cycle* environment if a good natural environment is not already present or is too expensive to build and implement.

Feng shui is so important to some strong believers, that they use it for healing purposes (although there is no empirical evidence that this practice is in any way effective) in addition to guide their businesses and create a peaceful atmosphere in their homes, in particular in the bedroom where a number of techniques involving colours and arrangement are used to achieve enhanced comfort and more peaceful sleep. In 2005, even Disney acknowledged feng shui as an important part of Chinese culture by shifting the main gate to Hong Kong Disneyland by twelve degrees in their building plans, among many other actions suggested by the master planner of architecture and design at Walt Disney Imagineering, Wing Chao, in an effort to incorporate local culture into the theme park.

At Singapore Polytechnic and other institutions, many working professionals from various disciplines (including engineers, architects, property agents and interior designers) take courses on feng shui and divination every year with a number of them becoming part-time or full-time feng shui (or geomancy) consultants eventually.

Feng Shui in the Southern Hemisphere

There is a divergence between some Feng Shui schools on the need or not to adapt the ancient Chinese theories when feng shui is used in the Southern Hemisphere. The differences between the two hemispheres are a fact of reality, but its influence on the feng shui not is unanimity among scholars and practitioners of Chinese technique.

The Feng Shui schools to the Southern Hemisphere defend the need for changes, that span the Feng Shui and Chinese Astrology 4 Pillars. Among the main arguments for changes to be made can be cited:

- The "Ba Gua" - octagon with a trigram on each side - is the cycle of the stations. In the Southern Hemisphere the seasons are reversed in relation to the Northern Hemisphere. So the Ba Gua should reflect these differences.

- The "Luo Pan" - Chinese compass with all formulas of Feng Shui summarized in a grid disc - was created to be used in regions that lack natural elements and landforms. Method of flying stars.

- The Coriolis effect causes the air currents and water rotate in opposite directions in the two hemispheres: counterclockwise in the Northern Hemisphere and clockwise in the Southern Hemisphere This effect causes a mirror in the distribution of energy on the surface of the globe..

- A new perspective, Feng Shui course, defends the adaptation of the Ba-gua Later Heaven Sequence for the Southern Hemisphere based on trigrams (and its correlation with the seasons) and the Northern Hemisphere Stars guide and the Hemisphere South: Polaris and Alpha-Crux. Feng Shui course created the Solar Method of the Four Seasons, unprecedented and valid method in both hemispheres. This perspective understands the profound Chinese philosophical and updated in Time and Space this important tool to create harmony and prosperity.

The validity of these statements can involve discussions and studies. The following article outlines some reasons and methods used by adopting the adjustments to the Southern Hemisphere.

Feng Shui in Brazil (for Example)

The application of feng shui depends on where we are on earth, the place of geography, near a river, where supposedly "energy flows", is moving or near a mountain where energy accumulates. In the case of people: where they are born, where they live.

Speaking in geographical coordinates, east and west remains, plus the equator acts as a mirror dividing Earth into two hemispheres, north and south.

In the Northern Hemisphere cold it is in the north - the Arctic, and the heat in the South the equator. Unlike the Southern Hemisphere where the heat is in the north, the cold is in sul_ Antarctica. The seasons also are reversed. When it is summer in the southern hemisphere, it is winter in the Northern Hemisphere. When it is autumn in the Southern Hemisphere, it is spring in the northern hemisphere, and vice versa. The I Ching mentions that we must turn to the light side, to meditate, i.e. sul in the Northern Hemisphere; which corresponds to turn north in the southern hemisphere. This is based on the position of the sun, which in the southern hemisphere rises in the east, it goes to the north and sets in the west. In the translation of the I Ching for the Portuguese it is also emphasized that one should observe the season referred to in the text and not the month in question, since the work was written in China, which fully meets in the northern hemisphere, and the months corresponding to the seasons are always different in the two hemispheres of the Earth. For example, the sign that represents the height of summer is the horse. Corresponds to heat, fire element, December, toward magnetic north, in the southern hemisphere; while the horse in the northern hemisphere corresponds to the month of June and the south.

The 5 elements (fire / summer, earth, metal / fall, water / winter, wood / spring) are related to the seasons, with directions, with the 12 signs (animals), with the months, days and hours, yielding a calendar.

When working on the floor plan of a building, the technique is used the "Bahzai", and in the case of people the technique of "Min-gua". The 8 trigrams of the I Ching will be related to magnetic coordinates, respectively, in the Southern Hemisphere, it goes for most of Brazil, including São Paulo: North 9, Northeastern 4, East 3, Southeast 8, south 1, Southwest 6, west 7, northwest _se 2 is a matrix (mathematics) 3x3, which is the plan, 360 degrees + (clockwise Northern Hemisphere) or - (anti-clockwise Southern Hemisphere); 5 is in the center, which is the number considered sacred.

2 Zhen	9 Qian	4 Tui
7 Kan	5 (69)	3 Li
6 Ken	1 Kun	8 Xun

"Magic Square"

The relationship between the 12 signs and the five elements originate to 60 binomials. On Summer 2006 is the year of the Metal Dragon in the Southern Hemisphere. The year of change occurs in the 1st Spring Month because the Lunar Year start on Tiger Month 1st Spring, in Summer 2008 is the year of the Water Horse (binomial 19). In 2009 is the Year of the Water Sheep. This date is calculated as the Northern Hemisphere.

Eight Principles

The identification and differentiation of syndromes according to the Eight Principles is one of the core concepts of traditional Chinese medicine diagnosis. The eight principles are as follows:

Exterior - Interior (li-biao 里表)

Sometimes referred to as Internal/External, this differentiation is not made on the basis of aetiology (cause) of disease but location. It can also give an indication of the direction the illness is taking, becoming more external or going deeper into the body. Exterior affects skin, muscles and jingluo (energy meridians). Interior affects the Zang Fu (internal organs) and the bones. The general symptoms for an exterior pattern are fever, aversion to cold, aching body, stiff neck, and a floating pulse. Onset is acute and the correct treatment will elicit a swift response. Exterior patterns usually involve the invasion of an external pathogenic factor, or if slow in onset can indicate painful obstruction syndrome (bi syndrome).

Cold or Hot (Han-re 寒热)

Hot/Cold describes the nature of a pattern and clinical manifestations usually in combination with Full or Empty conditions:

Full Heat

This is indicated by fever, thirst, red face, red eyes, constipation, scanty dark urine, full rapid pulse and a red tongue with yellow coating. It arises when there is an excess of Yang energies in the body. It can be caused by consuming hot energy foods, or long standing emotional problems causing for example liver qi stagnation. It can also be caused by invasion by an external pathogenic factor.

Empty Heat

Empty heat is characterised by afternoon fever, dry mouth, dry throat at night, night sweats, a feeling of heat in the chest and in the palms and the soles, dry stools, scanty dark urine and a floating and rapid pulse and a peeled tongue. It is usually accompanied by a feeling of restlessness and vague anxiety. The difference between full heat is that empty heat is cause by a deficiency of Yin rather than an excess of Yang.

Full Cold

Chilliness, cold limbs, no thirst, pale face, abdominal pain., aggravated on pressure, desire to drink warm liquids, loose stools, clear abundant urine, Deep-full-tight pulse and a pale tongue with thick white coating. Full cold is generated by an excess of Yin.

Empty Cold

Chilliness, cold limbs, dull-pale face, no thirst, listlessness, sweating, loose stools, clear-abundant urine, a deep slow or weak pulse and a pale tongue with a thin white coating. Empty cold arises from a deficiency of Yang.

Empty or Full (Xu-shi 虚实)

Full and Empty are also commonly called Deficient and Excess. This distinction is made according to the presence or absence of a pathogenic factor and the strength of the body's energies. Full is characterised by the presence of a pathogenic factor and the Qi is relatively intact. The Qi battles against the pathogenic factor which causes the excessive symptoms. Empty is characterised by absence of a pathogenic factor and weak Qi. The distinction between full and empty is made more than any other type of observation. Clinical manifestations of empty include chronic diseases, listlessness, apathy, lying curled up, weak voice, weak breathing, low pitched tinnitus, pain alleviated by pressure, poor memory, slight sweating, frequent urination, loose stools and empty pulse. Clinical manifestations of full patterns include acute diseases, restlessness, irritability, red face, strong voice, coarse breathing, pain aggravated by pressure, high pitched tinnitus, profuse sweating, scanty urination, constipation and excess pulse type. There are four types of emptu:

- Empty Qi
- Empty Yang
- Empty Blood
- Empty Yin

Yin or Yang (Yin-yang 陰陽)

Yin and Yang are general categories of the other six patterns: Interior, Deficiency and Cold are Yin, Exterior, Excess and Heat are Yang.

Three Treasures (Traditional Chinese Medicine)

The Three Treasures or Three Jewels (Chinese: 三寶; pinyin: sānbǎo; Wade–Giles: san-pao) are theoretical cornerstones in traditional Chinese medicine and practices such as Neidan, Qigong, and T'ai chi. They are also known as Jing Qi Shen (Chinese: 精氣神; pinyin: jīng-qì-shén; Wade–Giles: ching ch'i shen; "essence, qi, and spirit"). Despeux summarizes.

Jing, *qi*, and *shen* are three of the main notions shared by Taoism and Chinese culture alike. They are often referred to as the Three Treasures (*sanbao* 三寶), an expression that immediately reveals their importance and the close connection among them. The ideas and practices associated with each term, and with the three terms as a whole, are complex and vary considerably in different contexts and historical periods. (2008:562)

This Chinese name *sanbao* originally referred to the Taoist "Three Treasures" (from *Tao Te Ching* 67, tr. Waley 1958:225, "pity", "frugality", and "refusal to be 'foremost of all things under heaven'") and subsequently translated the Buddhist Three Jewels (Buddha, Dharma, and Sangha).

In long-established Chinese traditions, the "Three Treasures" are the essential energies sustaining human life:

- *Jing* 精 "nutritive essence, essence; refined, perfected; extract; spirit, demon; sperm, seed"

- *Qi* 氣 "vitality, energy, force; air, vapor; breath; spirit, vigor; attitude"

- *Shen* 神 "spirit; soul, mind; god, deity; supernatural being"

This *jing-qi-shen* ordering is more commonly used than the variants *qi-jing-shen* and *shen-qi-jing*.

In *Neidan* "internal alchemy" practice (Despeux 2008:563), transmuting the Three Treasures is expressed through the phrases *lianjing huaqi* 鍊精化氣 "refining essence into breath", *lianqi huashen* 鍊氣化神 "refining breath into spirit", and *lianshen huanxu* 鍊神還虛 "refining spirit and reverting to Emptiness". Both *Neidan* and Neo-Confucianism (Despeux 2008:564-5) distinguish the three between *xiantian* 先天 "prior to heaven" and *houtian* 後天 "posterior to heaven", referring to *Yuanjing* 元精 "Original Essence", *Yuanqi* 元氣 "Original Breath", and *yuanshen* 元神 "Original Spirit".

The (2nd century BCE) *Huainanzi* refers to *qi* and *shen* with *xing* 形 "form; shape; body".

The bodily form [*xing*] is the residence of life; the *qi* fills this life while *shen* controls it. If either of them loses their proper position, they will all come to harm. (1, tr. Englehart 2000:99)

The Taoist text *Gaoshang yuhuang xinyin jing* (高上玉皇心印經, "Mind-Seal Scripture of the Exalted Jade Sovereign", or *Xinyin jing* "Mind-Seal Scripture") is a valuable early source about the Three Treasures (tr. Olson 1993).

Probably dating from the Southern Song dynasty (1127-1279), this anonymous text presents a simple and concise discussion of internal alchemy (*neidan* 內丹). In particular, it emphasizes the so-called Three Treasures (*sanbao* 三寶), namely, vital essence (*jing* 精), subtle breath (*qi* 氣), and spirit (*shen* 神). (Komjathy 2004:29)

Frederic H. Balfour's (1880:380-381) brief essay about the *Xinyin jing* ("The Imprint of the Heart") contains the earliest known Western reference to the Three Treasures: "There are three degrees of Supreme Elixir – the Spirit, the Breath, and the Essential Vigour".

The (late 16th century) *Journey to the West* novel provides a more recent example when an enlightened Taoist patriarch instructs Sun Wukong "Monkey" with a poem that begins:

Know well this secret formula wondrous and true: Spare and nurse the vital forces, this and nothing else. All power resides in the semen [jing], the breath [qi], and the spirit [shen]; Guard these with care, securely, lest there be a leak. Lest there be a leak!

Keep within the body! (tr. Yu 1977:88)

References

- Taylor Latener, Rodney Leon (2005). The Illustrated Encyclopedia of Confucianism, Vol. 2. New York: Rosen Publishing Group. p. 869. ISBN 978-0-8239-4079-0.

- Xinzhong Yao (13 February 2000). An introduction to Confucianism. Cambridge University Press. pp. 98–. ISBN 978-0-521-64430-3. Retrieved 29 October 2011.

- Davis, Barbara (2004). Taijiquan Classics. Berkeley, California: North Atlantic Books. p. 212. ISBN 978-1-55643-431-0.

- Robinet, Isabelle (2008), "Taiji tu. Diagram of the Great Ultimate", in Pregadio, Fabrizio, The Encyclopedia of Taoism A–Z, Abingdon: Routledge, pp. 934–936, ISBN 978-0-7007-1200-7

- Megaw, Ruth and Vicent (2005), Early Celtic Art in Britain and Ireland, Shire Publications LTD, ISBN 0-7478-0613-6

- White, Lynn; Van Deusen, Nancy Elizabeth (1995), The Medieval West Meets the Rest of the World, Claremont Cultural Studies, 62, Institute of Mediaeval Music, ISBN 0-931902-94-0

- Werner, E. T. C. Myths and Legends of China. London Bombay Sydney: George G. Harrap & Co. Ltd. p. 84. ISBN 0-486-28092-6. Retrieved 2010-03-23.

- Waley, Arthur. 1958. The Way and Its Power: A Study of the Tao Te Ching and Its Place in Chinese Thought. Grove Press. ISBN 0802150853

- Wang, Mu. Foundations of Internal Alchemy: The Taoist Practice of Neidan. Golden Elixir Press, 2011. ISBN 9780984308255.

- Puro, Jon. "The Skeptic Encyclopedia of Pseudoscience, Volume 2: Feng Shui" (PDF). Antoniolombatti.it. Retrieved 30 October 2016.

Permissions

Index

www.ingramcontent.com/pod-product-compliance
Lightning Source LLC
Chambersburg PA
CBHW061935190326
41458CB00009B/2744